Symposium on
corrective rhinoplasty

Volume thirteen

Symposium on corrective rhinoplasty

Editor

D. Ralph Millard, Jr., M.D., F.A.C.S.

*Light-Millard Professor of Plastic Surgery and
Chief of the Division of Plastic Surgery,
University of Miami School of Medicine,
Miami, Florida*

Proceedings of the Symposium of The Educational
Foundation of the American Society of Plastic and
Reconstructive Surgeons, Inc., held at
Miami, Florida, January 15-18, 1975

with 980 illustrations and 2 color plates

The C.V. Mosby Company

Saint Louis   1976

Volume thirteen

Library of Congress Cataloging in Publication Data

Symposium on Corrective Rhinoplasty, Miami, Fla.,
    1975.
    Symposium on Corrective Rhinoplasty.

    (Proceedings of the symposium of The Educational Foundation of the American Society of Plastic and Reconstructive Surgeons; v. 13)
    Bibliography: p.
    Includes index.
    1. Rhinoplasty—Congresses. I. Millard,
David Ralph, 1919-   II. American Society of
Plastic and Reconstructive Surgeons. Educational
Foundation. III. Series: American Society of
Plastic and Reconstructive Surgeons. Educational
Foundation. Proceedings of the symposium; v. 13.
[DNLM: 1. Rhinoplasty—Congresses. WV312 S9892s
1975]
RD119.S94 1975   617'.523   76-16519
ISBN 0-8016-3413-X

TS/NK/B 9 8 7 6 5 4 3 2 1

Faculty

Jerome Adamson, Secretary of the American Society of Plastic and Reconstructive Surgeons, left me free to have the faculty I wanted, and over thirty experts came to mind. However, twenty guest faculty were eventually invited. Unfortunately, Frank McDowell, Ray Broadbent, Thomas Rees, and Richard Straith were unable to join us at this time.

Franklin L. Ashley, M.D.

Professor of Surgery, U.C.L.A. School of Medicine, Los Angeles, California

Gustave Aufricht, M.D.

Consulting Plastic Surgeon, Lenox Hill Hospital, New York, New York

William C. Conroy, M.D.

Attending Plastic Surgeon, Mountainside Hospital, Montclair, New Jersey

John Marquis Converse, M.D.

Lawrence D. Bell Professor of Plastic Surgery; Director, Institute of Reconstructive Plastic Surgery, New York University Medical Center, New York, New York

R. L. G. Dawson, M.B., F.R.C.S.

Consultant Plastic Surgeon to The Mount Vernon Center for Plastic Surgery, Norwood, Middlesex, The Royal National Orthopaedic Hospital, London, and The Royal Free Hospital, London, England

Reed O. Dingman, M.D., F.A.C.S.

Professor of Surgery and Head of Section of Plastic Surgery, University of Michigan School of Medicine, Ann Arbor, Michigan

Mark Gorney, M.D.

Associate Professor of Plastic Surgery, Stanford University School of Medicine; Executive Director, Plastic and Reconstructive Center, St. Francis Memorial Hospital, San Francisco, California

Lawrence V. Hastings, M.D., J.D.

Practicing Attorney and Assistant Professor of Medicine, University of Miami School of Medicine, Miami, Florida

Otto B. Kriens, M.D., D.D.S.

Professor of Plastic and Maxillo-facial Surgery, Bremen General Hospital, Bremen, Germany

John R. Lewis, Jr., M.D.

Institute of Aesthetic Plastic Surgery, Atlanta, Georgia

D. Ralph Millard, Jr., M.D., F.A.C.S.

Light-Millard Professor of Plastic Surgery and Chief of the Division of Plastic Surgery, University of Miami School of Medicine, Miami, Florida

Ross H. Musgrave, M.D., F.A.C.S.

Professor, Department of Plastic Surgery, University of Pittsburgh, Pittsburgh, Pennsylvania

Paul Natvig, M.D.

Associate Professor of Plastic and Reconstructive Surgery, The Medical College of Wisconsin, Milwaukee, Wisconsin

George C. Peck, M.D.

Associate Professor of Plastic Surgery, Temple University School of Medicine, Philadelphia, Pennsylvania

Rex A. Peterson, M.D.

Chairman, Department of Plastic Surgery, Arizona Crippled Children's Hospital, Phoenix, Arizona

Blair O. Rogers, M.D.

Attending Surgeon, Department of Plastic Surgery, Manhattan Eye, Ear, and Throat Hospital, New York, New York

Joseph Safian, M.D.

Retired from practice, Miami Beach, Florida

Jack H. Sheen, M.D.

Assistant Clinical Professor, Division of Plastic Surgery, Department of Surgery, U.C.L.A. School of Medicine, Los Angeles, California

Preface

This symposium was organized with the intention of exhausting the subject of corrective rhinoplasty. Our faculty was chosen carefully, and we are indeed fortunate to be able to present papers from so many outstanding experts. Each chose his own subjects. Discussion times at the symposium were set, but participants were free to raise questions at any time, since the purpose was to teach in depth an interesting and difficult subject. The format and order of discussion at the symposium have been retained in the book.

It was difficult to transpose the conference tapes into text at times when the speakers moved away from the microphone or mumbled in their natural dialect. What concerned me most, however, was our inability to figure out which participant was speaking during the discussions. Often they did not give their name or did it outside taping range. As my entire staff's memory could not recall each incident, the discussion has been credited to "participant" if necessary with our sincere apology. The only thing worse would be to credit people with something they did not say, and, alas, this too is a possibility.

I would like to thank the faculty members who so generously contributed their time to participate in the symposium and who prepared papers for publication. Their names are listed on the preceding pages. The symposium is also indebted to the participants who contributed to the discussions. And finally, I would like to acknowledge with thanks the people listed who made possible the televising of the live surgery or who provided other technical assistance.

Television director
Walter P. Garst, M.D.

Local arrangements chairman
Bernard Barrett, Jr., M.D.

Executive assistants
Lesley Cook
Connie Hard

Symposium assistants
Michael Bederman, M.D.
Gary Burget, M.D.
Malcolm Lesavoy, M.D.
Lawrence McCarthy, M.D.
Walter Mullin, M.D.
Howard Seider, M.D.
David H. Slepyan, M.D.

Taping of sessions
John Devine, Jr., M.D.
Lawrence McCarthy, M.D.

Photographers
Donald Barth
Otto B. Kriens, M.D.
David H. Slepyan, M.D.
Judith E. Slepyan, C.R.N.A.

Slide projectionists
Bernard Barrett, Jr., M.D.
Malcolm Lesavoy, M.D.
Walter Mullin, M.D.
Howard Seider, M.D.

D. Ralph Millard, Jr.

Contents

Color plates

Primary rhinoplasty

Chapter 1

Rhinoplasty surgery

John R. Lewis, Jr., M.D.

Lewis: I give 2 mg of haloperidol 2 hours before surgery and again 1 hour before surgery, and 10 mg of diazepam (Valium) ordinarily 2 hours before surgery. I give a hypodermic injection of 50 mg of meperidine (Demerol), 50 mg of hydroxyzine (Vistaril), and gr 1/200 of atropine 1 hour before surgery. However, this patient came to the operating room still wide awake, and I've given her at this point, in two divided doses, a total of 1 ml of Innovar intravenously and 1 ml of diazepam intravenously. Let's have a look at the patient's photographs (Fig. 1-2).

I'm going to start injecting with 2% lidocaine (Xylocaine) and epinephrine. This is the only place where I use full-strength 2% lidocaine with epinephrine, 1:200,000. I start the injection in the glabella and along the base and sidewalls. Then I like to wait 15 minutes after the injection to let the epinephrine take full effect. I also use a little bit of lidocaine in the supratip area. I feel that by the time I get to that point, practically all the swelling that I have produced by the injection is gone. Preoperatively, I do some other things too. I like to start several weeks ahead by giving my patients 500 mg of ascorbic acid, three times a day, and for 3 weeks ahead, 5 mg of vitamin K daily. They tend not to bleed or bruise as much, but I admit that a lot of things I use are probably not necessary. I also give 50 mg of hydrochlorothiazide (Hydrodiuril) 2 hours before the surgery to reduce the initial swelling about the eyes. If one keeps the initial swelling to a minimum, then usually they will not swell badly afterward.

I separate the upper part of the lower lateral cartilages from the upper laterals, inverting the

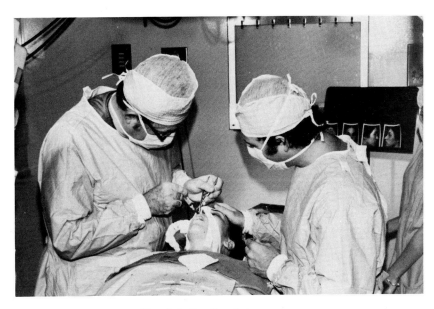

Fig. 1-1. Dr. Lewis in surgery.

3

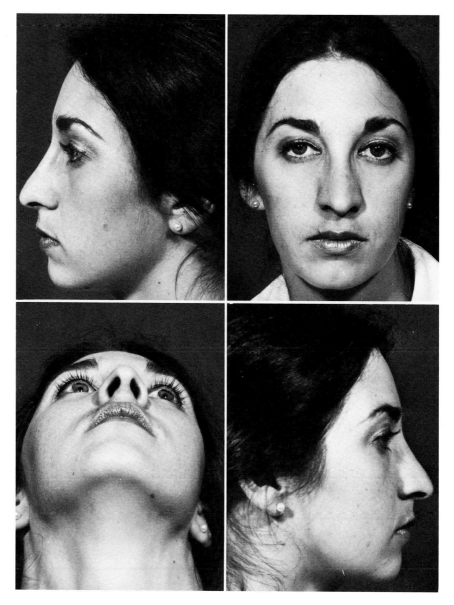

Fig. 1-2. Preoperative views of patient.

lower lateral for trimming. The supratip area is a little wide, as is the alar base. I do not do alar base resections on all noses, but perhaps in 35%. This is a profilometer developed by Dr. Claire Straith. It is a modification of a Joseph measuring instrument (rhinometer). Dr. Straith called it a profilometer, and I set the bridge angle from the glabella at 30 degrees. This nose is about 5.5 cm, so I'm going to do a bit of shortening. The tip angle (of the columella to the lip) was measured before I put in the local anesthetic, and I'm going to aim for 17 degrees. It is about 23 degrees with the swelling, but it's going to be about right if it ends up between 15 and 18 degrees. Then, when I measure along the side, I can get a quick indication of how much comes off the nasal bridge. I not only get a quick indication of how much I need to take off the bridge but how much I need to shorten it. Are you seeing that clearly?

Millard: Yes, that's coming through pretty well; I never did understand that instrument.

Lewis: I'll just use a no. 15 blade starting here going up through the lower lateral almost at the junction of the upper lateral, swinging around down toward the columella and undermining in a subcutaneous plane. I don't undermine all the way to the nasal base. I undermine what I need to undermine to allow the skin to shrink properly. I don't try to undermine beneath the periosteum. Then I reverse my knife and come across the top of the bridge. I'm going to do the marking now with the profilometer just to give myself a quick reference as to how much lowering of the bridge I want. In cutting the nasal bones and in rasping the nasal bones, I try to trim down and bevel the lateral edge so that there won't be a sharp protrusion that can be seen or felt. If I want to smooth things very well, I use a little diamond rasp (Peet rasp) at the end. At this point, I might try to show you the level of the nasal bridge because I tried to establish the level of my subglabellar notch. The bridge is still high because of the upper lateral cartilages and the septum, which I haven't trimmed as I have the nasal bones.

At this point, I like to separate the upper lateral cartilages from the septum, so I cut through the upper lateral cartilages right along adjacent to the septum. Normally one trims the septum before the upper lateral cartilages, but I know that the upper laterals are a little high, and I'm going to trim them first to get them out of the way for my septal trim. I have an Aufricht elevator with a fiberoptic light attached, which I use quite a bit. Now I'm going to trim along the top of the septum, contouring it, but not taking it very low because she doesn't have that much excess septum to spare along the dorsum. I'm through with the lowering, but I haven't done any shortening yet. At this point that's what I'm going to do. Now as I shorten the septum it has been cut almost straight, so I'm going to round it just a little into the tip. I'll start to taper down the top of the end of the septum and round out the tip. I'm going to do a little more trimming of the septum because otherwise my supratip area will be too high. I'm not trying to give her a Hollywood nose; I'm trying to give her a nose that looks nice and natural for her face.

I've got one finger trained to feel any irregularity along the bridge. I used my right index finger until I got it injured and lost some of the feeling in it, so I switched to my left index finger, which was really more convenient anyway.

At this point, I'm going to use a little Peet rasp to smooth down the nasal bones. At the end of the procedure (bridge osteotomy) I have my nasal bones and upper laterals and septum at the same level, but I want to leave them like this (center slightly higher than sides) so I have

a rounded bridge and not a flat top. It's like Dr. Straith used to say, "Raising two tent posts raises the top of the tent." Of course, I don't know if Dr. Straith ever went camping or knew about tents, but that's the way he described it. At this point, I'm going to use a chisel just to crack through the ridge of the nasal bones at the base of the nose. I'm going to aim out toward the rim at the inner canthus. I make a small incision in the vestibule and use a narrow elevator to elevate the tissue off the bone; then I use a chisel to cut through the nasal bone and find it works well also with a thick bone. Usually I don't even elevate the soft tissue when I use a narrow 3 mm chisel unless the bones are very heavy. On the other side, I'll do it with a saw, maybe in a little more classical fashion, and to show two ways to accomplish the base osteotomy. To tell you truthfully, I think I'm a little high on the nasal bone on the right side. I'm going to have to chisel some more off.

I now trim the upper edge of the lower lateral and the lower edge of the upper lateral cartilage, with the alar cartilage inverted into the nostril. I try not to sacrifice the mucosa at this point as I trim a little from the lower laterals. This is not a wide lower lateral, and most of what I'm doing is to loosen it so that it can adjust and drop down a little because it's pulling up a little toward the tip. I don't trim very far down toward the alar base because one can get that little retraction with dimpling of the sides of the ala. Now, whereas I've rounded the tip of the septum here, I also want to round the tip of the upper lateral cartilage. I also just trimmed this little triangle off the upper lateral cartilage beneath the mucosa. I can trim it off now or later as I want to. Now I think I'm ready to do the submucous resection (SMR), but I notice there is a little fullness here. On some noses you can just do one resection, and that's it. But in others I like to do a little piddling at the end to get it as perfect as I can. Can you see a small area of irregularity in the tip and along the bridge? It's actually a little high point in the upper lateral, which I'll trim slightly. I have a little extra mucosa on the upper lateral cartilages, not much, just a tiny little bit along the bridge.

This lady has a deviation of the septum and rather markedly enlarged lower turbinates, so I'm going to correct the septum and fracture the turbinates by breaking them medially and then laterally to push them outward against the sidewall. I occasionally take out a lower turbinate, especially in an old cleft lip nose where there is a very thick large turbinate obstructing the airway flow. I'm doing the SMR.

Now, at this point, I'm going to move the two nasal bones together and evaluate the symmetry. In feeling for irregularities along the bridge along the top of the septum I use a wet finger because I feel that this slides over these irregularities and gives me a more delicate touch. I now recheck with the profilometer to make sure my angles are correct. However, they might be off somewhat due to swelling. From the side you can see that her chin is just a little bit recessive. *Now,* I'm not trying to make everybody look alike, and furthermore she didn't mention her chin; so I really don't think that she needs an augmentation. I'm looking for triamcinolone (Aristocort) to inject into the turbinates.

I use Gelfoam and Vaseline gauze wrapped with Owen's gauze or parachute silk. I sprinkle it with Neosporin powder because it helps sterilize the nose, and I feel that it cuts down a bit on the odor. That is Gelfoam with Neosporin powder. The splint is sponge rubber, 1/4 inch thick with aluminum. I put a little extra gauze on top of the splint in the subglabellar area because I feel that if there is any tendency for a hematoma, this would be the spot. I use a small gold safety pin to hold the tape strap together. Nothing but the best for my patient! For my injection of triamcinolone, I use 20 mg, half on each side, into the lower turbinates. Actually I mix about 20 mg of triamcinolone or triamcinolone acetonide (Kenalog) into the local anesthetic, 12 or 15 ml total solution. I feel this cuts down a little on the edema postoperatively and minimizes postoperative discomfort.

Postoperatively I use elevation of the head, ice cold compresses to the eyes, an initial dose of diuretic to minimize the initial edema, and anti-inflammatory enzymes to minimize edema and ecchymosis. My patient should not have much postoperative pain.

Operation notes

Hospital: Victoria Hospital, Inc., Miami, Florida
Date: January 16, 1975
Surgeon: John R. Lewis, Jr., M.D.
Assistant: Michael Bederman, M.D.
Preoperative diagnosis: Deformity of nose, deflection of septum to the left with left nasal obstruction; marked hypertrophy of lower turbinates bilaterally with bilateral partial nasal obstruction.

Operation: Corrective rhinoplasty, left radical resection of septum, reduction of lower turbinates bilaterally.

Under local anesthesia, using 2% lidocaine (Xylocaine) with epinephrine, 1:200,000, incisions were made in a transcartilaginous fashion through the lower lateral cartilages close to the junction of the upper lateral cartilages. The incision was then extended through the membranous septum at the junction of columella to the lower end of the septum to the base of the columella. Undermining was carried out against the nasal bones and upper lateral cartilages up to the top of the nasal bridge. By measuring with the profilometer, the determination was made as to how much of the nasal bridge would be resected and how much shortening of the nasal tip would be carried out by shortening the septum and upper lateral cartilages. With the nasal saw, an osteotomy was carried out on the nasal bridge to the septum, and then, with a knife, the septum was trimmed. The upper lateral cartilages were freed from the septum on each side and were lowered with the bayonet scissors. The septum was then rasped smooth on each side, and the top of the septum was contoured with a knife. The lower end of the septum was shortened by excising a triangle base upward to shorten the central portion of the nose, and the top of the septum was beveled down in its distal 1 cm into the tip and rounded at the tip. The sidewalls were shortened by excising a triangle of upper lateral cartilage with a minimum of mucosa, base upward and rounding of the tip of the upper lateral cartilages. The alar cartilages were narrowed at the tip by excising a small triangle adjacent to the midline, and the alar cartilages were freed by undermining and were allowed to adjust. A small amount of cartilage was trimmed along the upper edge of the lower lateral cartilages. The nasal bones were then freed in the midline from each other and from the septum with the chisel, cracking them outward slightly. Then the nasal bones at the base were freed from the maxillae bilaterally, using a chisel on the left and a saw and chisel on the right. The septum was resected on the left, elevating the mucosa and resecting cartilage of the cartilaginous septum and bone of the bony (vomerine) septum, which deviated markedly into the left airway, causing an obstruction; the resection was carried out with the angled scissors and with the chisel and rongeurs. Further chiseling along the left side of the vomerine septum opened the airway more. The mucosa was then replaced, and the mucosa was not pierced on the right side and was preserved intact. The lower turbinates were fractured

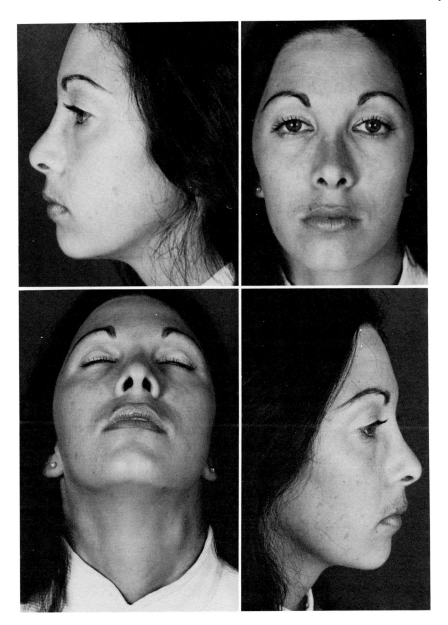

Fig. 1-3. Postoperative views of same patient. Early postoperative result reveals swelling in sides of base and in supratip area, which should subside. Airways are good.

internally, crushed to flatten the bony and spongy portions, and then fractured back laterally, flattening them outward against the sidewalls. The soft anterior portions of the lower turbinates were injected with corticosteroid, 10 mg of triamcinolone (Aristocort) on each side. The nasal bones were then moved with the thumbs medially, narrowing the nasal base. Further inspection of the nasal bridge and further trim of the upper lateral cartilages as well as the top of the septum were carried out, rounding and beveling the top of the septum into the tip. Then the mucosa, laterally and medially, was approximated, approximating the upper and lower lateral cartilages laterally and the septum to the columella. A bilateral alar base resection was carried out (about 4 mm width) and sutured with one buried suture of 4-0 Dexon, then a running suture of 5-0 Prolene. One 4-0 chromic suture was used on each side internally to further approximate the area of resection. Vaseline gauze packs were inserted, a padded nasal splint was applied, and a drip pad was applied under the nose. The patient left the operating room in good condition and awake. The bleeding was minimal and would be estimated at about 8 ml. (See Fig. 1-3.)

Chapter 2

Rhinoplasty surgery

George C. Peck, M.D.

Peck: Before doing surgery, I must look at the photographs (Fig. 2-2), evaluate the nasal tip, and draw the lines that are to be the sculpturing lines in the alar cartilage. I do this by first marking with pencil the inferior or caudal border of the alar cartilage. I draw the line from lateral to medial to the inferior margin of the dome and down into the medial crura. I then draw what will be the sculpturing incision, a gull-wing type incision, on the dorsum of the tip. In this case, since there is good projection, I will leave approximately 5 mm of alar cartilage in continuity in the alar rim, and as you can see here, I have drawn the line to represent the position of the sculpturing incision.

Surgery begins with the nasal tip. I prefer to do the tip before the nasal bridge because I feel that it is much easier to accommodate the bridge line to the tip than it is to try and accommodate the tip to the bridge.

Surgery is started with the intercartilaginous incision, which is made at the red-white line. The red-white line is that line made by the junction of the mucous membrane and skin, and it represents the line at which the alar cartilage and upper lateral cartilage meet. The incision begins laterally in the red-white line and moves medially to the dorsum of the septum. As the blade passes over the dorsum of the septum, it proceeds inferiorly to the septal angle. At this point, the blade is passed through the vestibular skin of the opposite side at the septal angle. The blade is passed around the septal angle separating the membranous columella from the septum. If the tip were to be elevated, the entire membranous columella would be separated

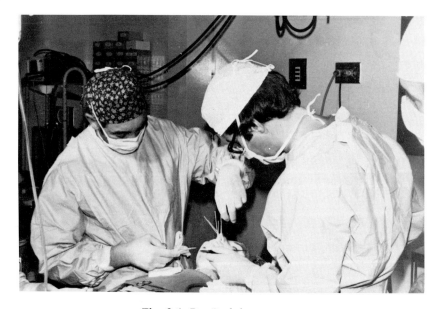

Fig. 2-1. Dr. Peck in surgery.

8

from the septal angle to the nasal spine. However, in this case the patient has an excellent nasolabial line, and no elevation of the tip will be made. In any event, the incision is carried down past the septal angle separating the membranous columella for at least 1 cm in order to give better mobility of the tip as I proceed to sculpture the alar cartilages. The same procedure is done on the opposite side, that is, an incision is made in the red-white line and carried from lateral to medial to meet the incision of the opposite side. I find in many of the secondary rhinoplasties that the intercartilaginous incision was made not at the red-white line but higher in the nasal vault. If this incision is made high in the vault, it will later be difficult to properly place the sculpturing incision. Therefore it is absolutely essential that the intercartilaginous incision be kept at the red-white line. With both incisions made, I have now mobilized the soft tissues of

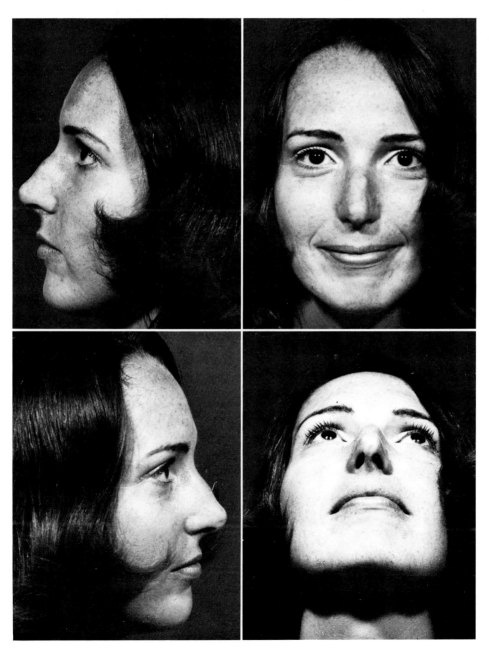

Fig. 2-2. Preoperative views of patient.

the nasal tip from the cartilaginous framework beneath. I am now undermining over the dorsum of the septum and the upper laterals so that I will have better mobility of the soft tissues of the tip as I proceed to the sculpturing incisions.

This particular patient has excellent nasal tip projection. The height of the nasal tip from the nasal spine to the tip is excellent and does not have to be reduced. Therefore the sculpturing incision will be confined to producing the sculpturing lines in the alar cartilage rather than attempting to reduce the entire pyramid of the nasal tip. We must always remember that the greater the volume of alar cartilage removed, the greater will be the nasal tip reduction in all planes of the nasal pyramid. It will then be understandable if we have a large nose, we would want to leave a very narrow rim of alar cartilage. In such a case, I would leave 2 or 3 mm of alar cartilage in continuity in the alar rim, and I would therefore remove a large volume of alar cartilage, which would subsequently reduce the nasal pyramid. However, in this patient, there is good projection, and I want to preserve the nasal tip height. I therefore want to leave as much alar cartilage as possible and at the same time to produce a sculpturing incision. This particular case is ideal for illustrating this concept, and this type of case is probably much more difficult than the large bulbous tip where I have a larger margin of error. I want to sculpture her alar cartilage, thereby producing the good aesthetic lines of the nasal tip, but at the same time not lower the projection of the nasal tip.

Millard: That sounds good, George.

Peck: As you can recall from the initial lines, the lower line represents the inferior margin of the alar cartilage, and the upper line represents the sculpturing incision. A double hook is then used to evert the alar margins. The suction tip is then introduced intranasally and into the dome area. The tip of the suction is then placed in the concavity of the intranasal dome area, and, by pressing against the vestibular skin with the suction tip internally and pressing externally with the middle finger, I am able to make an imprint on the vestibular skin that represents the sculpturing incision in the dome area. With the no. 15 blade an incision is now made at the imprint. I always begin at the dome so that I am sure of having cartilage remaining below. In this way it is impossible to wipe out or completely remove a dome, which would be a catastrophe. The incision now extends laterally, always remaining parallel to the alar rim, and it continues until there is no more alar cartilage to incise. I then go back to the dome and continue the incision from the dome down into the medial crural part of the dome for 2 or 3 mm. If I have properly positioned the incision, it will correspond to the sculpturing line that I had drawn prior to surgery on the external skin. A straight hemostat is then used to grasp the nasal lining, and with a blunt-pointed scissors, the skin is elevated from the fat and cartilage that will be removed. With a sharp-pointed scissors, the vestibular skin is now separated from the alar cartilage and contiguous fibrofatty tissue. I have now effectively sculptured the alar cartilage by removing the cephalad portion of alar cartilage and contiguous fibrofatty tissue. The same technique is then carried out on the opposite side, and at this point the nasal tip is complete. At the end of surgery I will again check the nasal tip lines, that is, the sculpturing lines, and if it is necessary to remove a little more cartilage, this can easily be done at that point.

With the sculpturing incisions in the tip complete, I now look at the bridge and determine what lines I want to create for the profile. In the bridge I am merely accommodating the bridge line to the new nasal tip. As I now examine the patient I can see that she has a slight nasal hump, with more prominence of the nasal hump on the left side.

Millard: George, will you get the cameras to get a profile?

Peck: The patient is now positioned so that we can see the profile line, and again we can see the slight hump that she has in this area. Since the hump is not large, I will elect in this patient to use a rasp rather than an osteotome. I always palpate the bony portion of the hump, and, as I do that in this patient, I find that she has very little bony component of the hump and the majority of the hump is cartilage.

Surgery on the hump begins by elevating the skin from the area of the hump. This is done by introducing the dull-pointed scissors into a pocket over the hump, and, by spreading the blades, I elevate the skin and soft tissues from the hump below. In the patient with a large bony hump, I feel that it is necessary to elevate the periosteum. However, in patients such as these, where there is very little bony component to the hump, I don't think it is necessary to do anything further than elevating the skin from the hump area. It is important to only elevate the skin from the area of hump removal, never elevate the soft tissues from the lateral nasal bones. The straight pull rasp is now inserted into the pocket, and I am rasping the bony component of the hump. After rasping the hump, I then inspect the profile line. By pressing down on the soft tissues of the tip I can delineate how much hump remains and how much has to be removed. The Aufricht elevator is then placed in the pocket between the skin and the hump, and, with the no. 15 blade, the cartilaginous portion of the hump is shaved and lowered. At this point I feel that my dorsal line appears about right; however, I know that when I infracture the nasal bones it is possible to get some changes. I therefore will always go back after the infracturing of the nasal bones for a final check of the profile line.

Previously I had mentioned that I never elevate the periosteum and skin from the lateral nasal bones, and the purpose is to prevent the nasal bones from dropping into the nasal vault. Contrary to what has been taught for so many years, when I do a lateral osteotomy and infracture, the maxillary ledge is not sufficiently wide to accommodate the nasal bones after they have been infractured. Therefore if I had elevated the soft tissues from the nasal bones, the nasal bones could then drop into the nasal vault, which produces a deformity that is very difficult to correct secondarily. I was able to prove this point by taking one of my postoperative patients on the second postoperative day. I removed the dental stent, which was immobilizing the nasal bones, and sent the patient to x-ray. There modified Waters views were taken and showed a definite air space between the maxillary ledge and the nasal bones, proving that the nasal bones were not resting on the maxillary ledge after infracturing as had been previously thought.

The lateral osteotomy is made with a 4 mm chisel. The chisel is inserted through a stab incision at the pyriform fossa, and, in a steplike manner, the lateral osteotomy is made in the nasal bone as I proceed cephalad. An 11 mm osteotome is then placed between the nasal bone and the septum. The nasal bone is then outfractured. Then, with my thumb, I infracture the nasal bone, and I have now completed the fracture. It is important to remember that the horizontal fracture line be made at an imaginary line across the inner canthi. If I produce a fracture line above the inner canthi, I will be fracturing

in heavy glabella bone, which can make an easy procedure a very difficult one. If we examine the supraorbital lines as they proceed down into the glabella, they are arching and curving down to the glabella and parallel at the imaginary line of the inner canthus. Good aesthetics shows that it is not necessary to narrow the glabella. It is important that the nose be narrowed at the point where the supraorbital lines meet in parallel, and this is always at or below the imaginary line across the inner canthus. After having made the lateral osteotomy infracture and outfracture on the opposite side, I have now completed the narrowing of the nasal bridge.

Millard: George, try to show the patient.

Peck: I am holding the head up; can you see the lines?

Millard: Fine.

Peck: I prefer to use the outfracture technique in many of the cases because the nasal bone will be fracturing at its weakest point, below the thick, heavy glabella bone. At this point I check the profile, and I can see that there is a slight suggestion of a hump, which is being produced by a high point in the septal cartilage. I now use my diamond rasp to rasp any irregularities, and then with the no. 15 blade I will shave down the dorsum of the septal cartilage to eliminate the high points. In checking, I see that I have some fullness over the upper lateral cartilages, and I will now remove some of the thick, fibrofatty tissue that lies between the skin and the upper lateral cartilage. This particular step is important in the heavy, bulbous nose, and it helps to thin the middle third of the nose from the front view.

The rhinoplasty is now essentially complete, and if it were necessary to do a submucous resection, it would be done at this point. In this particular patient, the septum is straight, and it will not be necessary to do a submucous septal resection. I now pack the nasal passageways with Adaptic and Oxycel cotton. I have not placed any sutures in the vestibular skin. However, if I had separated the membranous columella from the septum, I would have used one or two transfixion sutures with 2-0 chromic. In placing my packing I take care to make sure that I place the flap of vestibular skin made by the intercartilaginous incision and the intracartilaginous incision so that it lies evenly against the overlying skin. The nose is then tape-splinted, and a dental stent is applied in order to immobilize the fractured nasal bones.

Operation notes

Hospital: Victoria Hospital, Inc., Miami, Florida
Date: January 16, 1975
Operation: Rhinoplasty
Surgeon: George Peck, M.D.
Assistant: Gary Burget, M.D.
Preoperative diagnosis: Patient has a slight hump in the dorsal area, with the irregularity more prominent on the left side of the bony hump. Examination of the tip reveals a well-proportioned projection of the tip; however, there is some bulbousness of the nasal tip alar cartilages. The nasal bones are wide, and it will

be necessary to narrow the nasal bridge. The nasolabial angle is good and will not be changed.

The patient was prepared with aqueous benzalkonium (Zephiran) and draped. Before giving the local anesthetic of 2% lidocaine (Xylocaine) and epinephrine (Adrenalin), the patient was given intravenous diazepam (Valium) until she had slurring of speech. This required approximately 12 ml of diazepam.

Surgery began with an intercartilaginous in-

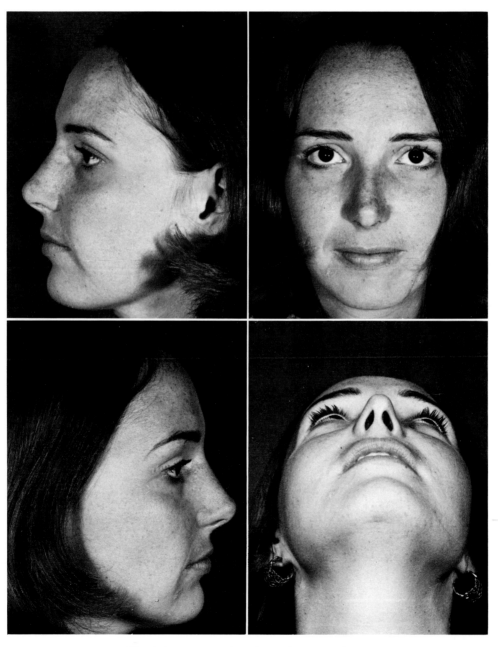

Fig. 2-3. Postoperative views of same patient.

cision separating the upper lateral from the alar cartilages and extending over the dorsum of the septum to the nasal angle. The membranous columella was then separated from the septum for approximately 1 cm. The same procedure was done on the opposite side, and, in this manner, the soft tissues of the tip were elevated from the cartilaginous framework beneath. With a double hook, the alar rim was everted and an intracartilaginous incision was made, leaving approximately 5 or 6 mm of alar cartilage in continuity in the alar rim. The skin was then elevated from the cartilage and fibrofatty tissue beneath. The cartilage and fibrofatty tissue were then removed, thereby producing the sculpturing incision. The same technique was used on the opposite side. The sculpturing incision lines correspond to the lines that had been previously outlined on the skin of the nasal tip. The skin was then elevated from the dorsum of the nose by blunt dissection, and the dorsum was rasped with a pull rasp. The cartilage of the dorsal hump was trimmed with a no. 15 blade. The profile was then acceptable. The lateral osteotomy was done using a 4 mm chisel placed at the pyriform fossa in a stab incision. No tunneling of periosteum was done, and, in a steplike manner, the lateral osteotomy was made with the 4 mm chisel. The steplike fracture was carried cephalad to a point representing the imaginary line across the inner canthi. With an 11 mm osteotome, the nasal bone was outfractured, and then, by digital pressure with the thumb, the nasal bone was infractured. The same procedure was carried on the opposite side, thereby producing a narrowing of the nasal bridge. Oxycel cotton and $1/2$-inch Adaptic gauze were used to pack the nasal passageways, with care being taken to properly position the vestibular flap made by the intercartilaginous and intracartilaginous incisions. The external nose was tape-splinted, and a dental stent was used to immobilize the nasal bones. (See Fig. 2-3.)

Chapter 3

Medicolegal aspects of plastic surgery, 1975

Lawrence V. Hastings, M.D., J.D.
Mark Gorney, M.D.

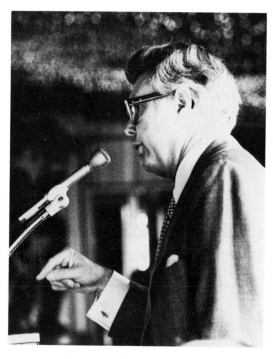

Lawrence V. Hastings, M.D.

PART I

Lawrence V. Hastings

Resolution of the present malpractice dilemma will require distinguishing facts from fantasies. For example, the tremendous strides in medicine and surgery made during the past 30 years have led many laymen to expect perfect results—or even miracles—and to deem anything less a mistake constituting malpractice. Plastic surgery carries an unusually high risk of this particular fantasy.

Historically, our legal system is based on liability for fault, not just a bad result. Presently, medical malpractice is based on deviation from the appropriate standard of care, not just a negligent mistake. Thus, while many are unaware of it, doctors are not legally liable for honest errors of judgment or for using treatment approved by a respectable minority of the profession though not the majority.

Unfortunately, some years ago the law appeared to unduly favor doctors in malpractice cases by such doctrines as the local community rule (whereby a doctor from another area could not testify as to the proper standard of care) and the conclusive evidence of negligence guideline (implying criminal rather than civil liability). Ethics and/or the so-called conspiracy of silence, which prevented a doctor from testifying against another doctor, compounded the problem. Perhaps as lawyers became judges and tried to effectuate a fairer balance, the pendulum swung too far, not only eliminating the local community rule but also permitting evidence not deemed enough to support a normal negligence verdict sufficient to support a malpractice verdict. If so, relatively minor changes in the law are indicated.

In addition, perhaps malpractice should require gross negligence rather than simple negligence in view of the special nature of the doctor-patient relationship and of the art of medicine itself. Or perhaps the law should encourage doctors to require written stipulations from patients that disputes will be the subject of arbitration with fixed monetary recovery limits.

But the recently proposed no-fault concept will not work in malpractice situations because less than perfect results are inherent in the practice of medicine: most of the time, bad or unexpected results are in no way attributable to neglience. A no-fault malpractice system would undoubtedly bankrupt insurance companies as well as doctors. Indeed, if the government were to pay all existing malpractice damage elements in all cases of bad results despite lack of deviation from the relevant standard of medical-surgical care, such socialized medicine or welfare concept would probably bankrupt the country.

According to an article in the January 9, 1975 *Wall Street Journal,* malpractice insurance companies' present lack of money is due in part to the 1973-1974 stock market decline, which wiped out the industry's surplus (built up over the prior decade), and is due in part to "management error," that is, poor business practices and analysis and investment policies. Nowhere in the article is anything said about high verdicts or large numbers of claims. Obviously thorough examination and study of insurance company and insurance commissioner statistics and reports is needed.

In conclusion, unless and until various doctors, insurance company representatives, and attorneys sit down together and manage to separate facts from fantasies, the malpractice dilemma will not disappear.

PART II

Mark Gorney

You know, everyone has been talking about the light at the end of the tunnel. Well, we saw that light at last and it turned out to be an oncoming freight train!

You have to be either blind or deaf not to know what is going on in the field of malpractice in 1975. What the doctor has just told us is informative as well as interesting, but the hour is late, and the lights are going out for all of us all over the country. The crisis is here! It's not tomorrow, it's now! We're faced with premiums that involve anywhere between 25% and 30% of your gross income within the matter of a year or two. Something has to be done! I don't want to prolong this any further, but I just want to remind you that about a year or two ago, when I was in charge of the Medical/Legal Committee, we did precisely as the good doctor has suggested. I organized three conferences, which I think you all know about. We finally had the doctors and the lawyers, both the trial and the defense, the hospital industry, the critical specialties, *everybody* talking to each other across the

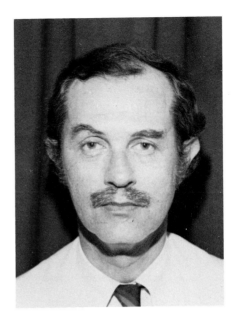

Mark Gorney, M.D.

table so we could address some of these problems by understanding each other's point of view between medicine and the law. Unfortunately, the AMA and the ACS shot me down. I was told, in so many words, that if you "lay down with the dogs, you get up with fleas." I think this is a somewhat unrealistic attitude to take when you're talking about a medical/legal crisis. I felt it would help if we could lean across the table and instead of calling each other dirty names, find out what the other guy is thinking. But apparently this is not to be. So we pass on to the next stage, which is today's crisis.

I was very interested to hear Dr. Hastings make the remarks about the insurance industry. I don't know how many of you remember; there was a play a few years back called Rashomon, a Japanese play, in which there are seven different versions of a rape as seen in the eyes of the "rapee," the witness, the husband, and so forth. Each one has a different story. It's fascinating to watch the same thing happen in the hospital corridors. I am stopped and told this long story of woe; but when I hear the other side of it, there is a whole other story. Same thing for the insurance companies; same thing for the attorneys. Everyone has a different story. But we're right smack in the middle because we're being dribbled on not only by the gross callousness and irresponsibility of the insurance companies, but also the greed and rapacity of the trial bar and by our own problems. Let's face it, gentlemen, we *do* have our own problems.

Behind the Godlike image and those fancy Gucci clothes, and those magic fingers, there is a man with hang-ups even as you and I. And the sooner we learn that, the better it is going to be for us. What we need is intensive education for the surgeon to realize that he is *not* God, to realize that he *does* have limitations. We also need relief right now; that's the thing we need most. We need relief from the legislatures and, above all, from backbreaking insurance premiums.

I am interested particularly in the remarks that were made about the insurance companies and the fact that their reserves have shrunk to this desperate low because of the slump in the stock market. I happen to have intercepted—I don't know why I said intercepted because it is public knowledge—there was an item in the trade journal of the insurance association out in California that was revealing. I learned that the casualty companies' reserves have shrunk to the pathetic figure of $13 billion. Now, that makes me want to lie down and cry! In some cases, it's shrunk down to $68 million—so that's really bad! That's why they have to double our insurance rates! Argonaut is part of a conglomerate, a company owned by Teledyne, and of course Teledyne looks at the cold red ink and says, "We've got to raise the doctor's rates; we've got to double them because we're not making enough money." The truth of this item was, "Yes, we're making money, we're just not making *enough* money." Actually, the losses in any program don't show until about the fourth or fifth year. But these people saw the handwriting on the wall. They collected about $15 million in California, paid out about $230,000, and then pulled the rug out from under us. Neat, huh? Well, I put this to you, gentlemen: insurance is supposed to be a semipublic trust, not a rip-off. You can't drive without insurance. The state legislature can step in and say to the insurance companies, "You *will* insure these drivers or you can't do business in this state." A few years ago, there was no workmen's compensation insurance, as none of the companies wanted to touch it. Then the state legislature came out and said, "You will issue these workers a reasonable rate or you can't do business." The same thing holds true for us also, gentlemen. A doctor can't work uninsured; it's socially irresponsible unless you have a contract with the Devil! It's socially irresponsible because you don't know what is going to happen to that patient, and if he *is* unjustly injured, not through your fault and not through anybody's fault, but if he becomes a vegetable, *somebody* should pay that patient adequate compen-

sation. So the source of it is insurance. My point, again, is that insurance is a semipublic trust. If they're in such dire straits that they cannot fulfill what I think is a public trust, if they can't do it, then the state *has* to step in and do it. They tell you, "Doctor, we have a loss experience of 150%." How many of you really know what that means? Loss experience means money taken in as premiums versus money actually paid out, *plus* those funds that they had set aside in reserves. The law says there shall be a certain proportion of those funds set aside, reserves versus claims, but it doesn't say what the *maximum* is. So you get sued, and they look at the case and say, "We will reserve one million dollars for this case." Okay, you can see very easily how in a few cases, you can run up to a loss experience of 150% if you start adding it up that way. They turn around and say, "Doctor, we've got a loss experience of 150%" and you say, "My God, raise my rates, I'll pay; I'll pay!" But the fact of the matter is that between the time that suit is filed and comes to court, 5 years have elapsed, and during that time, that million dollars is making 10% per annum compounded. Where is that money? You try to figure that out! Second, when the 5 years evolve and the case is either dropped or settled for $3,000 because it was a bum rap to begin with, what's happened to that money? No one asks that and no one tells you that. All they talk about is the red ink. Yes, the insurance rates are higher; the claims are higher. The awards are astronomical, particularly out where I live. But still in all, what they're showing you is the red ink; they're not showing the black. Obviously they aren't making *enough* money. But the thing that drives them nuts is the actuarial uncertainty—having to pay $3 or $5 in 1980 on every dollar of premiums taken in 1975.

I do think there are practical long-term solutions. We have to take the malpractice problem *out* of the courts and arrive at some other method of compensation. I don't like the term *malpractice;* there should be another term, perhaps *surgical misadventure,* which I think is better. There *are* longterm solutions. Workmen's compensation, binding arbitration, prescreening panels; there are all kinds of things. But for the time being, unless medicine (and I'm talking about organized medicine in the form of the ACS and the AMA) wakes up to the fact that we're in bad trouble, they will continue fighting a roaring forest fire with a little hand extinguisher. Between the time solutions are found and now, you're going to be out of pocket many thousands of dollars. I feel sorry for the young plastic surgeon struggling to set up a practice in a place where he's needed, and has to rake up that kind of money for malpractice insurance. He can't possibly! In New York we're in trouble; in Michigan, New York, North Carolina, Maryland, insurance is petering out. In California, on May 1, I'm going to have to come up with $35,000 extra just for the two men in my office. This kind of thing is intolerable. The best solution at this time might be for all the insurance companies to get the hell out! Then the problem will land right in the lap of the government, right in the lap of the legislature. Because one of these mornings, they are going to find out that there are no hospitals working; no doctor in his right mind is going to go to the hospital. And then, and only then, are we going to get to the bottom of this and find a solution—but quick! In the meantime, I urge every single one of you to pressure your state legislature and your federal legislature for relief. Because if you cry loud enough and don't wait for the AMA and the ACS to do it, you may be heard! *We,* the plastic surgeons, because *we're in trouble.* It's much later than you think!

Chapter 4

Early historical development of corrective rhinoplasty

Blair O. Rogers, M.D.

The age of corrective rhinoplasty began in 1887, when John Orlando Roe (Fig. 4-1), an otolaryngologist from Rochester, New York, described an intranasal operation confined to the tip of a so-called pug nose. With the title of "The Deformity Termed 'Pug Nose' and Its Correction by a Simple Operation,"[43] he essentially described an intranasal operation confined to the tip of the nose. His publication in 1891 of another paper, "The Correction of Angular Deformities of the Nose by a Subcutaneous Operation,"[44] was more

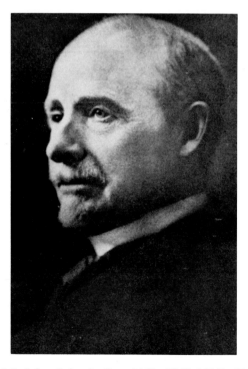

Fig. 4-1. John Orlando Roe, M.D. (1849-1915). (From Cottle, M. H.: Arch. Otolaryngol. **80:**22, 1964.)

truly the medical first, since it was a corrective rhinoplasty of the entire nose in which the nose was reduced in size throughout because of a prominent bony and cartilaginous hump and profile. Before listing the progressive development of corrective rhinoplasty after Roe's first paper, one might ask, When did corrective rhinoplasty have its very first beginnings? Was it back in the days of eighteenth-century Italy, as shown in this delightful Christmas card sent to me several years ago by the late Professor Sanvenero-Rosselli of Milan (Fig. 4-2)?

In all seriousness, its beginnings can probably be traced indirectly or tangentially to J. F. Dieffenbach (1792-1847). He was considered by many as the most skillful plastic surgeon in the mid–nineteenth century, whose reputation was so great that when he visited Paris all the hospitals were made available to him for his surgery.[35] For narrowing thick nostril walls, for example, he cut out small punched-shaped pieces of skin and cartilage, reducing their thickness by the tension of the skin closure (Fig. 4-3).

He also externally removed a vertical and horizontal piece of skin and subcutaneous tissue bilaterally, with the skin closure creating a reduction in the size of an overly large nose (Fig. 4-4). His method of raising a flattened or depressed nasal tip through an external incisional approach is seen in Fig. 4-5. The use of external incisions for any and all nasal corrective or reconstructive surgery was routine in his time, and any thought of an intranasal approach seems to have escaped the surgeons of that era. In his 1845 textbook,[9] he mentioned briefly a method of straightening a twisted or deviated nose, once again using external incisions, chiseling the septum loose from the palate

18

and the nasal bones loose from the face, and following this by fracturing the entire nose into a position of overcorrection.

Many of his techniques are the forerunners of corrective rhinoplasty, which began four decades later with Roe. The history of corrective rhinoplasty cannot, therefore, be divorced from the history of reconstructive rhinoplasty. Even today one is reminded daily how interwoven these two types of surgery are and always have been. A quote from Gillies and Millard's[14] classic textbook is appropriate here:

A great percentage of private practice is beauty surgery. It is here that perfection is a necessity. Reconstructive surgery is an attempt to return to normal; cosmetic surgery is an attempt to surpass the normal. No man is a plastic surgeon unless he becomes adept at both. Many never do and are a menace. It is easier to reduce than produce, but in plastic surgery it is nearly always necessary to remould after reduction. Thus anyone can cut off a bit of a nose or breast, but not so many can turn out a satisfying result.*

Dieffenbach's interest in the lining of a reconstructed nose is expressed in his 1845 book: "When the nostrils are too narrow or grown together, the operation (for correction) is fairly easy. To keep them open is difficult, however. If you cut out the skin or scars, you cause even more constriction."[9,35]

From the time of his predecessors, including Carpue, von Graefe,[52] and others in the early nineteenth century, the need for a framework of the reconstructed nose was apparent. Rousset,[55] in his 1828 Paris thesis, emphasized that reconstructed

---

*From Gillies, H. D., and Millard, D. R., Jr.: The principles and art of plastic surgery, Boston, 1957, Little, Brown & Co., p. 395.

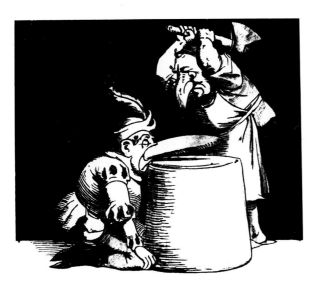

Fig. 4-2. Eighteenth-century caricature of a "corrective rhinoplastic" type of operation. (Courtesy Prof. Gustavo Sanvenero-Rosselli, Milan, Italy.)

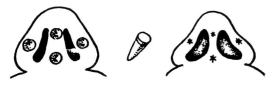

Fig. 4-3. Dieffenbach method of reducing thickness of nostril and columellar walls. (From Kolle, F. S.: Plastic and cosmetic surgery, New York, 1911, D. Appleton & Co.)

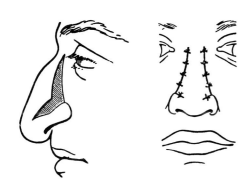

Fig. 4-4. Dieffenbach's method utilizing external excisions to reduce size of overly large nose with drooping tip. (From Davis, J. S.: Plastic surgery: its principles and practice, Philadelphia, 1919, P. Blakiston's Son & Co.)

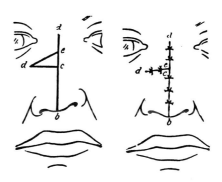

Fig. 4-5. Dieffenbach's method of correcting oblique nose with external incisions and excisions. (From Davis, J. S.: Plastic surgery: its principles and practice, Philadelphia, 1919, P. Blakiston's Son & Co.)

noses often collapsed, and therefore nineteenth-century surgeons used all kinds of supportive materials, including gold, lead, silver, aluminum, platinum, amber, celluloid, and caoutchouc implants as supports within the nasal cavity to hold the dorsum forward. All of these materials either were used as removable internal prostheses or were eventually extruded when implanted as buried material.

Until the 1860s, few if any attempts were made to create a living skeletal support for reconstructed noses. In 1864, however, Ollier,[42] after trying unsuccessfully to grow new bone in a newly reconstructed nose with several periosteal implants, finally brought down a forehead flap to the nose containing not only periosteum but also some bone as well. James Hardie,[15] in 1875, subsequently described his insertion of the denuded first and second phalanges of a finger into a saddle nose, and Koenig,[30] in 1886, cut out a fairly large piece of the outer table of the frontal bone, left it attached to a forehead flap, and transferred it to the reconstructed nasal dorsum.

Reconstructive rhinoplastic techniques in the latter quarter of the nineteenth century then began to develop a better and better sense of the aesthetic requirements of a reconstructed nose, until finally, in 1896, Israel[17] successfully transplanted a free bone graft taken from the anterior tibial surface and thus began the new age of free bone transplantation in reconstructive rhinoplasty. Soon thereafter, von Mangold,[62] in 1900, successfully used autogenous rib cartilages to correct saddle noses, inserting the transplants through glabellar incisions, thereby further ushering in the age of much more sophisticated reconstructive rhinoplastic surgery, which was soon to have its applications in corrective rhinoplasty as well. The work of Israel and von Mangold, who used longitudinal and glabellar incisions, respectively, to insert the transplants, was soon thereafter adapted by Joseph,[23] who, in 1907, reported his insertion of the transplant through an intranasal incision.

But let us return to the mid–nineteenth century; just before the publication of Roe's paper. Linhart,[32] some time before 1870, improved on Dieffenbach's technique to reduce thick nostrils by removing elliptical shaped segments of skin and cartilage to thin out the thick nasal wings (Fig. 4-6). Lossen,[33] in 1884, treating a deviated septum and nasal bones postoperatively, used an apparatus that exerted lateral pressure on the reset structures, a technique erroneously credited to Joseph. For the treatment of a markedly deviated nose,

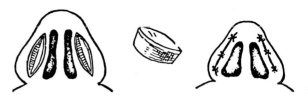

Fig. 4-6. Linhardt's method of reducing thickness of nostril walls. (From Kolle, F. S.: Plastic and cosmetic surgery, New York, 1911, D. Appleton & Co.)

Trendelenburg,[61] in 1889, advised using a postoperative pressure apparatus left on for several weeks to prevent the nose from returning to its former deviated position.

With this increasing overall concern for aesthetics in the shape of a reconstructed nose, we now can consider Roe's outstanding pioneering work. His concern with external scars caused by the commonplace external incisions produced by all of his colleagues can be seen in his very first paper of 1887: "Great care must, however, be exercised not to remove too much tissue, and also not to cut through into the skin, lest we may have afterward a scar or a dent in the external surface of the nose."[43]

In his 1887 paper, he described reducing bulbous nasal tips in five patients using an intranasal incision through which he dissected the lining loose, lifted the nasal tip up, and cut out the excess bulk. He crosshatched or trimmed the alar cartilages where they were deformed, and at the time of the operation he placed silver tubes in the nostrils and molded an external saddle or splint on the outside of the nose to hold it in its new shape until healing had set in. Fig. 4-7 shows a woman preoperatively and postoperatively with the improvement obtained after his operation for the so-called pug nose deformity.

As an otolaryngologist, before his 1887 paper,[5] Roe had previously written about nasal stenosis, a radical cure for hay fever, the relationship of nasal disorders to asthma, and various other topics not directly related to the nose, including esophagostomy, retropharyngeal abscesses, and laryngeal chorea. After his 1887 paper, he subsequently wrote more than a dozen papers[44-51] dealing with nasal deformities and deviations of the nasal septum, some of which may interest the reader who is absorbed with his contributions.

In his second paper in 1891, which was another medical first, he cosmetically reduced an entire nose, including the removal of a prominent bony

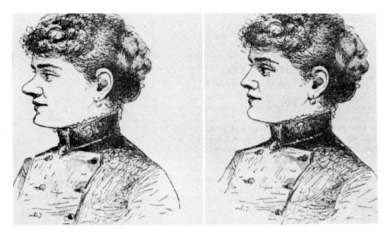

Fig. 4-7. Preoperative and postoperative photographs of patient treated by Roe for pug nose deformity. (From Roe, J. O.: Med. Rec. **31**:621, 1887.)

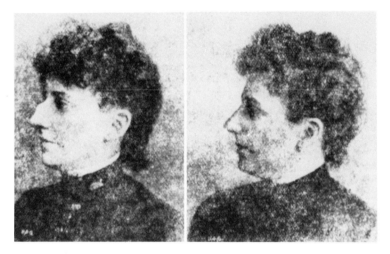

Fig. 4-8. Preoperative and postoperative photographs of patient treated by Roe to reduce overall size of nose. (From Roe, J. O.: Med. Rec. **40**:57, 1891.)

and cartilaginous hump through an intranasal subcutaneous approach (Fig. 4-8) 7 years before Jacques Joseph reported similar success using external incisions.[18,44] His operations were performed under local cocaine anesthesia. He undermined the skin widely, inserted an angulated bone scissors, and cut off enough of the hump until the dorsum was smooth. At the end of the operation he strapped the skin down with external pressure and a splint. There is no doubt on the part of medical historians today that these two papers of 1887 and 1891 have established Roe as the originator of corrective or cosmetic rhinoplasty, despite Joseph's claim to this title. In all fairness to Joseph, however, who came on the scene in 1898, no one would disagree (because of Joseph's accomplishments) if modern historians call him the overall father of corrective rhinoplasty.

One year later in 1892, Robert F. Weir[63] (1838-1927) of New York City (Fig. 4-9), a contemporary of Roe, who worked as Gurdon Buck's assistant,[59] described a new operation using intranasal incisions in which he stabilized newly fractured nasal bones in a more medial position by means of steel needles inserted transversely through the entire nose and held in place with clamps on either side of the nose. In another case, he operated on a young male socialite to reduce a large nose, but he employed an overly cautious bits-and-smidgens surgical approach, using four small separate operations in a difficult-to-please patient to accomplish what Roe, and subsequently several years later, Jacques Joseph of Berlin accomplished in a single operation. The only major contribution of Weir in this tedious case was his use of crescent-shaped incisions at the base of the ala nasae to reduce the width of the base and lower the nasal apex.

In this same paper he also described a technique common to the surgeons of his age of inserting a heterogenous transplant to correct a saddle nose. He used the breastbone of a freshly killed duck, which, after an initial satisfactory cosmetic result, had to be removed at the end of 8 weeks because it was the focus of a fulminating swelling and abscess.

The reader can be given an idea of the state of operating room asepsis by inspecting Fig. 4-10, a photograph of an operation performed in the year 1894 at Manhattan Eye, Ear, and Throat Hospital in New York City. Notice the absence of masks, gowns, and gloves, and the formal morning coat attire of the surgeons and the visitors in the gallery!

Czerny,[6] in 1895, used the upper lateral cartilages cut free from the septum, turned medially and upward and sutured back to back on themselves to elevate the dorsum of a saddle nose. This technique with many variations has been reported in subsequent decades by authors who have all too frequently thought their operation to be original without checking the older literature. Fig. 4-11

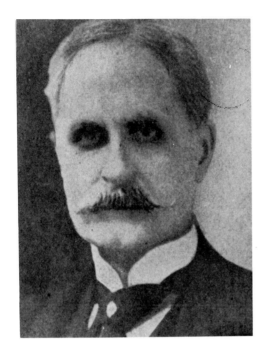

Fig. 4-9. Robert F. Weir (1838-1927). (From Aufricht, G.: Plast. Reconstr. Surg. **1:**3, 1946.)

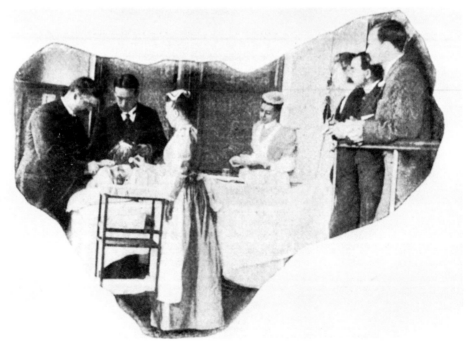

Fig. 4-10. Operating room in 1894, during nasal operation, at Manhattan Eye, Ear, and Throat Hospital, New York City. (From Manhattan Eye, Ear, and Throat Hospital Annual Reports, 1894.)

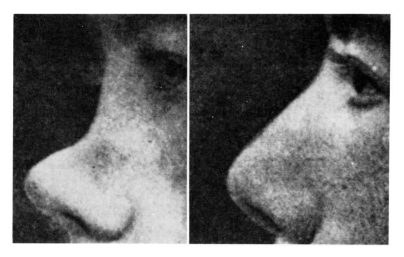

Fig. 4-11. Preoperative and postoperative photographs of patient treated by Roe for correction of saddle nose deformity. (From Roe, J. O.: Med. Rec. **51:**798, 1897.)

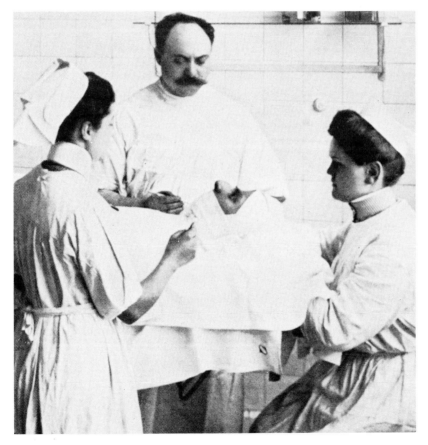

Fig. 4-12. Photograph of Jacques Joseph with two nurse assistants. (From Joseph, J.: Nasenplastik und sonstige Gesichtsplastik nebst einem Anhang ueber Mammaplastik, Leipzig, Germany, 1928, Verlag von Curt Kabitzsch.)

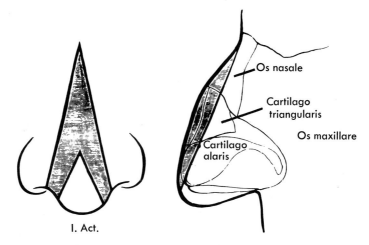

I. Act.

Fig. 4-13. Joseph's method of using external excisions to reduce size of overly large nose. (From Joseph, J.: Ueber die operative Verkleinerung einer Nase [Rhinomiosis], Berl. Klin. Wochenschr. **40**:882, 1898.)

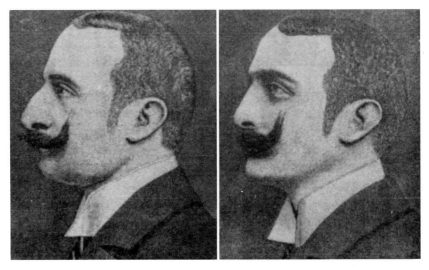

Fig. 4-14. Preoperative and postoperative views of first patient treated for reduction in size of nose by external incisions by Joseph in 1898. (From Joseph, J.: Berl. Klin. Wochenschr. **40**:882, 1898.)

shows preoperative and postoperative photographs of a patient in an 1897 paper of Roe in which a saddle nose was repaired by transplanting intranasal tissues to the cartilaginous dorsum "without aid of metallic or other artificial supports."[45]

In 1898, George Howard Monks[40] (1853-1933) described his technique of the removal of a bony hump and reduction in the size of a nose by use of a small incision made through the nasal tip skin just at the anterior border of the columella. Kolle and other surgeons who tried this technique found it practically impossible to perform any reasonably

good surgery with the scissors in the position illustrated by Monks, who apparently did not find it difficult to work through such a small columellar incision. In 1898, another historical milestone occurred when Jacques Joseph[18] of Berlin (Fig. 4-12), whose life is a fascinating one indeed,[41] excised externally an inverted V-shaped segment along the nasal dorsum through the skin, bone, cartilage, and mucosal lining, and the entire thickness of the nasal alae, and removed a wedge from the lower part of the septum to shorten and reduce an overly conspicuous nose all in one single operation (Fig. 4-13). Fig. 4-14 shows the preoperative and postoperative photographs of the "28-year-old [male] landowner" on whom Joseph performed this operation.

He published a second paper[19] in 1902 noting that he had then performed ten such cosmetic operations but was still using external skin incisions and excisions through which he removed the hump and shortened the nose. By 1904, despite the continued successes reported in America by Roe of the latter's use of intranasal incisions, Joseph[21] had to admit that he had finally come around to using intranasal incisions instead of his previously employed external skin incisions, and by that year he had performed forty-three operations. In another paper[20] in 1904 he described for the first time his external clamps and his right-angle nasal saws, and by 1905 he reported[22] that he had operated on 100 patients requiring corrective rhinoplasty. In another paper[35] in 1905 he emphasized the use of plaster casts and carefully taken photographs for studying each patient and the value of these items in assessing postoperative results.

He published his first extensive treatise[23] on rhinoplasty in 1907 in which he classified and described the individual operative steps for the correction of many types of nasal deformities. Other papers[24-27] led eventually in 1922 to a well-illustrated and lengthy treatise[28] on corrective rhinoplasty, and, finally, his monumental two-volume text[29] was published on this subject between the years 1928 and 1931.

Joseph Safian[56] and Gustave Aufricht[1] deserve great credit for bringing to the attention of English-speaking surgeons the accomplishments of Joseph. The text of Safian's 1935 book, *Corrective Rhinoplastic Surgery,* was so clearly and simply written that it helped in the more widespread adoption of many of Joseph's procedures. For all intents and purposes, Joseph originated most of the variations in intranasal operative techniques that we employ today, and he was responsible for the development of most of the rhinoplastic instruments we now use. Aufricht[3] wrote of him in his usual warm manner:

It was bewildering for a young surgeon to see that he [Joseph] had a special instrument for practically every step of a rhinoplasty. It almost seemed that one only had to have all those instruments and the operation was easy. . . . Some of the general surgeons thought that rhinoplasty was a very simple operation and that was the reason Joseph was reluctant to show it. It was said that Professor Axhausen, one of Germany's leading plastic surgeons, asked and received permission to observe Joseph's operation. He admitted afterward that

while rhinoplasty was surgically simple it took Joseph's special talent to perform it successfully.*

Aufricht,[1] in 1940, wrote that whereas Joseph used only adhesive and gauze dressings to splint his cases, occasional hematomas followed this inadequate type of postoperative splinting, and Aufricht, therefore, introduced his dental compound splint, which many of us use routinely today.

With the exception of Roe, Weir, Joseph, and a few others, corrective rhinoplasty started to come into its own only in the first decade of the twentieth century at a time when a few other cosmetic surgical procedures were being performed occasionally, some of them by men verging on the brink of quackery if not outright quacks.[53,54] The first specific book on cosmetic surgery was published in 1907 by Charles Conrad Miller,[37,38] a brilliant but tragic figure from Chicago, a quack whose accomplishments were reviewed in much more detail in two papers[53,54] published several years ago.

It was not uncommon in those days for some cosmetic surgeons to advertise in local newspapers. This did not help the cosmetic branch of surgery in gaining early acceptance and respectability by any stretch of the imagination. But many of us need not read the newspapers of 70 years ago to get the feeling or tone of such advertisements. They still exist today. For many years in New York City, the ad in Fig. 4-15 had been running in one of the city's leading cynical left-wing liberal newspapers, and the ad in (Fig. 4-16) ran in a New York City scandal sheet. And just to take a swipe at the other end of the political spectrum, the ad in Fig. 4-17 has been run off and on for years in the Paris edition of the International Herald Tribune.

Miller's[36] illustrations and photographs of surgery to reduce a hump nose deformity are perhaps the first in medical history to show us an actual corrective rhinoplasty being performed. Fig. 4-18 shows Miller's method of reducing a wide nasal tip by means of excising partial-thickness wedges of skin, cartilage, and mucosal lining from the nasal alae.[39] Several years before Miller's first surgical paper was published, injections of Vaseline for the correction of facial defects were described by Gersuny[13] in 1900. Vaseline injections were soon discarded because of unfavorable results and especially because of complications, including severe local tissue reactions and distant emboli, with some cases of fatal pulmonary emboli. In 1902,

---

*From Aufricht, G.: Plast. Reconstr. Surg. 1:3, 1956.

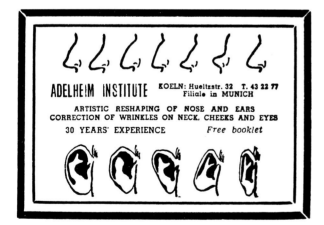

Fig. 4-15. Advertisement in New York daily newspaper of "plastic surgeon." (From New York Post, May 19, 1960.)

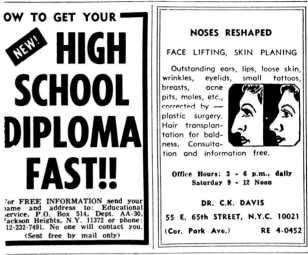

Fig. 4-17. Advertisement of European "plastic surgeon" performing corrective nasoplastic surgery. (From Paris edition, International Herald Tribune.)

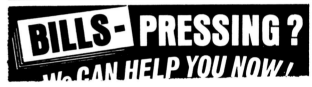

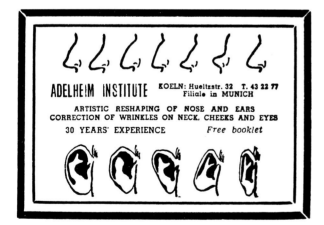

Fig. 4-16. Advertisement in New York City scandal sheet newspaper of "plastic surgeon" performing cosmetic surgery.

Eckstein[10] described the injection of low-melting-point paraffin. From that time onward for approximately 20 years or more many physicians injected paraffin with immediately good results, as seen in Fig. 4-19, showing a patient injected for the treatment of a nasal deformity by a surgeon on the staff of the Manhattan Eye, Ear, and Throat Hospital in 1904. Paraffin injections were finally discarded after many years of trial, however, because of local paraffinoma formation and distant complications, which included thrombosis, phlebitis, pulmonary emboli, and infarction. These injections of Vaseline and paraffin in the first two decades of the twentieth century served as one of the major drawbacks of this era, delaying the more rapid and accepted development of corrective cosmetic surgery in general and corrective nasoplastic surgery in particular because all too frequently good cosmetic surgeons such as Kolle[31] also fell susceptible to the blandishments of quick results obtainable through paraffin injections.

During this first twentieth-century decade, nasal prostheses of a surprisingly good quality

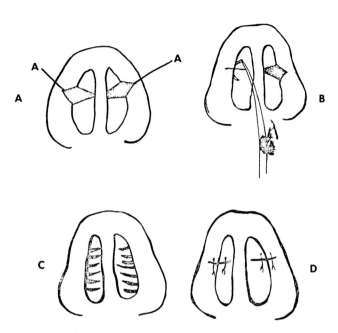

Fig. 4-18. Miller's method of excising wedges of tissue from alar cartilages and mucosa to reduce width of nasal tip. **A,** Diamond-shaped wedges for excision. **B,** Closure of wedge defects. **C,** Method to score lateral wings of alar cartilage to break stiffness and box shape of prominent nasal tip. **D,** Final closure of diamond-shaped defects. (From Miller, C. C.: Am. J. Derm. Genitourin. Dis. **11:**286, 1907.)

were available for those many cases of gaping facial and nasal defects due to syphilis of both the congenital and acquired variety. An example of one of these prostheses made in 1904 is shown in the advertisement in Fig. 4-20. Many of these prostheses were made of a celluloid compound or gutta percha and painted to resemble the normal skin of the nose.

Frederick Strange Kolle[31] (1871-1929) of New York City (Fig. 4-21) was the second author in medical history to describe cosmetic surgery in book form. His 1911 book, entitled *Plastic and Cosmetic Surgery,* was a large tome of 511 pages containing 522 illustrations. In this book he showed his readers the use of wedge excisions to narrow the alar base (Fig. 4-22), his excisions to reduce and narrow a box nasal tip (Fig. 4-23), his method to correct an overly retroussé nose (Fig. 4-24), his external excision of redundant columellar tissue to correct a hooked elongated nasal tip (Figs. 4-25 and 4-26), and his lateral external incisions on the nose for various other reduction procedures. Unfortunately he became victimized by the vogue of injecting paraffin and recommended it rather highly in his book. According to him, paraffin injections were developed partially as a replacement for the much-objected-to metallic and bony implants, which were often unsuccessful in an age in which the advantages of a protective antibiotic therapy were unavailable to those surgeons who had the amazing courage to perform such elective surgery without worrying about the consequences.

After Joseph's[23] recommendation for the inser-

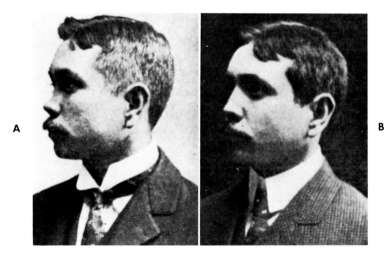

Fig. 4-19. A, Patient with saddle nose deformity. **B,** Improvement obtained in saddle nose deformity after injection of liquid paraffin. (From Manhattan Eye, Ear, and Throat Hospital Annual Reports, 1904.)

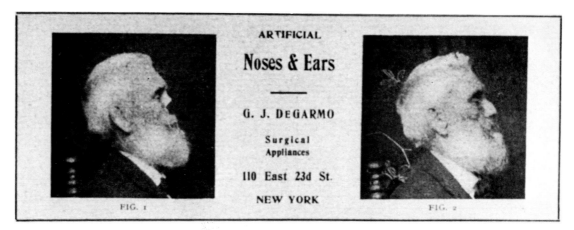

Fig. 4-20. Advertisement in 1904 demostrating available nasal prostheses for correction of gaping nasal defects. (From Manhattan Eye, Ear, and Throat Hospital Annual Reports, 1904.)

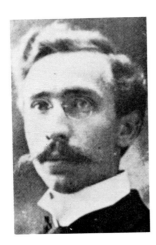

Fig. 4-21. Portrait of German-born American cosmetic surgeon Frederick Strange Kolle. (From Grigg, E. R. N.: The trail of the invisible light, Springfield, Ill., 1965, Charles C Thomas, Publisher.)

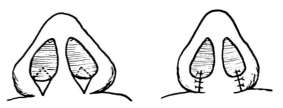

Fig. 4-22. Surgical technique to narrow alar bases. (From Davis, J. S.: Plastic surgery: its principles and practice, Philadelphia, 1919, P. Blakiston's Son & Co.)

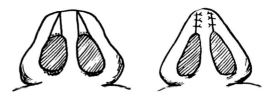

Fig. 4-23. External excisions to reduce and narrow box nasal tip. (From Davis, J. S.: Plastic surgery: its principles and practice, Philadelphia, 1919, P. Blakiston's Son & Co.)

tion of transplants through an intranasal incision rather than a glabellar incision, the controversy over the relative merits of the use of ivory versus bone versus cartilage was soon resolved by the majority of surgeons utilizing either fresh cartilage transplants, iliac bone grafts, or tibial bone grafts.

At the end of World War I, John Staige Davis, writing in his classic 1919 textbook of plastic surgery, like many men trained in those years in general surgery, had an attitude about cosmetic or aesthetic surgery that left a good deal to be desired.

He described corrective rhinoplastic surgery in this somewhat condescending fashion: "These trimming and shaping operations are extremely difficult, and a bad situation is often made worse by an unskillful operator or a poorly planned operation."[7] He unfortunately called the few corrective operations he described in his book "secondary rhinoplastic operations."

H. Lyons Hunt,[16] however, a plastic surgeon from New York City, writing several years later after the end of World War I, taking an aim at

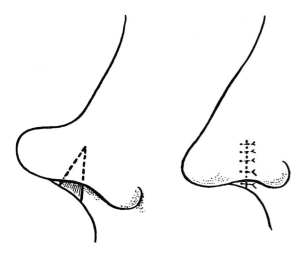

Fig. 4-24. Surgical method to correct overly retroussé nose by intranasal and intercolumellar excision of tissue. (From Kolle, F. S.: Plastic and cosmetic surgery, New York, 1911, D. Appleton & Co.)

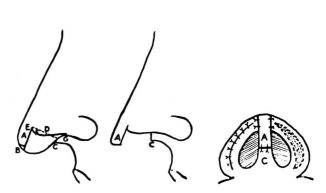

Fig. 4-25. External excision of redundant hooklike columellar tissue to correct elongated nasal tip. (From Davis, J. S.: Plastic surgery: its principles and practice, Philadelphia, 1919, P. Blakiston's Son & Co.)

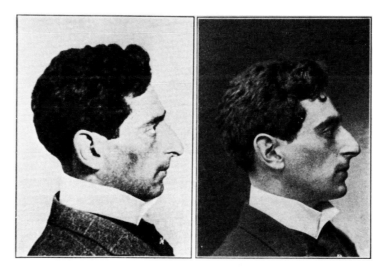

Fig. 4-26. *Left,* Preoperative photograph of an operatic baritone with "hooklike" prominent elongated nasal tip. *Right,* Postoperative results after operation shown in Fig. 4-25. (From Kolle, F. S.: Plastic and cosmetic surgery, New York, 1911, D. Appleton & Co.)

John Staige Davis' unsympathetic attitude about corrective surgery, stated:

The war ended. The injured returned. The reconstructive work of the plastic surgeons was now on exhibition. When it became known that plastic surgery was successful in returning these men to their places in civil life, a new call developed for this type of surgery. This time from those who from the cradle had suffered humiliation, and embarrassment because of irregular and distorted features. By those dependent upon their appearance for their living, a demand for cosmetic improvement was heard. This demand is by no means an unreasonable one, for there is a constantly increasing preference in the business and professional world for attractive and youthful employees.*

Hunt's book of *Plastic Surgery of the Head, Face and Neck* in 1926 was preceded a year earlier by J. Eastman Sheehan's *Plastic Surgery of the Nose*,[58] which was probably the first textbook devoted to corrective nasoplastic surgery, followed by other

_____
*From Hunt, H. L.: Plastic surgery of the head, face and neck, Philadelphia, 1926, Lea & Febiger.

excellent textbooks on corrective nasal surgery by Joseph[29] in 1928 to 1931, by Safian[56] in 1935, by Maliniac[34] in 1947, by Seltzer[57] in 1949, by Brown and McDowell[4] in 1951, by Denecke and Meyer[8] in 1967, and by Fomon[12] in 1970.

It might be appropriate to conclude with a quotation and a slight paraphrasing of the introduction to their book by Brown and McDowell[4] as follows:

Since the time of Joseph there have been many scholars and students who have added greatly to the procedures of corrective plastic surgery of the nose. [I would have liked] to include references to the reports of all who have contributed since Joseph, but space was not available for the long list.

The truth, as Socrates said, belongs to everyone, so that the trained plastic surgeon rightfully uses the basic procedures [of Dieffenbach, Roe, Joseph and others] and makes an original contribution in each patient that he is asked to care for. . . . [He] thus contributes to solving the main problem, which is restoration of [a more] normal contour to allow for [the best possible physical, emotional and psychologic response to his surgery on the part of each patient he is fortunate enough to treat. And we who consider ourselves corrective nasoplastic surgeons today all agree that this is indeed a very rewarding and satisfying branch of surgery for us to be fortunate enough to take part in from day to day].*

---

*From Brown, J. B., and McDowell, F.: Plastic surgery of the nose, ed. 3, Springfield, Ill., 1965, Charles C Thomas, Publisher.

REFERENCES

1. Aufricht, G.: Dental molding compound cast and adhesive strapping in rhinoplasty, Arch. Otolaryngol. **32**:333, 1940.
2. Aufricht, G.: The development of plastic surgery in the United States, Plast. Reconstr. Surg. **1**:3, 1946.
3. Aufricht, G.: Commentary on the paper: operative reduction on the size of a nose (rhinomyosis) by Jacques Joseph, Plast. Reconstr. Surg. **46**:181, 1970.
4. Brown, J. B., and McDowell, F.: Plastic surgery of the nose, ed. 3, Springfield, Ill., 1965, Charles C Thomas, Publisher.
5. Cottle, M. H.: John Orlando Roe, pioneer in modern rhinoplasty, Arch. Otolaryngol. **80**:22, 1964.
6. Czerny: Korrektur der Sattelnase durch Bildung eines Nasenrückens aus dem knorplig-knöchernen Seitendache der Nase, Chir. Kongr. Verhandl. **2**:214, 1895.
7. Davis, J. S.: Plastic surgery: its principles and practice, Philadelphia, 1919, P. Blakiston's Son & Co.
8. Denecke, H. J., and Meyer, R.: Plastic surgery of head and neck. 1. Corrective and reconstructive rhinoplasty, New York, 1967, Springer-Verlag New York Inc., p. 451.
9. Dieffenbach, J. F.: Die operative Chirurgie, Leipzig, Germany, 1845, F. A. Brockhaus.
10. Eckstein, H.: Ueber subkutane und submukose Hartparaffinprothesen, Dtsch. Med. Wochenschr. **28**:573, 1902.
11. Fomon, S., Caron, A. L., Bell, J. W., and Schattner, A.: Rhinologic versus orthopedic rhinoplasty, Arch. Otolaryngol. **62**:409, 1955.
12. Fomon, S., and Bell, J.: Rhinoplasty—new concepts: evaluation and application, Springfield, Ill., 1970, Charles C Thomas, Publisher.
13. Gersuny, R.: Ueber eine subcutane Prothese, Z. Heilkd. **1**:199, 1900.
14. Gillies, H. D., and Millard, D. R., Jr.: The principles and art of plastic surgery, Boston, 1957, Little, Brown & Co.
15. Hardie, J.: On a new rhinoplastic operation, Brit. Med. J., 1875, p. 393.
16. Hunt, H. L.: Plastic surgery of the head, face and neck, Philadelphia, 1926, Lea & Febiger.
17. Israel, J.: Zwei neue Methoden der Rhinoplastik, Arch. Klin. Chir. **53**:255, 1896; Plast. Reconstr. Surg. **46**:80, 1970.
18. Joseph, J.: Ueber die operative Verkleinerung einer Nase (rhinomiosis), Berl. Klin. Wochenschr. **40**:882, 1898; Plast. Reconstr. Surg. **46**:178, 1970.
19. Joseph, J.: Ueber einige weitere Nasenverkleinerungen, Berl. Klin. Wochenschr., p. 851, 1902.
20. Joseph, J.: Nasenverkleinerungen, Dtsch. Med. Wochenschr. **30**:1095, 1904.
21. Joseph, J.: Intranasale Nasenhöckerabtragung, Berl. Klin. Wochenschr., p. 650, 1904.
22. Joseph, J.: Weiteres über Nasenverkleinerungen, Münch. Med. Wochenschr. **52**:1489, 1905.
23. Joseph, J.: Beiträge zur Rhinoplastik, Berl. Klin. Wochenschr. **44**:470, 1907.
24. Joseph, J.: Nasenkorrekturen, Verhandl. Gesellsch. Dtsch. Naturforschr. u. Ärzte in Königsberg, pt. 2, vol. 2, sec. 2, p. 340, 1910.
25. Joseph, J.: Beiträge zur totalen Rhinoplastik, Münch. Med. Wochenschr. **51**:705, 1914.
26. Joseph, J.: Zur Gesichtsplastik mit besonderer Berücksichtigung der Nasenplastik, Dtsch. Med. Wochenschr., p. 35, 1919.
27. Joseph, J.: Beiträge zur totalen und partiellen Rhinoneoplastik nebst einem Vorschlage zur freien Hautüberpflanzung, Klin. Wochenschr. **14**:678, 1922.
28. Joseph, J.: In Katz and Blumenfeld, editors: Handbuch der speziellen Chirurgie, Leipzig, Germany, 1922, Verlag von Curt Kabitzsch.
29. Joseph, J.: Nasenplastik und sonstige Gesichtsplastik nebst einem Anhang ueber Mammaplastik, Leipzig, Germany, 1931, Verlag von Curt Kabitzsch.
30. Konig, F.: Eine neue Methode der Aufrichtung eingesunkener Nasen, Arch. Klin. Chir. **34**:41, 1886.
31. Kolle, F. S.: Plastic and cosmetic surgery, New York, 1911, D. Appleton & Co.
32. Linhart, W.: Beiträge zur Rhinoplastik, Würzb. Med. Z. **1**:37, 1860.
33. Lossen: Hüters Grundriss der Chirurgie, vol. 2, 1884, p. 85.
34. Maliniac, J. W.: Rhinoplasty and restoration of facial contour, Philadelphia, 1947, F. A. Davis Co.
35. McDowell, F., Vallone, J. A., and Brown, J. B.: Bibliography and historical note on plastic surgery of the nose, Plast. Reconstr. Surg. **10**:149, 1952.

36. Miller, C. C.: Surgical treatment of hump nose, Med. Brief **34**:160, 1906.
37. Miller, C. C.: Cosmetic surgery: the correction of featural imperfections, Chicago, 1907, Oak.
38. Miller, C. C.: Cosmetic surgery: the correction of featural imperfections, ed. 2, Chicago, 1908, Oak.
39. Miller, C. C.: Outstanding alae nasi, Am. J. Derm. Genitourin. Dis. **11**:286, 1907.
40. Monks, G. H.: Correction, by operation, of some nasal deformities and disfigurements, Boston Med. Surg. J. **139**:262, 1898; Plast. Reconstr. Surg. **48**:485, 1971.
41. Natvig, P.: Some aspects of the character and personality of Jacques Joseph, Plast. Reconstr. Surg. **47**:452, 1971.
42. Ollier: De l'ostéoplasie appliquée à la restauration du nez, Gaz. Hôp. Paris **37**:349, 1864.
43. Roe, J. O.: The deformity termed pug nose and its correction by a simple operation, Med. Rec. **31**:621, 1887; Plast. Reconstr. Surg. **45**:78, 1970.
44. Roe, J. O.: The correction of angular deformities of the nose by a subcutaneous operation, Med. Rec. **40**:57, 1891.
45. Roe, J. O.: Correction of depressed and saddle back deformities of nose by operations performed subcutaneously without aid of metallic or other artificial supports, Med. Rec. **51**:798, 1897.
46. Roe, J. O.: Case of fracture and depression of anterior wall of maxillary antrum, with restoration of depressed wall, Trans. Am. Laryng. Assoc., 1898, p. 203.
47. Roe, J. O.: Correction of nasal deformities by subcutaneous operations, Am. Med. Quart. **1**:56, 1899.
48. Roe, J. O.: New operation for restoration of columna and anterior portion of nasal septum, Trans. Am. Laryng. Assoc., 1902, p. 221.
49. Roe, J. O.: Removal of obstructions and cicatricial contractions of nose by plastic method, Trans. Am. Laryngol. Assoc., 1903, p. 257.
50. Roe, J. O.: The correction of nasal deformities, Laryngoscope **18**:782, 1908.
51. Roe, J. O.: Nasal deformity as cause of nasal obstruction corrected by subcutaneous method, Trans. Am. Laryngol. Assoc., 1915, p. 285. 1915.
52. Rogers, B. O.: Carl Ferdinand von Graefe (1787-1840), Plast. Reconstr. Surg. **46**:554, 1970.
53. Rogers, B. O.: A chronologic history of cosmetic surgery, Bull. N.Y. Acad. Med. **47**:265, 1971.
54. Rogers, B. O.: A brief history of cosmetic surgery, Surg. Clin. North Am. **51**:265, 1971.
55. Rousset: Thèse sur la rhinoplastie, thèse de Paris, 1828. Cited by Nelaton, C., and Ombrédanne, L.: La rhinoplastie, Paris, 1904, G. Steinheil.
56. Safian, J.: Corrective rhinoplastic surgery, New York, 1935, Paul B. Hoeber, Inc.
57. Seltzer, A. P.: Plastic surgery of the nose, Philadelphia, 1949, J. B. Lippincott Co.
58. Sheehan, J. E.: Plastic surgery of the nose, New York, 1925, Paul Hoeber Co.
59. Stark, R. B.: Friendship of three giants, Plast. Reconstr. Surg. **40**:599, 1967.
60. Szymanowski, J. von: Handbuch der operativen Chirurgie, Braunschweig, Germany, 1870, F. Vieweg u. Sohn.
61. Trendelenburg: Verhandl. Dtsch. Gesellsch. Chir. **19**:82, 1889.
62. von Mangold: Heilung der Sattelnase durch Knorpelübertragung, Chir. Kongr. Verhandl., p. 470, 1900; Verhandl. Dtsch. Gesellsch. Chir. **29**:460, 1900.
63. Weir, R. F.: On restoring sunken noses, N.Y. Med. J. **56**:449, 1892.

Chapter 5

More recent concepts of nasal development

Otto B. Kriens, M.D., D.D.S.
Walter Ritter, D.D.S.*

HISTORICAL REVIEW

According to the first descriptions of the nasal development by von Baer[1] in 1828 and by Rathke[18] in 1832, the frontal process occupies almost the entire width of the embryonic face. At its stomodeal margin the frontal process was inferred to develop a medial and lateral process on each side. They were assumed to grow around the nasal pits and fuse ventrally. It was surmised from the external appearance that the frontal process is separated by a slitlike furrow from the maxillary process of each side in much the same way branchial arches were believed to be separated, that is, by a membrane of endodermal and ectodermal epithelium. These early studies were performed under magnifying glasses. With the improvement of the microscopes in the middle of the last century, more detailed and precise illustrations were published[3,8,15] (Figs. 5-1 and 5-2).

For many years the development and fusion of the facial processes were given undue attention. The reason may be the understanding of the facial processes as more or less autonomous processes similar to those of the branchial arches. Each process was erroneously assumed to be related to a specific nerve or artery. Fusion of the processes was supposed to occur across these epithelial walls. This conjecture was perhaps arrived at also because of the similarity of the location of the furrows and of several facial anomalies, for example, the cleft lip, the oroauricular cleft, and the oroocular cleft.

For many decades it has been discussed whether clefts in the face are primary in nature, that is, a nonfusion of facial processes, or secondary, that is, a rupture of the epithelial wall after insufficient mesodermal penetration.[6,25] Morian[13] and Pollitzer[17] published evidence that several facial clefts do not correspond to the embryonic furrows, and Frangenheim[4] postulated a yet-unknown cleft to explain the pathomorphology of the lateral nasal cleft. In 1942 Töndury[24] said that the formation of the processes is less important than the elimination of the furrows, a statement that emphasizes the importance of mesectodermal development below the surface of the eminences of the developing face.

Evidence against the concept of processes and furrows consists of findings in favor of mesectoderm developing below the neural plate.[16] It helps to form the supportive structures. Furthermore, growth in the prechordal region was found to be nonmetameric.[5,26] Studies revealed that the nasolacrimal duct does not correspond to the topography of paranasal clefts.[17] Among the clinical observations unexplainable by the von Baer-Rathke concept are the median clefts of the nose, the median cleft face syndrome, unilateral nasal aplasia, monorhinic conditions with a lateral proboscis, and the lateral nasal cleft.

STAGES OF DEVELOPMENT

The development of the nose can be divided into three successive stages, which overlap. Each is likely to have its characteristic developmental disturbances. These stages are (1) the undifferentiated mesectodermal stage, during which the em-

*Professor of Dentistry, Zahn-, Mund-, und Kieferklinik, University of Muenster, Muenster, Germany.

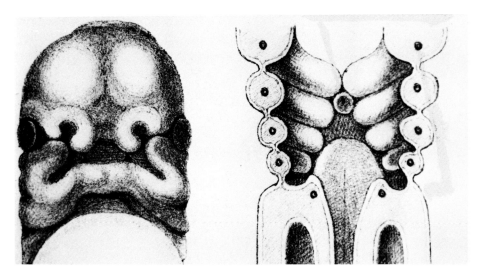

Fig. 5-1. Embryonic face and branchial arches. At stomodeal border of frontal process two crescent-shaped eminences develop around nasal pits. Frontal process is divided from maxillary ones by a slitlike furrow, which was believed to resemble epithelial membrane between branchial arches. (From His, W.: Unsere Koerperform und physiologische Probleme ihrer Entstehung, Leipzig, Germany, 1874, Vogel.)

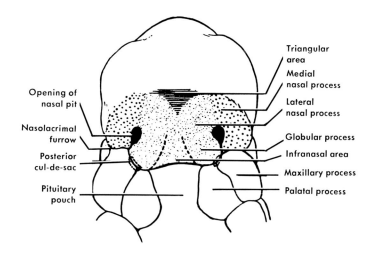

Fig. 5-2. Drawing of embryonic face by Peter, who still adhered to von Baer-Rathke concept in 1909. (From Peter, K.: Atlas der Entwicklung der Nase und des Gaumens beim Menschen, Jena, Germany, 1909, Fischer.)

bryonic face and especially the nose can be regarded as a growing epithelial mold, (2) the stage of the nasal capsule, and (3) the stage of the final differentiation of the primordial mesectodermal derivates into perichondrial and endochondral bone as well as into cartilage and fibrous tissue.

The undifferentiated mesectoderm

On the eighteenth day the optic placode appears as the first sensory organ anlage. It is followed by the appearance of the otic placode at about the twenty-first day. Finally, about the thirtieth day, the olfactory placodes can be observed on the ventral aspect of the telencephalic prominences. The nasal placodes are induced by mesoderm and prosencephalic tissue.[23] The human embryo measures about 6 mm crown-rump length at this time.[22] Rapid mesectodermal growth leads to an "invagination" of the nasal placodes. Their cells are elongated and can readily be distinguished from the adjacent epithelial cells on cross sections. Induction initiates the development of

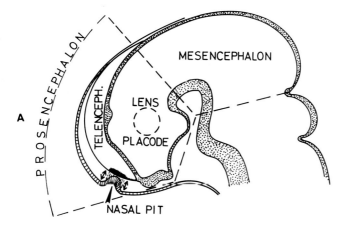

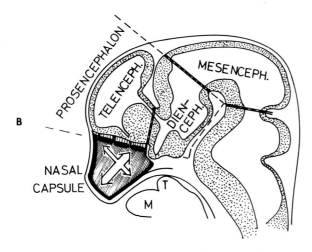

Fig. 5-3. A, Sagittal section through embryonic head at about thirty-fifth day. Nasal pit develops on anteroventral convexity of prosencephalic hemisphere. **B,** Three-dimensional expansion of nasal capsule below prosencephalon is indicated by arrows.

the olfactory nerves in the area of the placodal epithelium. The other epithelium is "carried" forward by the increment in tissue of the developing face, and regular surface epithelium is formed in the remaining nasal cavity (Fig. 5-3, *A*).

The nasal capsule

The early traces of the developing nasal capsule have been observed in the human embryo by Slaby[21] at about the thirty-fifth day. The nasal capsule appears as a condensation of its blastema. Cartilage cells are visible in the blastema about the fortieth day. Soon after the olfactory nerves have developed (about the forty-fifth day), the area of the cribriform plate of the nasal capsule forms.

Although the nasal capsule apparently forms from one common blastema, it starts to grow from different centers of chondrification. The various portions of the nasal capsule increase in size and "mature" at different periods of time. While in one portion the primordial cartilage is still growing, it may begin to be resorbed or replaced by endochondral or perichondrial ossification in other areas.[20,22] Thus an optimal stage of development of the nasal capsule is never attained.

The nasal capsule is made up of the septum sagittal in the midline (Fig. 5-4, *B*). It is continuous with the tectum nasi or roof, the later dorsum of the nose (Fig. 5-5). The lateral wall (paries nasi) has its own center of chondrification. The developmental borderline between the tectum and the paries nasi appears to be a branch of the nasoethmoidal nerve. The cribriform plate is an important structure cephalad. The two elongated ventral openings are closed anteriorly by the transverse lamina (Fig. 5-4, *A*). It connects the lateral wall with the ventral margin of the septum. The nasolacrimal duct passes over the transverse lamina ventrally and enters the nasal cavity anterior to it. The paraseptal cartilages (Fig. 5-4, *C*) at both sides of the ventral margin of the septum begin at the posterior border of the transverse lamina. Also posterior to the transverse lamina, the incisive foramen is formed with the fusion of the palatal shelves.[20,22]

The septum probably contains several older structures, for example, the paired rostral portion of the trabeculate lamina, which is the narrow primordial cranial base in the midline of the chondrocranium. The septum is also believed to contain the interorbital septum, and the medial wall of the paired anlage of the nasal capsule.[21]

The bony skeleton of the nose

Most of the surface of the nasal capsule is eventually covered by perichondral bone. The sites of the first perichondral bone formation are over the tectal cartilage, over the lateral wall with its own center of chondrification, and on the ventral side of the transverse lamina (Fig. 5-6).

Animal experiments have revealed that the contour of the perichondral bone can differ considerably from that of a dysplastic nasal capsule and thus may camouflage a developmental malformation of the chondrocranial stage, such as a choanal atresia.

A much lesser portion of the nasal bone is formed by endochondral ossification, for example, the posterior region of the nasal septum. The explanation may be that endochondral growth facilitates a rapid growth of the primordial skeleton, and only perichondral ossification seems to cope

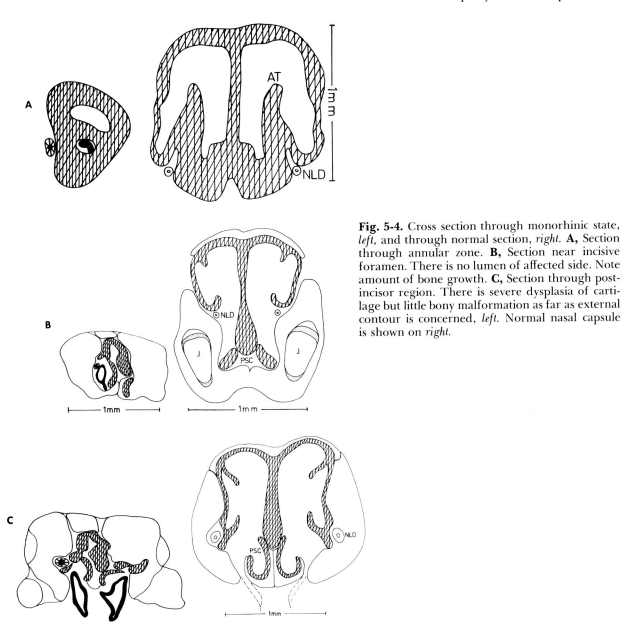

Fig. 5-4. Cross section through monorhinic state, *left,* and through normal section, *right.* **A,** Section through annular zone. **B,** Section near incisive foramen. There is no lumen of affected side. Note amount of bone growth. **C,** Section through post-incisor region. There is severe dysplasia of cartilage but little bony malformation as far as external contour is concerned, *left.* Normal nasal capsule is shown on *right.*

Fig. 5-5. Rostral region of nasal capsule. Semischematic illustration of various cartilaginous components existing during development. There is a close principal resemblance of these portions of the chondrocranial skeleton among vertebrates despite variations in species. There is no maximal or optimal stage of development of nasal capsule: it starts to develop confluently from various centers of blastema. Later at different periods portions may be replaced by bone, permanent cartilage, or fascia or may disappear.

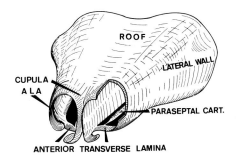

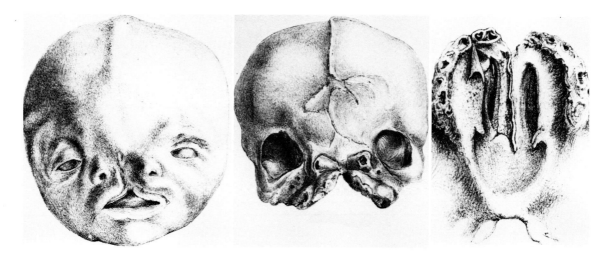

Fig. 5-6. Median cleft face syndrome. Nasal capsule has remained paired by median dysraphia. Perichondral bone formation has occurred over rostral portions of malformed nasal capsule. (From Witzel, O.: Arch. Klin. Chir. **27:**893, 1882.)

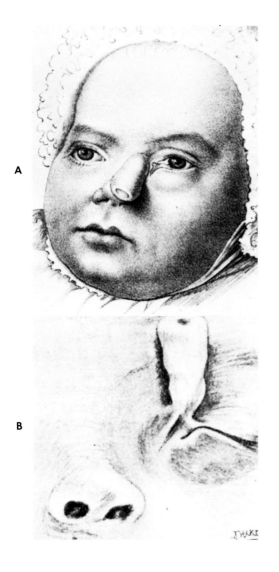

Fig. 5-7. A, Lateral proboscis with normal contralateral nose in 5-week-old boy. (From Landow, M.: Z. Chir. **30:**544, 1890.) **B,** Lateral proboscis with normally configurate nose and proboscis. (From Kirchmayr, L.: Dtsch. Z. Chir. **81:**71, 1906.)

with it. Few areas of the nasal capsule are transformed into fibrous tissue, for example, the intercartilaginous fascia in the tip. The anterior (that is, rostral) portion of the nasal capsule remains cartilaginous.

MALFORMATIONS OF THE EXTERNAL NOSE
The nose in holoprosencephaly

As early as 1882 Kundrat described the relationship of nasal and cerebral malformation in a monograph on arhinencephaly, published in Graz, Austria. He classified the various hypoteloric conditions (cyclopia, ethmocephaly, cebocephaly) and dealt with the deficient development of the brain. In cyclopic infants the vestige of the nasal primordia is located above the one eye. No nasal cavity has developed in these arhinencephalic individuals. The external nose is but a median proboscis.[9,11] Cyclopic infants, however, have a nearly normal upper lip, although blastema of the frontal process cannot have helped to form the philtrum region as normally. Even if only half of the nose is malformed, no cribriform plate exists. Only a lateral proboscis hangs down from the supraorbital

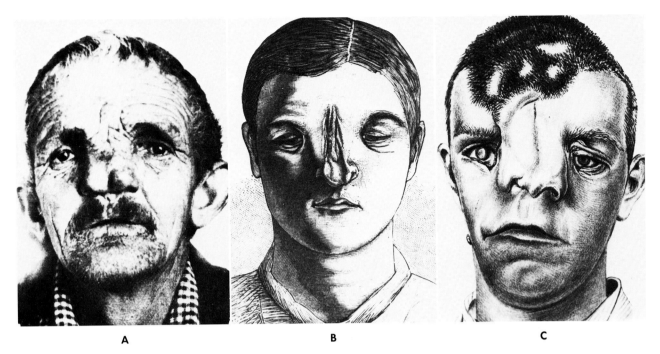

A   B   C

Fig. 5-8. Various degrees of median cleft nose. **A,** Bifid nasal tip and midphiltrum sinus. (From Bumba, J., and Lucksch, F.: Arch. Path. Anat. **264:**554, 1927.) **B,** Median nasal cleft with hypertelorism. (From Nasse, D.: Arch. Klin. Chir. **49:**767, 1895.) **C,** Median cleft face syndrome with lateral nasal cleft, coloboma of right lower lid, hypertelorism, and gyrated skin. (From Lexer, E.: Arch. Klin. Chir. **62:**360, 1900.)

rim or the medial portion of the upper lid. The ipsilateral upper lip is usually normal (Fig. 5-7). A lateral proboscis may contain a cartilage, an epithelial lining inside, and even excretory glands. Kirchmayr[10] reported a case with two normal nares and a lateral proboscis dangling on a peduncle from the inner angle of the upper lid (Fig. 5-7, *B*). With such a supernumerary nasal anlage, the cribriform plate is expected to be normal. These anomalies are believed to be caused by disturbances during early development, during the stage of undifferentiated mesectoderm, when the face resembles a growing epithelial mold adjacent to the prosencephalon.

The median cleft nose

The cerebral underdevelopment in cyclopia, ethmocephaly, and cebocephaly is not compatible with life; however, patients with hypertelorism have a high incidence of normal mentality. The median cleft face syndrome or facial dysrhaphia is characterized by a median cleft nose (bifid tip, median cleft), possible cleft of the upper lip and alveolus, and possibly an occult cleft of the cranium.

The median cleft nose reveals the paired anlage

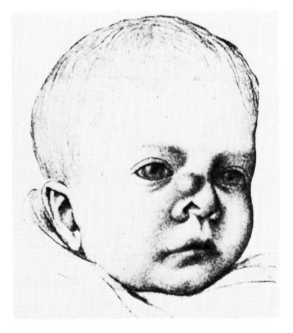

Fig. 5-9. Lateral nasal cleft in 2-week-old child. Nodule over dorsum of nose was read as muscle, cartilage, and fibrous tissue. (From Frangenheim, P.: Beitr. Klin. Chir. **65:**54, 1909.)

of the nasal capsule. There may be only a bifid tip, or, in more severe cases, a cleft in the dorsum and a Y-shaped nasal septum (Fig. 5-8). The nasal cavity is never open; the cleft is covered by normal skin. It is deepest at the tip and becomes shallow toward the root of the nose and the membranous portion of the septum. The extent and the particulars of the median cleft nose trace the disturbance to the early development of the nasal capsule.

The lateral nasal cleft

A triangular-shaped notch in the alar cartilage (lower lateral) characterizes the lateral nasal cleft. Its pathomorphogenesis cannot be explained by the classical theory, since a cleft should occur only ventral to the nares, if at all. For this reason Frangenheim[4] postulated an unknown embryonic cleft, which might explain the constant appearance of the lateral nasal cleft (Fig. 5-9).

ANIMAL EXPERIMENTS
Material and method

Various maxillofacial anomalies have been induced by the administration of 130 rads to pregnant mice on the seventh day and 20 hours after conception by Ritter.[19] The fullterm offspring were killed and the heads serial sectioned in the frontal plane. This material was kindly made available for the study of nasal dysplasias. The serial sections were transcribed on cardboard, which was then saturated in hot paraffin, cut out, and mounted so as to render a three-dimensional reconstruction of the nasal capsule. The fetuses examined were affected by different degrees of hypoplasia and dysplasia.

Monorhinic condition

The reconstructed model of a monorhinic nasal capsule reveals a severe hypoplasia and dysplasia rostral to the annular zone (Fig. 5-4). Posterior to it, however, the cartilage becomes even more hypoplastic and severely malformed. Besides the fact that the monorhinic nasal capsule is smaller than half of a normal nasal capsule, the various structures can hardly be distinguished. It seems that the ipsilateral paraseptal cartilage is connected with the lateral wall. The epithelial lining of the "naris" terminates shortly cephalad to the annular zone.

This murine monorhinus resembles somewhat the configuration of a proboscis. It seems that the annular zone is more resistant to hypoplasia than others.

One-sided hypoplasia

Similar to the condition of the hemiaplasia just described, the nasal capsule of a one-sided hypoplasia was most severely affected posterior to the annular zone. The hypoplasia of the ipsilateral nares was moderate. Although the marginoturbinate of the mouse was missing, the various portions of the rostral framework could be identified around the almost normal wide opening. Posterior to the annular zone, however, there was no ventral opening of the nasal capsule, which appeared to be normal on the other side. The affected nasal capsule forms a dyplastic cartilage tube, which narrows cephalad. It does not have turbinate structures, which can be seen on the opposite side. The paranasal cartilage is noticeably smaller and is located in close proximity to the ventral border of the hypoplastic lateral wall.

A most striking finding is a cleft in the rostral portion of this nasal capsule on the affected side, which extends in much the same way into the alar region as in man. It seems to be the cleft the existence of which was postulated by Frangenheim[4] on account of the uniform shape of the lateral nasal cleft.

Our knowledge of the nasal capsule, particularly of its malformations, is sparse. With a similar development of the chondocranium in mammals, teratologic experiments and the tedious reconstruction of models from serial sections promise to disclose some of the unsolved questions of the pathogenesis of nasal deformities.

SUMMARY

The first concept of nasal development was based on observations of the surface of the embry-

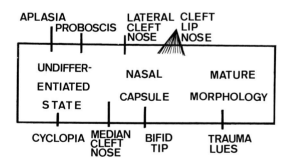

Fig. 5-10. Diagrammatic correlation of congenital nasal malformations of three main developmental structures of nose: embryonic blastema, fetal chondrocranial nasal capsule, and differentiated tissues. Type and severity of malformations coincide with affected developmental stage of nasal and adjacent areas (e.g., cleft lip nose with and without cleft lip).

onic head. Decades of dispute passed by about what happens in the bordering zones or furrows between the processes. Experimental and clinical evidence has been brought forth to regard several successive stages during nasal development. Disturbances of the early prosencephalic development are likely to cause severe malformations. In the primordial nasal capsule other specific nasal anomalies may occur, which again have their bearing on the bone laid down. Animal experiments, however, indicate that there is no definite correlation between the two; on the contrary, the perichondral bone growth seems to compensate for the dysplasia and hypoplasia observed in the chondrocranial nasal capsule. (See Fig. 5-10.)

REFERENCES

1. Baer, K. E., von: Ueber die Entwicklungsgeschichte der Tiere. Beobachtungen und Reflexion, vol. 1, Koenigsberg, Germany, 1828.
2. Bumba, J., and Lucksch, F.: Ein Fall von Doggennase, Arch. Path. Anat. **264:**554, 1927.
3. Dursy, E.: Zur Entwicklungsgeschichte des Kopfes des Menschen und der höheren Wirbeltiere, Tuebingen, Germany, 1869, Laupp.
4. Frangenheim, P.: Zur Kenntnis der seitlichen Nasenspalten, Beitr. Klin. Chir. **65:**54, 1909.
5. Froriep, A.: Einige Bemerkungen zur Kopffrage, Anat. Anz. **21:**243, 1902.
6. Hochstetter, F.: Ueber die Bildung der inneren Nasengänge oder primitiven Choanen, Anat. Anz. 6(suppl).:145, 1891.
7. Hochstetter, F.: Ueber die Art und Weise, in welcher sich bei Saugetieren und beim Menschen aus der sogenannten Riechgrube die Nasenhöhle entwickelt, Z. Anat. Entwicklungsgesch. **113:**105, 1944.
8. His, W.: Unsere Korperform und physiologische Probleme ihrer Entstehung, Leipzig, Germany, 1874, Vogel.
9. Josephy, H.: Ueber Rüsselbildung bei Zyklopie, Arch. Path. Anat. Physiol. Klin. Med. **206:**407, 1911.
10. Kirchmayr, L.: Ein Beitrag zu den Gesichtsmissbildungen, Dtsch. Z. Chir. **81:**71, 1906.
11. Landow, M.: Ueber einen seltenen Fall von Missbildung der Nase nebst einigen Bemerkungen über die seitliche Nasenspalte, Z. Chir. **30:**544, 1890.
12. Lexer, E.: Angeborene median Spaltung der Nase, Arch. Klin. Chir. **62:**360, 1900.
13. Morian, R.: Ueber die schräge Gesichtsspalte, Arch. Klin. Chir. **35:**145, 1887.
14. Nasse, D.: Zwei Fälle von angeborener medianer Spaltung der Nase, Arch. Klin. Chir. **49:**767, 1895.
15. Peter, K.: Atlas der Entwicklung der Nase und des Gaumens beim Menschen, Jena, Germany, 1909, Fischer.
16. Platt, J. B.: The ectodermic origin of the cartilages of the head, Anat. Anz. **8:**273, 1893.
17. Pollitzer, G.: Zur normalen und abnormen Entwicklung des menschlichen Gesichtes, Z. Anat. Entwicklungsgesch. **116:**332, 1952.
18. Rathke, H.: Ueber die Bildung und Entwicklung des Oberkiefers und der Geruchswerkzeuge der Säugetiere, Abhandl. z. Bildungs- und Entwicklungsgesch. der Menschen und Tiere, vol. 1, 1832, p.95.
19. Ritter, W.: Kraniofaziale Dysplasien und Störungen der Zahnentwicklung, Stuttgart, Germany, 1968, Gustav Fischer Verlag.
20. Schmidt, G.-Ph.: Zur Morphogenese des Schädels der Albinomaus, Dozent-Thesis, Munich, Germany, 1975.
21. Slaby, O.: Die fruhe Morphogenese der Nasenkapsel beim Menschen, Acta Anat. **42:**105, 1960.
22. Starck, D.: Embryologie, ed. 3, Stuttgart, Germany, 1975, Georg Thieme Verlag K. G.
23. Tuchmann-Duplessis, H., Auroux, M., and Haegel, P.: Illustrated human embryology, vol. 3, Nervous system and endocrine glands, New York, 1974, Springer-Verlag New York, Inc.
24. Tondury, G.: Ueber den Bauplan des fotalen Schädels, Rev. Suisse Zool. **49:**168:1942.
25. Veau, V.: Hasenscharten menschlicher Keimlinge auf der Stufe 21-23 mm S. St. L., Z. Anat. Entwicklungsgesch. **108:**459, 1938.
26. Veit, O.: Ueber das Problem Wirbeltierkopf, Kempten, Germany, 1947.
27. Witzel, O.: Ueber die angeborene mediane Spaltung der oberen Gesichtshälfte, Arch. Klin. Chir. **27:**893, 1882.

Chapter 6

Anatomy of the nose

Paul Natvig, M.D.

Standard anatomic nomenclature for structures of the nose is well documented in the *Nomina Anatomica*. It behooves us to use these terms. However, clinical nomenclature for parts and for regions of the nose has been introduced, and it is necessary to acquaint ourselves with this.

Descriptions here will be an admixture of standard and clinical nomenclature. For this discussion the anatomy is by necessity abbreviated and limited to practical applications that relate to aesthetic rhinoplasty. Detailed descriptions of anatomy and histology of the nose are available to the reader in many volumes.

EXTERNAL NOSE

The external nose is triangular in shape and supported by a skeleton of bone and cartilage, which is covered by periosteum, perichondrium, muscles, subcutaneous fat, and skin externally. It is lined with periosteum and perichondrium and covered by skin and respiratory mucous membrane.

The root of the nose is above and its base is below, overhanging the upper lip (Fig. 6-1). Between the root and the base is a rounded bridge with the highest portion of the bridge known as the dorsum. In the base are two openings, the nostrils or nares, which are separated by the columella (Fig. 6-2).

From the dorsum the sides slope posteriorly and inferiorly on both sides and terminate at the cheek and the base. The inferior and posterior portion of the nose is wider and more convex and forms the alae of the nose. The alae terminate at the cheek surface in grooves known as the nasal sulci (Fig. 6-3).

Between the perpendicular plate of the ethmoid bone and the vomer the quadrilateral septal cartilage is attached, which, collectively, is the nasal septum (Fig. 6-4). The inferior portion of the nasal dorsum or bridge is supported by the septal cartilage. Its upper part is sometimes grooved in the midline. This portion of the septal cartilage is in continuity (although cemented with periochondrium) with the lateral nasal cartilages. The upper borders of the lateral nasal cartilages (upper lateral cartilages) lie beneath the inferior border of the nasal bones with the maximum overlap by the nasal bones in the midline and lesser overlap laterally where there is attachment to the frontal processes of the maxillae. The lower borders of the lateral nasal cartilages are connected with the upper margins of the lateral crura by connective tissue. However, the superior margins of the lateral crura of the major alar cartilages usually overlap the lower edge of the lateral nasal cartilages. In the midline the lateral nasal cartilages in their upper two thirds are connected with periochondrium to the dorsal edge of the septal cartilage

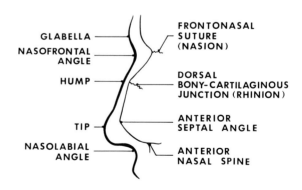

Fig. 6-1. Diagram of sagittal section of nose with part of septum and frontal bone. (Modified from Bernstein, L.: Arch. Otolaryngol. **99**:69, 1974. Copyright 1974, American Medical Association.)

but in the lower third are separated by connective tissue (Fig. 6-5).

The paired (never symmetric) nasal bones lie between the two frontal processes of the maxillae (sometimes erroneously called nasal processes) (Fig. 6-6). The frontal processes of the maxillae are part of the bony pyramid of the nose.

The alar tip and columella of the nose is supported by the paired major alar cartilages (lower lateral cartilages). The major alar cartilages have a lateral and medial crus (Fig. 6-7). Most of the medial crura are within the columella. Superior to and in continuity with the columella is the membranous septum, which bridges with the base of the cartilaginous septum. The minor alar cartilages are lateral to the major alar cartilages and are sometimes in several pieces with connective tissue connections to the lateral crura. The inferior borders of the lateral crura are not parallel with the rims of the alae but ascend toward the cheek.

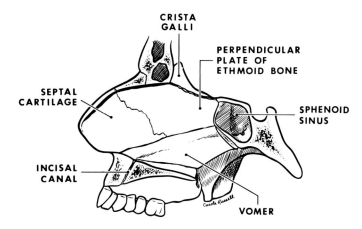

Fig. 6-4. Sagittal section, medial view of nasal cavity.

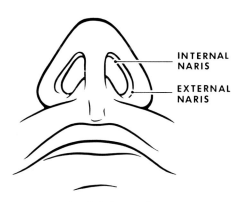

Fig. 6-2. Base of nose.

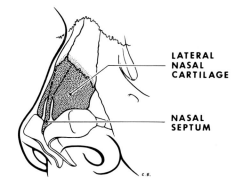

Fig. 6-5. Diagram of nasal bones and lateral nasal cartilages showing relationship of connective tissue attachment of lower part of lateral cartilages to septum.

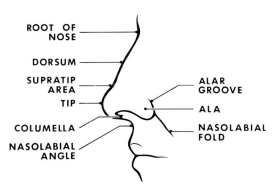

Fig. 6-3. Diagram of some areas of nose.

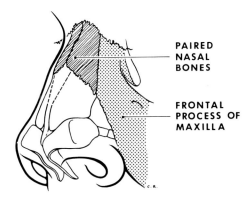

Fig. 6-6. Relationship of nasal bones to frontal processes of maxillae.

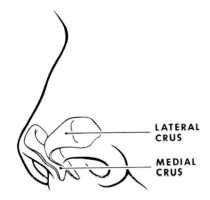

Fig. 6-7. Major alar cartilages.

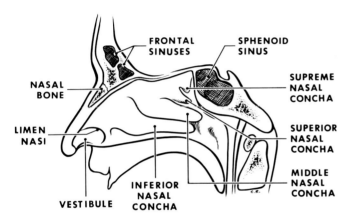

Fig. 6-8. Sagittal section, lateral view of nasal cavity.

INTERNAL NOSE

The vestibule, which is immediately inside and above the rims of the nostril, is a skin-lined cavity rich with sebaceous glands and numerous hairs known as vibrissae. The upper borders of the lateral crura of the major alar cartilages coincide with the inferior borders of the lateral nasal cartilages where there is a graceful fold of the lining. This fold is known as the *limen nasi* (formerly called *limen vestibuli*). It is at this level or just slightly above where there is transition between the skin and the mucosa.

The lateral walls of the nasal cavity are occupied by the conchae (Fig. 6-8). The middle and superior conchae (and sometimes supreme conchae) are parts of the ethmoid bone. The inferior conchae are separate bones.

The mucous membrane is pseudostratified ciliated columnar epithelium and is differentiated into convex and concave mucosa. The convex mucosa is thick and highly vascularized, and the veins form networks that have been compared with cav-

ernous erectile bodies. The concave mucosa is thinner, contains fewer glands and blood vessels, and is fused with periosteum by one layer of connective tissue.

In the roof of the nasal cavity lies the olfactory area, which extends for a short distance down onto the septum and the lateral walls. The olfactory mucous membrane has a yellowish brown color. Branches of the olfactory nerve enter the cranial cavity, where they are known as olfactory filia traversing the cribriform plate of the ethmoid bone.

BLOOD SUPPLY

The external carotid system richly supplies the external nose and nasal cavity. The facial artery, which arises from the anterior wall of the external carotid, ascends across the inferior border of the mandible upward and forward, supplying branches to the upper and lower lip and terminating as the angular artery near the medial canthus. Branches from the superior labial artery ascend to the lower border of the alae of the nose and septum and then anastomose with nasal branches of the ophthalmic artery from the internal carotid system. Further, the facial artery ascends at the lateral border of the nose, supplies the lateral parts of the nose and approximal cheek regions, and anastomoses with infraorbital artery of the maxillary. The facial artery anastomoses with branches to the ophthalmic artery, where it ends again as the angular artery.

Internally the nose receives its blood supply from the posterior nasal branches of the sphenopalatine artery and the descending palatine artery. The descending palatine artery in the pterygopalatine canal gives off the inferoposterior nasal branches, which enter the nasal cavity and supply the inferior conchae and the proximal regions of the lateral walls of the cavity of the nose. The main branch of the descending palatine artery, which travels through the nasopalatine foramen, is known as the major palatine artery. This artery runs anteriorly in the submucosa of the hard palate, and its terminal portion, the nasopalatine branch, ascends through the incisive canal. Here it enters the nasal cavity, where it anastomoses with the septal branches of the sphenopalatine artery. This artery is the last of the terminal branches of the maxillary artery and supplies a large part of the nasal cavity.

The sphenopalatine artery passes from the upper part of the pterygopalatine fossa through the sphenopalatine foramen and into the nasal cavity. Near the roof of the nasal cavity the artery separates into lateral septal branches. The posterolateral nasal artery divides on the lateral wall into numerous branches, which supply the superior and middle conchae and the adjacent nasal mucous membrane. Some of the smaller branches perforate the lateral nasal wall and reach the mucosa of the maxillary sinus. The posterior septal artery goes to the nasal septum over the roof of the nasal cavity and then descends downward and then forward along the septum. After supplying the branches to the nasal septum this artery anastomoses with the nasopalatine branch of the major palatine artery. Part of the blood supply to the dorsal part of the nose is from the terminal facial branch of the ophthalmic artery. The facial branch of the ophthalmic artery terminates as the nasal dorsal branch, which descends onto the lateral surface of the nose and anastomoses with the angular artery. The nasal artery also anastomoses with the infraorbital artery.

The venous drainage of the nose parallels the arterial supply of the nose.

NERVE SUPPLY

The nerves of the external nose are divided into sensory from the fifth cranial nerve and motor from the seventh cranial nerve. The external nasal ramus from the ophthalmic nerve is behind the nasal bones. It comes to the surface between the nasal bones and the lateral nasal cartilages and supplies sensory branches to the dorsum and tip of the nose. The lateral nasal and alar walls are supplied by the branches of the infraorbital nerve of the second division of the trigeminal nerve.

The inferoposterior parts of the nasal cavity (the mucosa and septum) are innervated through the sphenopalatine ganglion. This ganglion, in addition to sensory fibers from the maxillary division of the trigeminal nerve, receives parasympathetic fibers from the great superficial petrosal nerve from the geniculate ganglion of the facial nerve and sympathetic fibers from the deep petrosal nerve and reaches the ganglion as the vidian nerve. The ganglion in the pterygopalatine fossa is near the sphenopalatine foramen, which makes it accessible for the application of topical anesthesia. The sphenopalatine foramen is just behind and above the posterior end of the middle turbinate. Sensory fibers from the lateral wall of the nasal cavity pass through the ostia to supply the sinus mucosa.

MUSCLES

Movements of the nose by facial muscles of expression are innervated by the seventh cranial nerve. The skin of the nose and the nasal tip are elevated by the angular head of the labii superioris quadratus (the levator labii superioris alaeque nasi). This muscle arises from the frontal process of the maxilla at about the level of the medial palpebral ligament as a narrow band of muscle fiber and runs deeply downward and inserts principally into the skin of the ala of the nose. Some of the fibers pass around the lateral circumference of the nostril and reach the posterior border and interlace with the nasal muscle. Some muscle bundles pass into the upper lip and they end in the region of the philtrum, where they are interwoven with fibers of the orbicularis oris muscle.

The nasal muscle arises from the eminences of the lateral incisors and canines of the maxillae at the base of the alveolar processes. Fibers ascend toward the wings of the nose. This muscle has two parts. The alar part is the dilator muscle of the nostril and ends in the ala. The transverse part of the nasal muscle (the compressor muscle of the nostril) passes over the lower part of the bridge of the nose to join the nasal muscle of the opposite side. The alar or lower part of the nasal muscle ends at the lateroposterior circumference of the nostril. Medial fibers extend to the posterior end of the mobile septum, and the lateral fibers terminate in the skin of the nasal alae. Above, the muscle fans out upwardly and medially into a thin, wide aponeurosis and joins with that of the opposite side. The nasal muscle hence forms a slinglike band for coverage of the cartilaginous portion of the bridge of the nose.

AREAS OF THE NOSE WITH CLINICAL APPLICATION

Bony pyramid. The bony pyramid is represented by the paired nasal bones and the frontal processes of the maxillae (Fig. 6-9).

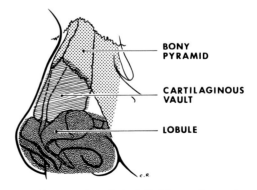

Fig. 6-9. Three major clinical divisions of nose (see text for accurate description of lobule).

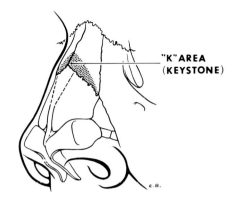

Fig. 6-10. Support or "K" area of nose.

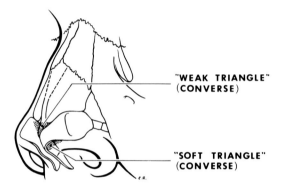

Fig. 6-11. Converse's triangles of nose.

Cartilaginous vault. The cartilaginous vault is made up of the paired lateral nasal cartilages and that part of the upper cartilaginous septum to which it is attached (Fig. 6-9).

Lobule of the nose. The lobule is collectively the tip, alae, columella, and the membranous septum and the internal structures they envelop (lateral and medial crura of the major alar cartilages and the minor alar cartilages). There is no bone or other cartilage continuity. On palpation this unit or lobule is movable and associated with the septum and lateral nasal cartilages only by connective tissue attachments. The skin of the lobule is thicker than the upper two thirds of the nasal skin and contains more glandular structures (Fig. 6-9).

"K" area. The "K" area or keystone area (first named by Cottle) is that area in the midportion of the nose where the inferior parts of the nasal bones overlap the superior parts of the lateral nasal cartilages (Fig. 6-10).

Weak triangle of the nose. The weak triangle of the nose described by Converse is a connective tissue aponeurosis over the septal angle lying be-

tween the major alar cartilages and the inferior parts of the lateral nasal cartilages (Fig. 6-11).

Soft triangle of the nose. The soft triangle of the nose described by Converse is an area inferior and lateral to the junction of the lateral and medial crura. At the inferior margin of the triangle (alar rim), skin abuts skin. When the soft triangle is visible externally, it is known as a facet. Facets of the nose are analogous to lapidary ornamentation of precious gems. Many facets are aesthetically pleasing, but some are less pleasing and may require surgical modification (Fig. 6-11).

Mobile septum. The mobile septum is the most inferior part of the septum, which is the membranous septum and columella.

Valves of the nose. The valves of the nose are formed by the junction of the lateral nasal cartilages with the septum. Respiration moves the inferior parts of the lateral nasal cartilages to and from the septum. The valves direct streams of air into the internal nose, which are narrow on inspiration and wider on expiration.

JACQUES JOSEPH AND A PHILOSOPHY OF AESTHETIC RHINOPLASTY

Jakob Lewin Joseph of Berlin (1865-1934), better known as Jacques Joseph, is the father of modern aesthetic rhinoplasty (Fig. 6-12). In studying reports of the multiple techniques of aesthetic rhinoplasty, one finds that Joseph said it all before. That other surgeons before Joseph wrote about aesthetic rhinoplasty does not detract from Joseph's methods. He was the imaginative innovator-investigator and independently developed almost all of the intranasal techniques we use today.

The most perplexing operation in plastic surgery is the aesthetic rhinoplasty. Yet it is not technically difficult and not time-consuming. For the patient and the surgeon a poor result is disastrous. But a nose maintained or restored in function and beautifully carved is one of the most gratifying of all surgical procedures.

To the artist, the operation is simple. To the artless surgeon it can be a dilemma; he may possess great knowledge but is bereft of imagination, taste, and skill.

To draw a similarity between Leonardo da Vinci and Jacques Joseph may seem venturesome because Leonardo ascended to the highest level of human achievement. Yet the parallel underscores the importance of the artist in the surgical operation, aesthetic rhinoplasty. Had Leonardo been a rhinoplasty surgeon there is little doubt that anyone would ever have been his equal.

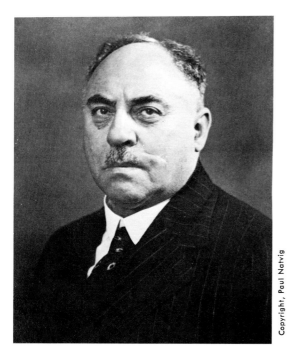

Copyright, Paul Natvig

Fig. 6-12. Jacques Joseph (1865-1934), father of modern rhinoplasty.

It is useless to speculate that Leonardo used better brushes, pigments, palettes, or panels, or had better light by which to paint, since we can assume he did not. Leonardo was saturated with artistry, intellectual curiosity, and innovation; he was an innate genius. Leonardo studied anatomy and dissected cadavers in subterranean vaulted chambers. He made great numbers of notes in mirror-image cursive and hundreds of sketches in preparation for major works.

Joseph sketched, made notes, and studied anatomy. He made moulages of the nose, dissected cadavers, carved, and learned about variations of the anatomy of the nose. Friedrich Kopsch, the German anatomist, once said to Joseph's grand-nephew, a medical student in Berlin, "Helmut, you should be only half as good as your uncle, because even after he has been out of school for a long time, he still works with me and dissects skull, after skull, after skull, and knows every little artery and every little nerve in the face."

Joseph prepared well. He resolutely sought knowledge, but more, he was an artist. Joseph accomplished superior aesthetic results in rhinoplasty; he did not hold steadfast to a mechanical procedure. Whether the surgeon makes variable sizes of intranasal incisions, intercartilaginous or intracartilaginous, rim incisions, or a combination thereof, whether one uses a scalpel, an elevator, chisel, or saw, it is not at odds with the original Joseph teachings. His methods have certainly excited others to make minor modifications, and the very nature of the surgical operation calls forth altered and individual execution, which is style. Yet the surgeon must not invest a nose with a new form that looks the same for each patient or so carve on a nose that it bears the travesty of his maldirected knife.

What, then, must be the end result of this symposium? The plastic surgeon, the rhinoplasty surgeon, must study the old, learn about the new, and accept the challenge to be an artist.

REFERENCES

1. Bernstein, L.: Applied anatomy in corrective rhinoplasty, Arch. Otolaryngol. **99:**67, 1974.
2. Converse, J.: The cartilaginous structures of the nose, Ann. Otol. **64:**220, 1955.
3. Cottle, M.: Corrective surgery, nasal septum and external pyramid, Chicago, 1960, American Rhinologic Society.
4. Dingman, R.: Personal communication, 1974.
5. Joseph, J.: Nasenplastik und sonstige Geischtsplastik nebst Mammaplastik, Leipzig, Germany, 1928-1931, Curt Kabitzsch.
6. Natvig, P., Sether, L., Gingrass, R., and Gardner, W.: Anatomical details of the osseous-cartilaginous framework of the nose, Plast. Reconstr. Surg. **48:**528, 1971.
7. Personal papers of Professor and Mrs. Jacques Joseph in possession of the author.
8. Sicher, H.: Oral anatomy, ed. 6, St. Louis, 1975, The C. V. Mosby Co.
9. Sicher, H.: Personal communication, 1974.
10. Straatsma, B., and Straatsma, C.: The anatomical relationship of the lateral nasal cartilage to the nasal bone and the cartilaginous nasal septum, Plast. Reconstr. Surg. **8:**443, 1951.

Chapter 7

Nasal physiology
surgical and medical considerations of the obstructed airway

William C. Conroy, M.D.
Howard E. Hock, M.D.*

Of all deviations from the normal in nasal physiology, obstruction of the airway is the most distressing to the patient. Its origin may be traumatic or surgical on one hand or purely medical on the other. The rhinoplasty surgeon must be conversant with all facets of the problem, since, when the reason for alteration of normal structures is aesthetic, no lasting abuse of normal function is acceptable.

FUNCTIONS

The two chief purposes of the nose are those of olfaction and protection of the respiratory tract by moistening, heating, and cleaning the inspired air.

Impelled by negative intrapharyngeal pressure, the stream of air enters the nose through two nozzles or nares, which direct it high and medially in an arc passing the olfactory sensors to the nasopharynx. Medially a straight wall or septum is provided to allow the bulk of the air to pass smoothly. Dynamic, erectile, streamlined masses protrude from the lateral walls to modify the air as required. It is probably more than a coincidence that noses with acute nasolabial angles are usually humped, whereas obtuse nasolabial angles rarely have strong bridges. If one accepts that the stream of air is directed at right angles to the plane of the nostrils, it can be seen that it is far more logical and physiologic to redirect the air below the new dorsum in rhinoplasty by an inferior septectomy

than to injure a straight septum to provide room after infracture of the nasal bones. The millimeter or so of room gained probably does no good, since the overly patent airway, as seen in septal deflections, is reduced by hypertrophy of the turbinates. Turbinates require a relationship to the septum to provide required nasal resistance and to allow them to efficiently modify the inspired air.

SURGICAL CONSIDERATIONS

The turbinates and the septum are the two keys to the nasal airway.

The turbinates and their linings, rich in glands and cilia, are influenced by many factors, including environmental temperature, emotions, and ingestion of alcohol and condiments, in addition to pathologic agents to be described below. Rhinomanometric studies have demonstrated a nasal cycle of alternate nasal patency and congestion varying from 20 minutes to a few hours in 80% of patients tested, providing a consistent resistance to the total respiratory pathway of about 30%, a resistance necessary for proper pulmonary function. The turbinates are affected by posture. At sleep the dependent turbinates are engorged, possibly due to a nasopulmonary reflex. The above facts are important to the unilaterally obstructed nose, since half of the time such a patient cannot breathe through the nose without medication, and naturally such a patient will prefer to sleep on the obstructed side.

Septal deviations cause the air column to be directed against the sidewalls with resultant drying, crusting, and interference with the ability of

*Attending Physician, Otolaryngology, Mountainside Hospital, Montclair, New Jersey.

the cilia to move the mucous mantle back to the nasopharynx. Bernoulli observed that when air, a fluid, moves from a tube of higher caliber to one of lower caliber, velocity increases, giving annoying turbulence and a drop in pressure leading to sidewall edema. This is usually noted on the convex side or that away from the tip displacement.

However, it should be remembered that significant obstruction is rarely due to septal deflection alone. On routine ear, nose, and throat examinations it is common to find virtually complete unilateral obstruction sometimes with moderate contralateral obstruction in a patient who insists that he has no trouble with nasal respiration, whereas others complain bitterly with little obstruction evident.

MEDICAL CONSIDERATIONS

In discussing medical causes of obstruction in order of frequency, it should be noted that the most common cause of nasal airway obstruction is acute inflammatory change associated with viral or bacterial nasal infection and, occasionally, with paranasal sinus infection. Bacterial infections respond promptly to appropriate antimicrobial therapy and establishing adequate drainage. Viral infections tend to be self-limited and run their course in 7 to 10 days for the most part. Chronic nasal congestion that has persisted for many months is not likely to be caused by infection. When this occurs, one must look for an underlying cause of nasal congestion other than infection, and, in order of decreasing frequency, this is due to allergy phenomena, chronic nasal irritation secondary to excessive use of topical decongestant medication, and, finally, a miscellaneous etiologic grouping, including (1) emotional factors and (2) reaction to systemic preparations such as reserpine (Serpasil) or similar preparations, which reduce the autonomic effect of the sympathetic nervous system, allowing an excessive contribution by the parasympathetic system with the associated vascular dilatation, congestion, and increased glandular secretions characteristic of parasympathetic stimulation of the nasal mucous membranes. One also sees an overaction of parasympathetic activity for a number of reasons, for instance, increased estrogen effect during pregnancy. Increased estrogen activity reduces the activity of the enzyme acetylcholinesterase necessary for rapid breakdown of the active acetylcholine produced at the parasympathetic postganglionic nerve endings in the nasal submucosa. The increased resultant parasympathetic activity is a common cause of nasal stuffiness

with the administration of estrogenic hormones or, in certain instances, during pregnancy with increased estrogenic activity. Less commonly, alterations in thyroid function, emotional activities resulting in hypothalamic parasympathetic stimulation, sensitivity to temperature extremes, and, more uncommonly, vasodilators such as ethanol may be a factor.

TREATMENT

Optimal treatment of nasal congestion on the basis of hypertrophic oversecreting membranes requires identification of the causative factors, which vary a great deal from one patient to another. The treatment of bacterial infection is usually straightforward and accomplished, for the most part, with fairly prompt resolution of the nasal congestive effects. Treatment of viral inflammatory changes requires supportive measures such as topical or systemic decongestant medications, humidification of the air when the nose is bypassed and mouth breathing is part of the problem, analgesics for the known headache tendency associated with mucosal engorgement, particularly at the sinus ostia, and symptomatic treatment according to the particular symptoms of the patient. Allergy problems are best managed by identification of the allergens with either avoidance or hyposensitization, although this is occasionally accomplished with some difficulty. Patients who have brief seasonal distribution of their allergic symptoms tend to respond well to antihistamine medication or, under certain circumstances, steroid medication, either topically or systemically, and are usually not a problem. Patients who have more constant allergy symptoms, suggesting hypersensitivity to a large number of allergens, are controlled with more difficulty, and prolonged use of various medications, particularly topical decongestants and corticosteroids, can result in a worsened medical state.

VASOMOTOR RHINITIS MEDICAMENTOSUM

If one has the need for altering the parasympathetic imbalance chemically in hope of lessening nasal congestion, there are several available approaches, none of which are entirely satisfactory in a difficult patient who proves refractory to most forms of treatment. For a self-limited condition that can reasonably be expected to run its course in 10 days or less, the best relief of the nasal congestion, usually the result of histamine, serotonin, and slower-acting vasodilators, can be obtained by topical vasoconstrictors, which, for the most part, are sympathomimetics that tend to exert a vaso-constricting action. Parasympathetic inhibitors tend to exert a less vigorous effect. Continued use of sympathomimetic drugs results in a refractory state of the arterioles in which they become less responsive to sympathetic control. This is seen, for instance, in the overuse of sympathomimetic topical preparations when the patient increases the frequency and strength of the agent but finds a gradually lessening effect in regard to decongesting the nasal airway. This is described as vasomotor rhinitis medicamentosum and occasionally is the factor that prolongs nasal congestion when the initiating inflammatory reaction has subsided, but continued use of sympathomimetic agents prolongs the nasal congestive problem.

In allergy problems, antihistamine preparations combat the histamine release from the mast cells in the tissue and the associated serotonin release, which causes vasodilatation, increased secretions, and the typical allergic reaction. Corticosteroids that can be taken systemically in the form of oral preparations in a diminishing dosage technique, parenteral injection of short-acting or, more suitably, long-acting steroids and, under certain circumstances, where hypertrophy of the inferior turbinates appears to be the predominant obstructing factor, direct injection of repository steroid material into the inferior turbinates is often beneficial. Topical steroids in the form of dexamethasone (Decadron) in a nebulizing cartridge (Turbinaire) are often beneficial and lessen the amount of steroid systemically distributed in the patient. Steroids have been particularly useful in combating the inflammatory changes associated with overuse of decongestant sprays and drops.

TURBINATE SURGERY

In more refractory situations in which hypertrophy of the inferior turbinates seems to be the primary obstructing factor, as is commonly the case, direct attention to the turbinates can be beneficial in restoring a more patent airway. The turbinates can be cauterized to result in a scarring of the tissue and less capacity for the ballooning hypertrophy and the marked nasal congestion that are associated with this turgescent property of the inferior turbinate. More recently, cryosurgery has been utilized to destroy chronically inflamed turbinate mucosa. Studies indicate that the turbinate is replaced with a less scarred, more normally functioning epithelium, often with relief of symptoms.

SPHENOPALATINE GANGLION SURGERY; VIDIAN NERVE SURGERY

Two techniques are available in an attempt to interrupt parasympathetic hyperfunction when more specific causes of chronic nasal congestion have been ruled out. One technique is cryosurgical destruction of the sphenopalatine ganglion in which a cryosurgical probe is applied just posterior to the middle turbinate and an attempt is made, with the cryosurgical unit, to freeze and destroy the sphenopalatine ganglion or, at least in theory, the bulk of the immediate postganglionic parasympathetic fibers. This has met with some degree of success, although cryosurgical application to the inferior turbinate is beneficial in lessening chronic nasal congestion and may play a role, along with the destruction of this sphenopalatine ganglion or its immediate postganglionic fibers, in lessening nasal congestion.

A surgical procedure that results in interruption of the vidian nerve in the vidian nerve canal has been frequently used with varying degrees of success. The vidian nerve in the vidian nerve canal contains preganglionic parasympathetic fibers and postganglionic sympathetic fibers. The rationale for the procedure suggests that excessive stimulation of the parasympathetics is resulting in nasal congestion and that destruction of the parasympathetic and sympathetic innervation interrupts the autonomic control, which is out of balance, so to speak, and allows intrinsic mechanisms and, perhaps, a residual sympathetic innervation, which reaches the nasal mucosa by other paths, to establish a control of the nasal mucosa less dominated by parasympathetic stimulation.

RHINOPLASTY EFFECTS

Intranasal respiratory obstruction after rhinoplasty has properly been a hotly debated subject, with most discussion directed to what approach interferes as little as possible with the internal valve and what tip-reducing technique will avoid post-rhinoplasty alar collapse.

The limen vestibuli, or internal valve, is the projection of the upper lateral cartilage inside the alar cartilage and the accompanying furrow of the intercartilaginous area. The airway dramatically narrows at this point, and one can note slight opening of the olfactory fissure on normal inspiration and wide opening on forced inspiration when the accessory nasal respiratory muscles are brought into play. Dilation of the nasal passage is accomplished by contraction of the transverse portion of the nasalis muscle acting in conjunction with the angular head of the quadrati labii superioris (internal valve) and the dilator naris posterior (external valve). None of these muscles arise or insert in cartilage, attaching instead to an aponeurosis or skin. We have never seen obstruction traceable to the intercartilaginous incision, but this valve action can be destroyed by synechia where mucoperichondrium has been abused. Undermining as little as necessary and undermining in the subperiosteal and subperichondrial plane protects these valves.

Shortening the forward projection of the nasal tip a few millimeters can be accomplished by simply lowering the septum. More than this requires removal, at least in part, of the dome. In large setbacks, Conroy has removed the dome and entire lateral crus with meticulous preservation of mucoperichondrium and careful splinting in a large number of operations without ever seeing an alar collapse. Likewise we have never seen an alar collapse without mucous membrane or vestibular skin loss. One does not convert a box to a triangle without attenuating the dome cartilage to the point of collapse. Its continuity is of small importance physiologically but may be important aesthetically. The dome consists of two layers of skin rolled and opposed much as Detroit does with the edge of a fender for strength. In our experience this has been enough.

Postrhinoplasty nasal obstruction after the use of posterior and anterior packing used to control the sixth- or seventh-day postoperative hemorrhage is a real entity predicated on pressure necrosis. Treatment of this worrisome complication by vigorous noseblowing to expel all clots and light packing has solved this problem in our experience.

Finally, it is suggested that, just as we have surgical and medical diseases of the skin in which the plastic surgeon is considerably more competent in treating the former and the dermatologist the latter, a similar situation exists with nasal obstruction, and the rhinoplasty surgeon, whatever his origin, would do well to value the services of the competent rhinologist and his largely nonsurgical approach to breathing problems.

Chapter 8

Preoperative consultation
a different concept

Ross H. Musgrave, M.D., F.A.C.S.
William S. Garrett, Jr., M.D., F.A.C.S.*

One of the major problems confronting the plastic surgeon in whatever aesthetic procedure he performs is the difference between the patient's expectations of the finished product and the physician's ability to produce the same result. We have all been confronted by the patient whose preconceived concept of a desired result differs greatly from what would really suit him or her best or even from what it is humanly possible for the surgeon to produce with the patient's tissues. The prospective patient who has this totally preconceived idea of an ideal nose and who seeks consultation carrying a number of photographs of fashion models or celebrities has traditionally been considered a difficult personality. In such a situation the possibility of the patient's selecting the type of nose that would best fit other features or that is obtainable with his or her nasal structure is, at best, chancy. Therefore unless communication lines are extremely well established preoperatively, the surgeon is frequently unable to obtain a result that pleases the patient, who subconsciously has lodged in his or her mind something vastly different. I, for one, happen to be upset by the patient who arrives with such a collection of photographs, and inform him or her at the initial consultation that my chances of achieving this result, that is, the idealized nose, are slim. Rees[5] goes so far as to state, "Perhaps the most commonly observed psychological contraindication to surgery is in the patient who brings to the surgeon photographs of a celebrity he or she would like to resemble."

*Clinical Assistant Professor of Surgery (Plastic), University of Pittsburgh School of Medicine, Pittsburgh, Pennsylvania.

All too often the patient arriving with these photographs (of a finely chiseled model's nose) has thick, heavily pored skin with almost a bulbous tip. In this situation it is next to impossible to achieve a delicately defined sculpted photogenic look. However, the family, often the mother, is apt to be more realistic and more likely to absorb the surgeon's carefully worded warnings. Even though the experienced surgeon is aware that some improvement can be offered, he learns to be cautious with this type of person, and will frequently refuse to accept him or her as a patient.

The matter of communication, or lack of communication—a matter which has recently surfaced legally under the euphemistic title of "informed consent"—is an old one. Our predecessors in the field of aesthetic surgery have used varied preoperative communication techniques in an attempt to make their patients and the patients' families better informed and have a more realistic expectation of the finished product. These approaches have ranged from moulages to silhouettes to glossy prints that have been doctored with pencil or crayon. They have included markings on the patient's skin or blocking out the hump with a profilometer or the surgeon's index finger, and they have, in some instances, included multiple mirror techniques, not unlike the clothing salesman who is trying to get the prospective wearer to make up his mind which suit to select. Some physicians have resorted to penciled sketches, and for those who are artistically talented or trained, this method has proved satisfactory. However, it takes a skilled artist to capture the patient's features and sketch them with any degree of accuracy and then to pictorially demonstrate the proposed changes in nasal contour. Other surgeons use blackboard and chalk, which, of course, provides easy erasure.

The simplest course to follow, it would seem, is to show before-and-after photographs of some of one's previous cases. This is what many prospective patients expect, and, in fact, they are frequently perturbed if they are denied this privilege. A number of experienced plastic surgeons have been successfully following such a practice for

years. As long as it is carefully pointed out to the potential patient and the family that no two noses are exactly alike and that the photos shown are not necessarily representative of their particular type of nose (but merely an example of how a rhinoplasty can change the whole appearance of one's face), this method is probably a safe and a satisfactory one. If this course is followed, I would caution the younger surgeons that the before-and-after photos should *not* be produced as the first

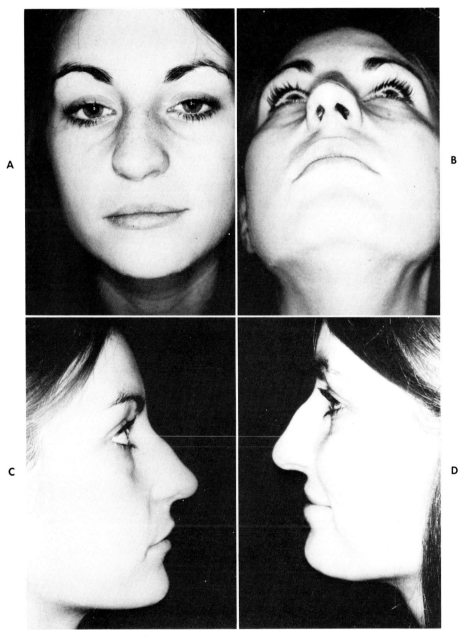

Fig. 8-1. A, Full-face preoperative view. **B,** Submental preoperative view. **C,** Right profile preoperative view. **D,** Left profile preoperative view.

item on the consultation agenda. Rather, after some rapport has been established, and after the details of the technical aspects explained, that is, length of the operation, the stay in the hospital, the anesthetic agent, the blackeyes, the splints, the sutures, the packing, if any, the sort of discomfort to expect, then and only then should the surgeon attempt to delineate for the person what type of nose he or she would look best with as a finished product. For the plastic surgeon to start off the interview after the first cheery greeting with a series of before-and-after photographs is akin to the Avon Lady or the Fuller Brush Man who wants to catch the attention of the potential customer with a quick-flash glimpse of the product!

I realize there has been much controversy about the inadvisability of showing any before-and-after photographs, since it has been pointed out by Gorney and others[1,4,5] that this practice may be misconstrued to imply some type of warranty. Not only has this controversy been discussed at length, but it has also crept into print (particularly by Alexander[1]). A carefully worded rebuttal to the Alexander monograph was recently written by Goin.[3] Included in the same issue was a summation by DeMere,[2] who stated that in his opinion, photographs may be of considerable benefit to patients and their parents, but if the intent is to convince the patient or parent of the skill of the plastic surgeon and to imply that he will get a similar result, a less good result could lead to a verdict against the surgeon in a subsequent lawsuit.

I no longer show patients before-and-after photographs of previous patients. Instead, for the past 10 years we have been showing the patients their own photographs, which are in reality 2 × 2 Kodachromes projected in a Kodaslide Table Viewer with a frosted-glass 8-inch screen. At the time of the first visit and after examining the patient, I discuss the various details of the proposed surgery, preferably with the patient alone. I then have my office assistant take four 35 mm Kodachrome color transparencies before the patient leaves (Fig. 8-1). The four views are full face, a submental view, and two profile views, with an attempt made to take one profile view with the patient smiling and the other with the patient's features in repose, since this certainly alters the configuration of the tip and of the lip-columella angle. Before leaving the office, the patient is also given a small booklet that contains questions and answers about plastic surgery and is asked to read the section on rhinoplasty before returning for the second visit with mother, father, husband, or friend.

The fee is also discussed at the time of the first visit, and a specific date, approximately 3 weeks later, is made for the patient to return with his or her family to view the projected slides. As Rees[5] so aptly stated, "This hiatus between consultations can be of great value for both surgeon and patient. The passing time allows seeds of suggestions and questions planted at the first interview to generate and sometimes brings forth valuable information at the second interview." I request the patient to jot down any questions unanswered or not understood at the time of the first interview on the back cover of the information booklet. As a rule, the return visit is arranged to accommodate the person who is paying for the surgery, usually the husband or father. For us, this means late afternoon or early evening office hours one day a week. It is surprising what a difference it can make in the attitude of the man (who usually is to pay for the surgery) not to have to take time off from his work to come meet his wife's or daughter's proposed plastic surgeon.

When the patient returns with his or her family, the Kodachrome slides are projected on the table-viewer screen (Fig. 8-2, *A*), and I point out the features that are problem areas or that will deserve attention in the subsequent surgery. I then mark out with a black felt-tipped pen on the glass screen the proposed changes on all four views, showing the front view first, the submental view second, and then the two profile views (Fig. 8-2, *B* and *C*). This process may be repeated over and over, wiping the glass screen clean with a paper tissue (Fig. 8-2, *D*). Disproportions in forehead or chin are also pointed out.

The father who arrives in a belligerent mood and who frequently assures the surgeon "his daughter is beautiful and doesn't need this foolish surgery" is usually amazed at what he sees projected on the screen. This projection method is also of great value for the patient who is adamant that all he or she wants is to have the hump removed. It can easily be demonstrated for the family and patient, that removing *only* the hump frequently does not improve the patient's appearance but ofttimes would make the nose seem more unattractive. As I discuss such details as the small scars that result from alar base incisions, I can sketch these in lightly on the frosted glass screen. During this portion of the interview, I constantly assert that the appearance that results from my sketching is what I would be aiming for in my surgery but that plastic surgery is not like carving in wood or marble or sculpting in clay. I reiterate to the pa-

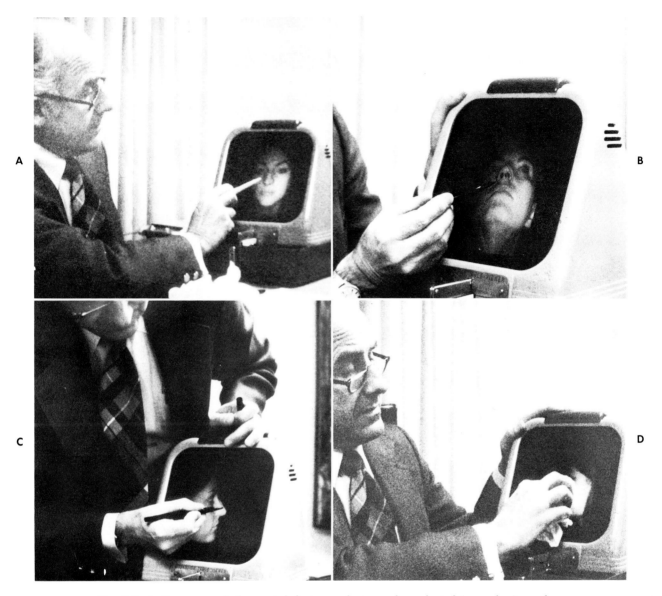

Fig. 8-2. A, Surgeon pointing out defects on photograph projected (rear view) on glass screen of table viewer. **B,** Black felt-tipped pen used to mark out proposed outlines of correction of same patient as in Fig. 8-1. **C,** Proposed profile being sketched. **D,** Markings on glass screen can be easily erased with paper tissue. Process can be (and usually is) repeated several times.

tient that what I am sketching is merely to give a rough concept of the postoperative result. I further state that we are dealing with human structures, which, after surgery, heal with scar tissue, a factor that can distort the nose from the contour we thought we had achieved in the operating room. As Alexander[1] so well summarized, "We are dealing with living tissues subject to all the restrictions and limitations of traumatized tissue, however slight that trauma may be. The healing pro-

cesses which ensue do not follow a standard or uniform pattern."

In summary, then, we have presented our method of preoperative communication, a method that, incidentally, we have used successfully not only for rhinoplasties, but for most, if not all, aesthetic procedures. In our practice it has become a valuable asset in communicating with the patient and the patient's family in a manner that is quick and relatively inexpensive and that demonstrates

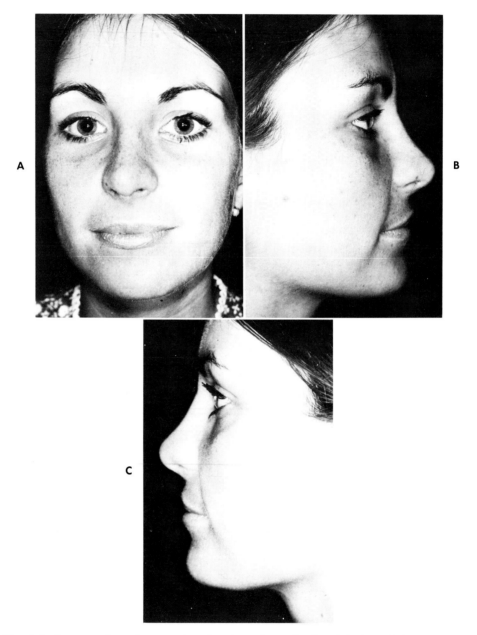

Fig. 8-3. Postoperative photographs of patient shown in Fig. 8-1. **A,** Full-face postoperative view. **B,** Right profile postoperative view. **C,** Left profile postoperative view.

what we seek to achieve for the prospective patient. Like the blackboard and chalk method Gorney[4] describes, the markings are temporary and are erased immediately. Furthermore, the color transparency is not altered, since the markings are on the frosted glass. We have had fewer problems and happier patients since using this method (Fig. 8-3). In our minds it is more meaningful for the patient to see his or her own features as they might be altered, rather than some carefully selected photograph of some total stranger, even if at first glance the other patient's nasal deformity seemed to be similar.

REFERENCES

1. Alexander, J.: Challenges in esthetic plastic surgery, Plast. Reconstr. Surg. **52**:337, 1973.
2. DeMere, M.: Views of several prominent attorneys on the pre-operative showing of photographs of results in other patients, Plast. Reconstr. Surg. **54**:90, 1974.
3. Goin, J. M.: On showing photographs pre-operatively to patients, Plast. Reconstr. Surg. **54**:90, 1974.
4. Gorney, M.: Psychiatric and medicolegal implications of rhinoplasty, mentoplasty and otoplasty. In Masters, F. W., and Lewis, J. R., Jr., editors: Proceedings of symposium on aesthetic surgery of the nose, ears, and chin, St. Louis, 1973, The C. V. Mosby Co.
5. Rees, T., and Wood-Smith, D.: Cosmetic facial surgery, Philadelphia, 1973, W. B. Saunders Co.

Chapter 9

Preoperative evaluation for rhinoplasty

Rex A. Peterson, M.D.

Nasoplasty has been likened to cleft lip plastic surgery in that both are considered among the most demanding and fascinating operations in plastic surgery. Why? Because in nasoplasty, as in cleft lip surgery, the ultimate long-term success of the operation depends not only on the judgment, experience, empathy, skill, aesthetic sense, gentleness, and precision of the surgeon, but also on the planning that precedes the incisions. Some surgeons possess such keen powers of observation and innate ability that the mental computations for preoperative nasoplasty evaluation may be automatically instantaneous, almost a reflex comparable to the reactions and signal-calling improvisations of a highly skilled football quarterback. Others need more planning, and all could benefit by it.

Preoperative evaluation for nasoplasty should be more than just adequate. It should be an essential important first step in the surgical process. Here, as in the operation itself, superficiality should be excluded in favor of intense study and concentration so that the end product is as perfect as is possible for the surgeon involved.

The thorough observation and record of the characteristics of not only *the nose,* but of the *person with the nose* can only lead to improved results in nasoplasty because they establish the basis for precise action in surgery. To gain understanding of the rhinoplasty patient, eight key questions are recommended. These can be worked into the conversation of the consultation at the appropriate times and are not necessarily asked in the sequence presented here.

THE PATIENT AS A PERSON

1. Why do you want your nose operated on? (What's wrong with it?)

   The response to this question is a key to the patient's personality, motives, self-image, and reasonableness regarding the anticipated surgery.

2. Have you ever had a broken nose?

   Documentation of prior injuries and condition for medicolegal purposes.

3. Do you have any trouble with your nose?

   Breathing?
   Allergies?
   Sinus problems?
   Nosebleeds?
   Documentation of physical complaints.

4. Do you have pain in your nose?

   Beware of psychiatric problems if the answer is "yes." Rarely is there a physical reason for chronic nasal pain. If one operates on a patient having a complaint of pain in the nose, one should be prepared to hear the complaint repeatedly after the patient is well.

5. Have you ever seen another doctor about operating on your nose?

   Documentation of prior conditions, examinations, and surgery for medicolegal purposes. Exposes individuals with complaints against doctors. Indicates whether the patient is a shopper.

6. How is your general health?

   Provides the opportunity to learn the significant information for "Review of Systems," use of medications and medical allergies. Is important in evaluation for the use of sedative, analgesic, and anesthetic medications.

7. What would *you* like done for your nose?

   Promotes communication of patient's desires. Are they realistic?

8. Do you understand everything I have told you about the operation?

   This question and the response provide the basis for informed consent regarding the methods of surgery and treatment, the anticipations of the patient and surgeon, the potential hazards or complications, and the inability to guarantee results. It may well be best presented in writing with all other necessary information of adequate informed consent.

THE PERSON AS A PATIENT

Evaluation for nasoplasty through examination of the *person as a patient* must include more than study of the nose. The following should be considered.

Gender. Femininity should be a goal in rhinoplasty on women, who often complain of too large a nose in the projection of the osseocartilaginous profile, the tip or alae, and excess width of both. This usually implies nasal reduction to gain a contour consistent with contemporary ideas of feminine beauty.

Masculinity should be preserved in the nose of a man seeking rhinoplasty, providing a heterosexual behavior exists. One should not consider a tipped-up retroussé profile or a petite nose in men. A straight dorsal profile line seems more desirable.

Ethnic type. One must consider also the racial and ethnic background of the patient and must have a clear understanding that the patient desires an alteration of nasal contours consistent with another racial type, before making a radical conversion to a stylized nose. (An Italian does not ordinarily want to resemble an Irishman, and vice versa.) More often, the patient wishes a nose consistent with the image of beauty within the patient's own ethnic and racial heritage, unless there is a desire for assimilation and acceptance into another culture.

Age. At 13 or 14 years, girls are often not too young physically for rhinoplasty, but they may be too immature emotionally to cope with the procedures of local anesthesia, sedation, and postoperative care. If they are physically as large in stature as their mothers and possess a large nose, reduction of which would give a psychologic benefit, the surgeon may find them apt and cooperative patients. However, girls usually respond better to the anxieties of surgery at 16 years or older.

Boys reach maturity later than girls, and surgery should usually be delayed until 18 or older. One should consider the potential hazards of contact sports to the male nose, and preoperative discussion should include a thorough discussion of injury of the nose in sports, masculine activities, and altercations.

The teen years are best for rhinoplasties because of the youthful turgor of the skin. The twenties and thirties are good years also, but less so. After 40 years, the skin loosens and follows the attraction of gravity, and raising the tip of the nose may be less successful.

However, advanced age, even into the seventh decade, is no contraindication to nasoplasty, because the surgeon can overcome the loss of elasticity of the nasal skin through an open-flap rhinoplasty (Chapter 12) consisting of a rhinoplasty and a flap lift of the nasal skin.

Body type. Height, weight, and body type should be considered. Generally, tall people need longer noses, large people need larger noses, and short people need smaller noses; a tall, slender woman should not have a short, tilted pixie nose.

Facial structure. Facial configuration is one of four types: round, oval, rectangular, or triangular. Generally, an upturned, short nose is attractive on a round face, a slender, straight nose is good for the oval face, a strong nose matches a rectangular face, and a triangular face may need the strength of a chin augmentation to go with a nasal reduction of an appropriate profile and width. The size of the face relative to total body size should also be considered.

Nasal anatomy. The rhinoplastic surgeon must possess a knowledge of external and internal nasal anatomy and physiology, so that function may not be lessened by an aesthetic rhinoplasty and may be improved by submucous septal resection, septoplasty, or turbinate resection if necessary.

EXTERNAL NASAL EXAMINATION

A systematic examination and evaluation of the external and internal nasal structures should include skin, external bones, external cartilages, nares, mucosa, septum, and turbinates.

Skin. Young, thin skin is best. Thick, sebaceous skin will preclude a desired good result. Inelastic, aged skin may not contract to a smaller nasal architecture. Hence, the surgeon should note if the skin is thick or thin, sebaceous or fine, mobile or taut, to advise the patient if a fine result may be achieved.

External bones. Observation of the width, projection (profile or dorsum), and alignment (or deviation) of the external bones should be made.

External cartilages. Are the lateral cartilages large? Is there an osseocartilaginous hump? Is there cartilaginous deviation? What are the size and shape of the alar cartilages? Are the medial crura short or long (columellar length)? Are the lateral crura large and wide or fine and narrow? Are the alae thin? Are there indentations above the lateral crura? Is there arching of the alae, or are the lateral sidewalls thick and redundant?

Nares. Are the nares equal, flaring, narrow or wide, vertical or horizontal, long or short?

INTERNAL NASAL EXAMINATION

The internal nasal examination should be as systematic and thorough as the external examination and should be conducted with a speculum and head lamp or head mirror to eliminate parallax.

The patient's breathing at quiet respiration and forced respiration should be noted. A thumb lightly applied from below each naris in turn will allow the examiner, without a rhinomanometer, to estimate the volume of flow through each nostril. An enquiry as to how this relates to the patient's usual breathing gives one an idea of the state of function.

Mucosa. The condition of the mucosa of the leading edges of the inferior and middle turbinates should be noted with regard to color, edema, crusts, inflammation, synechiae, discharge, or metaplasia. Allergic rhinitis is revealed by pale bluish, boggy membranes with a glary, clear, stringy discharge. Allergic rhinitis is important to note, as those with this problem will complain of difficulty in breathing after surgery. Seasonally allergic patients (not in season) and patients with food allergies may appear normal, whereas urban patients with allergy may have a red, granular appearance of the nasal mucosa from chronic exposure to air pollutants.

After initial examination of the nasal mucosa, a 2% solution of ephedrine (or other topical decongestant of choice) is sprayed in the nose with a pressure atomizer inserted through a nasal speculum. The allergic patient in season may require packing with cotton dipped in 4% to 10% cocaine. If mucosal shrinkage does not then occur, the attention of a rhinologist or allergist should be sought.

Patients in the height of a seasonal allergic response should have surgery deferred pending medical control or subsidence of their allergies. Those with chronic allergic rhinitis should be considered for systemic steroid therapy immediately before and after surgery.

After shrinkage, the nasal vestibule and mucosa should be examined further to observe the presence of polyps, ulcerations, synechiae, or scars.

The relative size of the inferior and middle turbinates after shrinkage is noted. There may be a compensatory hypertrophy of the turbinates when the septum is deviated to the other side.

Septum. Septal deviations, cartilaginous and osseous, should be studied. Are they low, high, anterior, or posterior?

The area of osseocartilaginous junction is of particular import: the anterior nasal spine, maxillary crest, vomer, vertical plate of the ethmoid, and nasal dorsum. Hypertrophy of the turbinates with impaction on the septum is noted.

The breathing test of each naris is repeated after mucosal decongestion to determine the part played in the nasal obstruction by the mucosa.

In septal deviations, the mechanism of the trauma should be understood. A blow on the left side of the nose by a good right hook may deviate the nasal bones and dorsal part of the septum to the right and displace the quadrilateral cartilage out of the vomerine groove to the left, causing a spur or shelf obstruction in the left nasal passage. Correction requires resection of the vomerine and sometimes the ethmoid plate deviation posteriorly and release of the quadrilateral cartilage from the vomer and vertical plate of the ethmoid. Often the cartilage will then swing to the midline. Resection of quadrilateral cartilage is not usually necessary or desirable.

A more direct blow from the front may cause a similar injury plus a fracture or telescoping of the quadrilateral cartilage on the vertical plate of the ethmoid and an angulation or C-curvature of the quadrilateral cartilage. The presence of high (close to the dorsum or profile) deviations in the quadrilateral cartilage and ethmoid plate is most important in evaluating the probability of a successful correction of an externally and internally deviated nose.

Deviations occurring in childhood or youth are often severe and may be accompanied by bony hypertrophy of the vomer and turbinates. One must be prepared to reduce the turbinates on the concave side of the septum to allow replacement of the septum to the midline.

In turbinate hypertrophy of lesser duration that responds to decongestants, surgical reduction is not usually necessary.

THE QUANTUM EVALUATION

Much attention has been given to the quantum evaluation in preparation for nasal surgery. This ordinarily refers to the methods that aid the surgeon in determination of the amounts and location of tissues to be reduced or altered in rhinoplasty.

Moulages and plaster of Paris casts or models are of insufficient value for consideration. A rhinoplasty is by no means comparable to shaving down and sanding a plaster model. Profilometers likewise have little connection with reality. Cephalometry is of value only for osseous and dental structure.

Professional photography, with color slides and

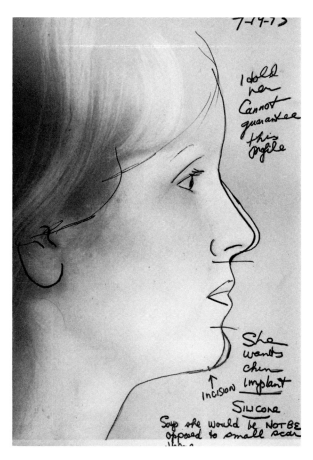

Fig. 9-1. Life-size lateral preoperative photo of K. M., age 25, indicates exact areas and finite amount of nasal reduction. Observe that nasolabial angle is ideal. Patient requested and may well benefit from chin augmentation. Sketch was made on reverse of photo and may be studied from both sides by placing on x-ray view box. Frankfort line and line of facial plane are seldom necessary to determine desired aesthetic profile. Photo and sketch have been used as a method of communication between plastic surgeon and patient.

glossy black-and-white prints, is the superior modality for the quantum evaluation.

The same photographer, camera, film, background, camera-to-patient distance, tripod height, patient height, lighting, patient's attire, views, and film processing should prevail in every photo sitting to ensure uniform photographic results.

Color slides should be composed horizontally so they may be trimmed for composite before-and-after slides. This permits horizontal composition in the final dual mounts of each view.

The glossy black-and-white prints should be at least 4 × 6 inches so they can be readily seen in the operating room. A life-size lateral and basal or worm's-eye view are desirable for accurate preoperative planning.

These are most effectively used by placing them on an illuminated x-ray view box (as described by Becker in 1946 and Gonzales-Ulloa in 1962) in a reverse position and sketching the desired nasal reduction and aesthetic contouring in a superimposed position. The life-size lateral view indicates the exact areas of desired reduction, the nasolabial angle, the length of the nasal profile compared to other portions of the face, and the projection of the chin and dentition as well as the nose. The life-size worm's-eye basal view reveals the shape of the tip, size and shape of the nares, the width of the alar bases, and the columellar length. One may accurately plan the rhinoplastic alterations from these photographic studies (Figs. 9-1 to 9-3).

The surgeon may draw the Frankfort line and facial plane on the reverse of the life-size lateral view to assist in planning the operation.

These photographs (particularly the life-size lateral view) are most valuable in arriving at communication with the patient. After the initial consultation, the photos are obtained, and the patient

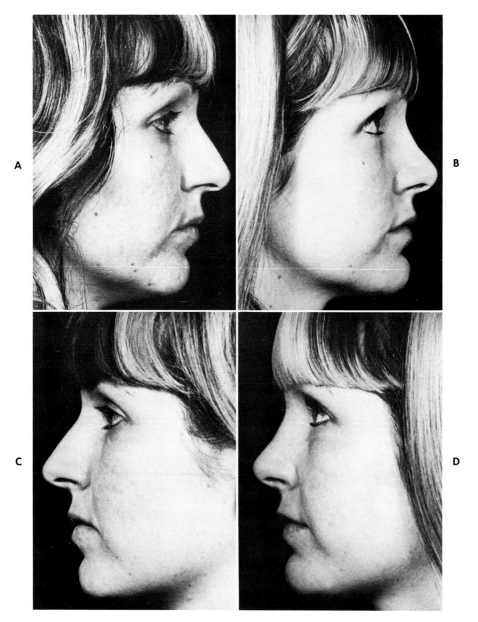

Fig. 9-2. Composite preoperative and postoperative photos of K. M., standard six views, reveal that result of operation can be close to preoperative plan. Rhinoplasty and silicone chin implant were accomplished. **A,** Preoperative right lateral view. **B,** Postoperative right lateral view. **C,** Preoperative left lateral view. **D,** Postoperative left lateral view.

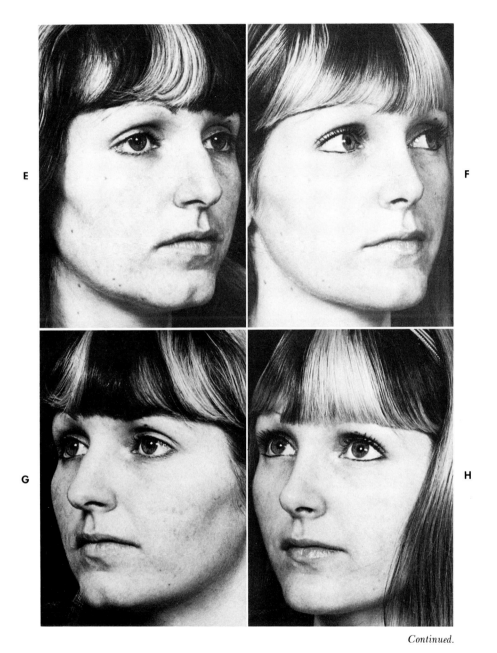

Continued.

Fig. 9-2, cont'd. E, Preoperative right oblique view. **F,** Postoperative right oblique view. **G,** Preoperative left oblique view. **H,** Postoperative left oblique view.

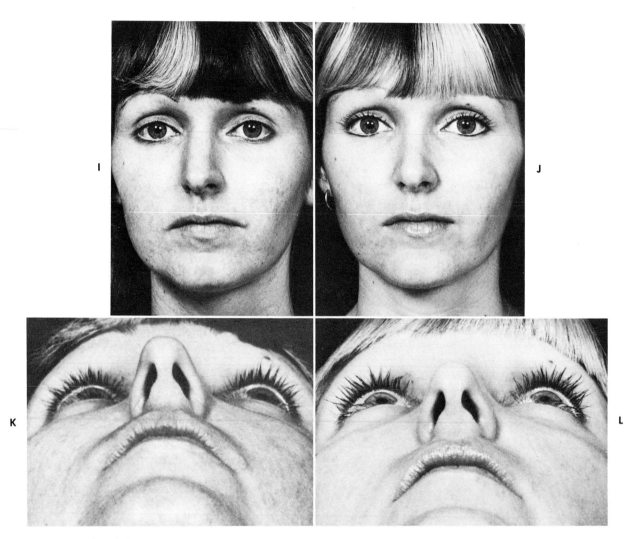

Fig. 9-2, cont'd. I, Preoperative anterior view. **J,** Postoperative anterior view. **K,** Preoperative basal view. **L,** Postoperative basal view.

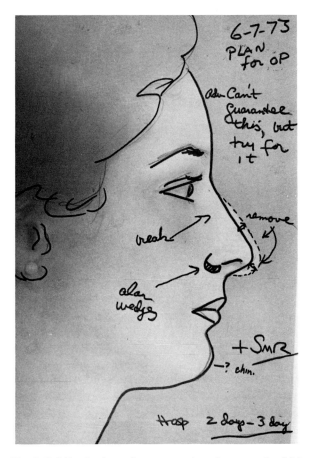

Fig. 9-3. Life-size lateral preoperative photograph of 23-year-old patient for planning nasal reduction and achieving communication with patient regarding plastic surgeon's aesthetic goals and surgical method. Photo and sketch may be studied from both sides by placing it on x-ray view box. Patient has a large, long Italian nose. Nares are large. Alar cartilages are large medially and laterally and protrude caudally in columella.

is given a second appointment to discuss them with the surgeon. The surgeon may indicate with the planning sketches on the photo reverses what is to be attempted, with a note in writing that "The profile so sketched is a preoperative plan, and no guarantee is given that it can be achieved in the operation." This information may be written on the photograph in the patient's presence, and the date recorded. By revealing the surgical goal to the patient, one learns whether it is acceptable, whether the patient's own image of the nose coincides with the photographic fact, and exactly what the patient would like accomplished.

Properly presented, this method of communication of surgeon's and patient's goals does not appear to represent a medicolegal hazard; in fact, it may well be an important facet of informed rhinoplasty consent.

A third preoperative visit may be desirable if a long interval has elapsed between the initial consultation and the date of surgery, to review the operative plan, methods, anesthesia, risks, and to answer questions. Thorough preoperative evaluation, documentation of the examinations and discussions, interest in and dedication to the patient's well-being, adequate planning, and communication of goals are all ingredients of a successful rhinoplasty.

REFERENCES

1. Becker, O. J.: Aids in rhinoplastic procedures, Ann. Otol. Rhinol. Laryngol. **55:**562, 1946.
2. Gonzalez-Ulloa, M.: Quantitative principles in cosmetic surgery of the face (profiloplasty), Plast. Reconstr. Surg. **29:**186, 1962.

Chapter 10

Anatomy of a rhinoplasty

Joseph Safian, M.D.

A little over a half century ago, I presented my first paper on rhinoplasty before a medical society in New York.

About 25 years later, in 1947, I published "A Critical Review of the Recent Literature on Rhinoplasty."[2] It was prompted by a rash of publications describing new methods and new procedures in rhinoplasty. They were all based on deceptive concepts of aesthetic rhinoplasty[3] and produced a great many surgical defects.

And now after 50 years, a review of some current literature and practice of rhinoplasty indicates that some surgeons completely disregard the anatomic guidelines that are essential for success in the practice of aesthetic rhinoplasty.

One important thing to remember is that whenever a change is made in the surface anatomy of any part of the human body, an anatomic abnormality is produced and a defect is created, and the nose is particularly vulnerable to a change in its anatomy because it is a conspicuous part of the surface anatomy.

We must also realize that the anatomy of a big nose is exactly the same as that of a small nose. The only difference is in the size and shape of the eight component parts that make up the external nose. Since no anatomic difference is involved, we are privileged only to reduce the size and modify the shape of these parts but never to change the anatomy or the anatomic relationships of these parts. We may never either totally or even subtotally resect any one of these parts, nor may we create a situation whereby the skin and lining membrane of the nose come in contact and become attached to each other. Such a situation does not exist in a normal nose. Nature has provided that these two membranes be separated by either bone or cartilage throughout the entire structure of the nose.

It is equally important that the normal structure of the nasal cartilages never be changed by crushing, morselizing, or crosshatching. Such tissues are alien to the human anatomy. They can be reduced in size or modified in shape only when they are in their normal state.

A paper entitled "Five Most Important Points in Reduction Rhinoplasty"[6] states, "the lower lateral and upper lateral cartilages, if they bulge convexly, usually . . . will be found to be flat within the nose and [will] not require total ext[i]rpation. They can be removed without hazard." This statement obviously violates the anatomic guidelines of aesthetic rhinoplasty.

Another violation of anatomic principles is the attempt to shorten the nose by excision of a triangular segment of the cartilaginous septum just above its lower border.[1,7] The apex of this triangle is to be close to the anterior nasal spine. The two sides of this triangle are to be brought together with sutures. It is obvious that the authors have produced an isoceles triangle, no two sides of which are of equal length, and therefore the sides cannot be brought together without producing a defect. In this instance it will appear along the dorsum of the nose.

Another paper, with complete disregard of normal anatomy, presents "A New Method for Correction of the Prominent Nasal Tip."[5] The authors propose that the lower half of the columellar cartilage be amputated and the upper half freed from its surrounding tissues. Then by pulling down on the remaining portion of the columellar cartilage, part of the lateral crus would be pulled down into the space left by the amputated portion of the columellar cartilage. There certainly are simpler and more effective methods of reducing a prominent nasal tip without changing the normal anatomy.

Another recently published paper deals with three methods of nasal tip correction.[7] The description of these methods is so vague that I could not determine which method applies to what. However, if any one of these methods has consistently proved successful and satisfactory, the other two might best be discarded.

In recent years some surgeons have adopted a method of rhinoplasty that advocates the nasal tip reduction as a first step of the rhinoplasty. The procedure in this reduction consists of an almost total submucous resection of the lateral crus, leaving but a narrow strip of cartilage to support the alar rim. This procedure takes account neither of the size or shape of the existing nose nor of the one contemplated by the reduction rhinoplasty. It merely eliminates some fullness of the nasal tip above the alar rim, and it is the same in every case. In addition, the extensive submucous resection of the lateral crus produces the type of anatomic abnormality previously mentioned, in which the skin and lining membrane of the nose come in contact in the area of submucous resection. They become firmly attached to each other, and, as the scar tissue contraction progresses, an indentation is most likely to appear in this area.

It is standard surgical procedure that in making external incisions, they are placed within the lines of Langer, and that in separating tissues, it is best done in the normal lines of cleavage. It is therefore rational that the incision for exposing the nasal framework should be in the intercartilaginous space and not through the body of the lateral crus.

To produce a normal-looking, aesthetically desirable nose, the eight component parts of the external nose are reduced in size or reshaped in harmonizing proportion to one another. To achieve this goal, Professor Joseph and his followers depended on surgical craftsmanship. The same results can rarely be produced by amateur carpentry.

The size and shape of the nasal tip depend almost entirely on the size and shape of the alar cartilages and particularly on that of the lateral crus. In the operating room, I have often pointed out how exactly the lateral crus reflects the aesthetic defect of the nasal tip and how accurately it can be corrected when the lateral crus is properly exposed.

In converting a bulbous tip into one that has aesthetic value, the surgeon has the opportunity to display his artistic vision and skill by reducing the size of the lateral crus and reshaping it in an infinite number of subtle variations, so that each operated nose acquires some aesthetic individuality. The only problem presented here is how to gain proper access to the lateral crus to carry out the necessary changes.

About 1932 I developed the split cartilage tip technique of rhinoplasty.[4] This has produced most gratifying results for me during the succeeding 40 years of my practice. It is the only change in the Joseph technique that I found beneficial. It is also the only procedure, to my knowledge, that delivers the entire lateral crus in the form of a pedicled flap into the hands of the surgeon. He can then, by direct vision, convert it to whatever size and shape his judgment dictates. The reshaped crus, freed from its overlying skin, with its lining membrane attached and intact, snaps back into position to resume its function of shaping and supporting the nasal tip. The undermined skin readily shrinks and drapes itself smoothly over the reduced size of the nasal tip. Neither the anatomy nor the anatomic relationships of the area structures is in any way changed from the normal.

The average rhinoplasty is not a difficult procedure. It consists of only four easily performed surgical steps. But it is important that these four steps be performed in proper sequence and by proper coordination.

The method of intranasal rhinoplasty originated by Professor Joseph and the sequence of his procedures are most rational. He first resected the hump or the dorsal convexity. He then performed the lateral osteotomy and infractured. He thus established the basic structure of the corrected nose in proper proportion to the patient's face. Shortening of the nose or tip tilting was the next step. Judging the degree of the nasolabial angle was accurate because the permanent profile line had been established. At this point he realized, and it is true, that no matter how little or how much the tip was raised, its shape and forward protrusion changed. And it was only then that the tip could be properly fashioned to harmonize with the new nose and the patient's other features.

I followed the Joseph procedures throughout the years of my practice with only the change I mentioned in the nasal tip reduction method.

All but one of my rhinoplasties were performed under local anesthesia. After the lateral osteotomy, I always infractured. A small gauze dressing was applied with a modified Joseph clamp over it to prevent the accumulation of blood under the skin. It was not intended as a retention apparatus for the narrowing of the nasal bridge. The clamp and all other dressings were discontinued after 48 hours. I used no packing postoperatively unless

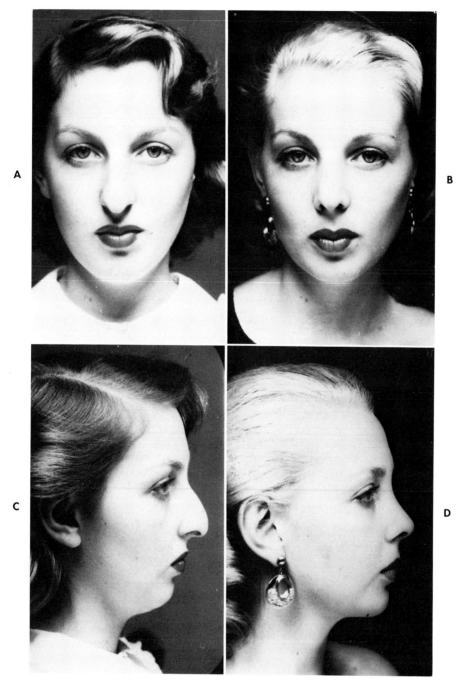

Fig. 10-1. A, Full-face preoperative view. **B,** Full-face postoperative view. **C,** Right profile preoperative view. **D,** Right profile postoperative view.

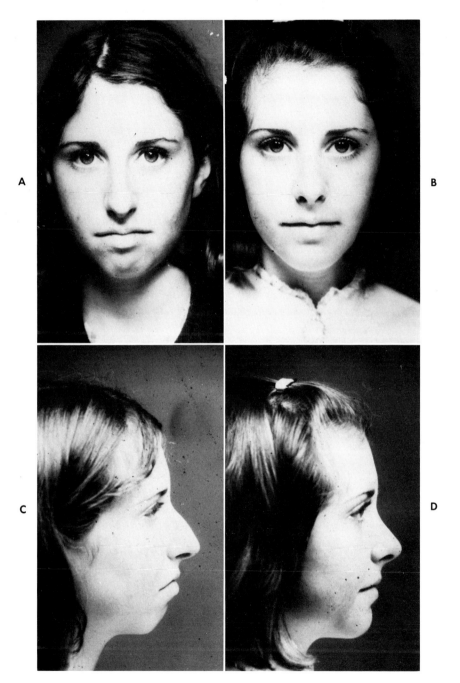

Fig. 10-2. A, Full-face preoperative view. **B,** Full-face postoperative view. **C,** Right profile preoperative view. **D,** Right profile postoperative view.

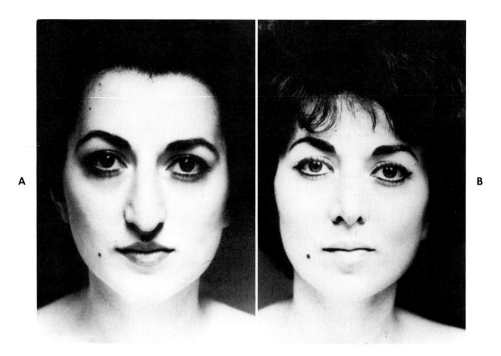

Fig. 10-3. A, Preoperative view. **B,** Postoperative view.

a submucous resection of the septum was performed at the same time.

This simple routine produced most gratifying results without any change in the normal anatomy of the nose (Figs. 10-1 to 10-3).

REFERENCES

1. Parkes, M. C., and Brennan, H. G.: High septal transfixion to shorten the nose, Plast. Reconstr. Surg. **45**:487, 1970.
2. Safian, J.: A critical review of the recent literature on rhinoplasty, Plast. Reconstr. Surg. **2**:463, 1947.
3. Safian, J.: Deceptive concepts of rhinoplasty, Plast. Reconstr. Surg. **18**:127, 1956.
4. Safian, J.: The split cartilage tip technique of rhinoplasty, Plast. Reconstr. Surg. **45**:3, 1971.
5. Spina, V., Kamakura, L., and Paillakis, J.: A new method for correction of the prominent nasal tip, Plast. Reconstr. Surg. **51**:416, 1973.
6. Tamerin, J.: Five most important points in reduction rhinoplasty, Plast. Reconstr. Surg. **48**:214, 1971.
7. Webster, R. C., White, M. F., and Courtis, E. H.: Nasal tip correction in rhinoplasty, Plast. Reconstr. Surg. **51**:384, 1973.

Discussion

Musgrave: Are there any questions?

Rogers: Dr. Safian, perhaps in order to start a controversy, in view of some of the results seen in surgery at national meetings, would you advise a young, resident surgeon today to only apply a clamp and a gauze dressing for 48 hours in a routine nasoplasty?

Safian: Not necessarily a clamp, but any pressure, either metal pressure or what they're using now, just for 48 hours to prevent hematoma. If they depend upon that pressure to narrow the nasal bridge, then they are mistaken. If they did not narrow that bridge originally at the time of the operation properly, it will not stay that way.

Rogers: Could I ask a question for discussion whether Gus Aufricht or some of our other senior men would agree with that in the teaching of residents today, in teaching a routine rhinoplasty?

Aufricht: Joseph never used a pack or splint on his noses. He put on the splint a week or 10 days later. As a matter of fact, he was very careful in emphasizing, "Don't put any pressure on the skin because it might get damaged." I started with the splint in New York because I operated in a number of small hospitals, and I was afraid of hematoma formation, which might be hard to remedy. Then I developed the splint made of dental molding wax. I cannot say the results depended on the splint because Joseph got marvelous results without the splint. So whatever the resident wants.

Safian: I agree with you fully that the application of the clamp is not for the purpose of narrowing the bridge. I use it as a deterrent to hematoma. The only difference in the way you do one part of this operation is that you perform an outfracture before you do the infracture. Right? I never do that. There is nothing wrong with doing the outfracture, but I feel and it has been my experience that I've been able to infracture every single case without any difficulty. And the advantage of that procedure, that one little procedure is this: I produce a nasoglabellar suture fracture at that point because a partially impacted fracture cannot help to maintain the bones in proper position. I do it on this basis. If a person gets hit on the nose and gets an infracture, he's got a crooked nose. It doesn't come out by itself unless you use an elevator. On that same principle, I feel that if I infracture the nose at the nasofrontal suture on each side, it will stay there, so I don't have to use any retention apparatus at all. My noses remain narrow, and you cannot depend on any pressure device. Dr. Aufricht is right in what he does because he outfractures and he has to maintain the lateral walls of the nose for a longer period of time until either fibrous or bony union forms to maintain it in that position. At least this has been my experience.

Aufricht: Joseph, we're not competing!

Safian: No, no, no!

Millard: The only one enjoying this more right now, more even than any of us, is Jacques Joseph himself!

Safian: I hope so!

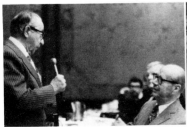 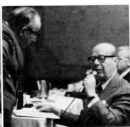 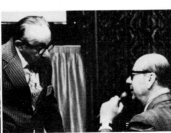

Dr. Safian and
Dr. Aufricht

69

Chapter 11

Total concept of rhinoplasty

Gustave Aufricht, M.D.

Professor Joseph, in his momentous book *Nasenplastik und Sonstige Gesichtsplastik,* noted that until the middle of the nineteenth century, reconstruction of nasal defects constituted by far the major and most interesting part in the history of plastic surgery. That this was so is understandable, since the nose, the most obvious and prominent part of the face, was purposefully mutilated during wars and was the object of ancient punitive injuries. (In India noses were cut off to punish such crimes as adultery.) Regardless of what caused the defect, reparation was of paramount importance to the victim, since the nose is such an expressive and conspicuous facial feature.

During the late nineteenth and early twentieth centuries, when modern cosmetic rhinoplasty was being developed, the attention of the plastic surgeon as well as of the public was focused for several decades on the correction of nasal deformities alone. A patient sought the services of a plastic surgeon to reduce the proportions of an oversized nose, to straighten a hump nose, or to shorten a long nose—nothing more—and the surgeon would comply, changing the contours and proportions of the nose alone. Some aimed at achieving a replica of the stereotyped nose (for example, straight and turned up), whereas others tried to fit the nose to its surrounding features.

With increasing experience in nasal correction and more awareness of its effect on the face overall, it gradually became evident that features other than the nose also contribute to symmetry and attractiveness and that they too are amenable to surgical correction. What is the use of making a straight, short nose when the patient is left with a markedly receding chin? If the nose is not fitted to the face, the result might be even more conspicuous than the preoperative defect. Nature has its own aesthetic standards: a hump on the nose sometimes compensates for the weakness of a receding chin; removal of the hump without adding prominence to the chin could well weaken the face.

The chin thus became the next facial contour of surgical interest; it also is a character feature. Although one clearly cannot and should not judge human character and disposition from appearance, there are nevertheless certain stereotypes impressed on the public's mind. A receding chin is often believed to symbolize weakness; a prominent chin, especially when combined with a long, humped nose, may be considered to indicate strength; a slightly protruding chin in combination with a nose of normal proportion can be pleasantly provoking and, in a woman, even coquettish.

Occasional augmentation of the chin alone was being done at the beginning of this century. Esser in Germany used costal bone for the purpose; Lexer transplanted a ball of abdominal fat; Eckstein injected hard paraffin; Joseph used ivory. These corrections, however, were done for the chin alone, without consideration of the nose. Joseph even reported a patient with a hump nose and a receding chin in whom he augmented the chin without straightening the nose. In another case he performed minor corrections on the alae nasi while simultaneously augmenting the chin with an ivory implant.

Until about the third decade of this century, no surgeon aimed at simultaneous correction of the nose and the chin for aesthetic purposes. At this time, however, they realized that these two features should be considered in the combined contour relationship. In 1922, in Berlin, I implanted a piece of ivory in the nose to create a dorsal hump and simultaneously placed a piece in the chin to augment its prominence. This procedure was done

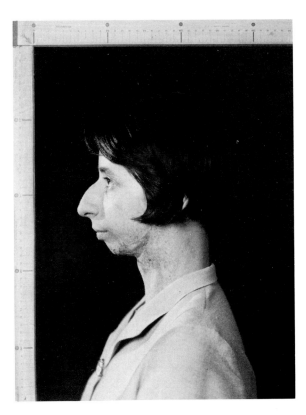

Fig. 11-1. Burn scar contracture of chin and neck. Note skin graft to relieve scar contracture, large hump nose, and receding chin.

on a Russian refugee actor, not for aesthetic purposes but to disguise his identity for political reasons.

My first case of combined rhinoplasty and mentoplasty using the osteocartilaginous hump from the nose for the augmentation deserves mention. The patient was a young woman with an extensive burn scar on the chin and neck from a childhood injury. The scar had been treated with x rays by another physician to soften and smooth its surface. I first relieved the scar contracture on the neck with a full-thickness skin graft in December, 1928 (Fig. 11-1).

About a year later I performed a rhinoplasty on her. During the procedure, after I had removed the exceptionally large osteocartilaginous hump in one piece, it occurred to me that the canoe-shaped convex specimen would lend itself distinctly to augmenting the patient's receding chin. I dipped the specimen in an alcoholic antiseptic solution (a procedure I no longer use), washed it with normal saline, removed the mucous membrane from the inside, and trimmed the ends to size. From a submental incision, I prepared a pocket in front of the mandible and inserted the osteocartilaginous specimen.

It healed per primam. The graft had taken.

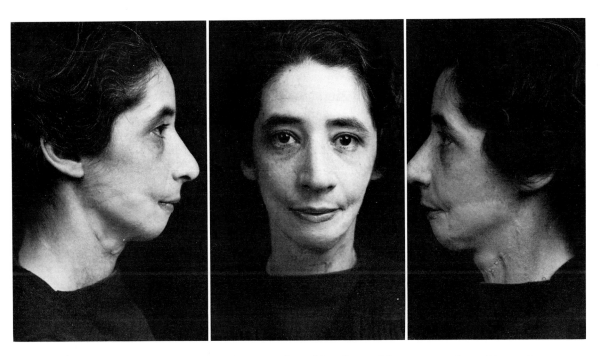

Fig. 11-2. Same patient as in Fig. 11-1 after rhinoplasty, chin augmentation with nasal hump, and replacement of burn scar with a pectoral flap. (From Cronin, T.: Burn contractures of the neck. In Lynch, J. B., and Lewis, S. R., editors: Symposium on the treatment of burns, vol. 5, St. Louis, 1973, The C. V. Mosby Co.)

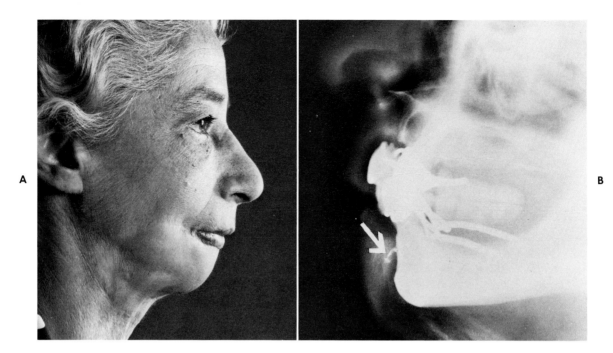

Fig. 11-3. A, Same patient as in Figs. 11-1 and 11-2, 30 years later. **B,** X-ray film shows that osteocartilaginous graft is intact. Note that graft was placed unintentionally too high. It would have been better at tip of mandible.

This operation, performed on November 12, 1929, to my knowledge was the first instance of my or anyone's using a transplant from the nose to the chin. Subsequently I completely removed the scar and radiation-affected areas and replaced the defect with a pectoral flap (Fig. 11-2). I followed this case for 28 years, and the transplant has remained intact (Fig. 11-3).

Encouraged by this early experience, I began increasingly to combine rhinoplasty with chin augmentation, using nasal tissues. I have utilized not only the hump but also the septal cartilage, pieces of the lower lateral cartilage, and practically all nasal skeletal tissues. With this method the surgeon can add almost 1 cm to the prominence of the chin. If there is no nasal material available, I use a silicone rubber implant. The results of combined nasal and chinplasty have been favorably accepted. When I first began to use this procedure, I usually had to persuade the surprised patient to comply with my suggestion of combining nose and chin surgery; but 10 to 15 years later the patient himself often asked if something could also be done for his chin. The profession in general is doing more and more simultaneous chin augmentation, although not necessarily with nasal tissues.

On further study of the overall face and potential corrections, my attention became directed toward the upper lip. I had occasionally grafted rib cartilage to the front of the maxilla to raise a sunken upper lip in the so-called dish face deformity (Fig. 11-4), but it was a bit later that I became interested in correcting minor but objectionable contour imperfections in connection with nasal deformities.

After the eyes, lips are the most expressive facial feature. They consist of sensitive voluntary muscles and partake in the expression of all emotions, such as happiness, anger, and fear. The lips lend definite characteristics to the face, even in repose.

The upper lip on a classic head occupies a third of the vertical dimensions of the lower third of the face, according to Schadow's Canon (Fig. 11-5). The upper lip in whites usually originates from the columella at about the middle of the long axis of the nostril. The vertical proportion of the upper lip and its prominence in relation to the nose and lower lip vary. In extreme cases these proportions can be aesthetically objectionable, and often they can be surgically corrected. Gradually I paid more and more attention to the simultaneous correction of upper lip contours and rhinoplasty.

By the early 1960s it became common, almost routine, to combine rhinoplasty with simultaneous correction of the upper lip and chin augmentation.

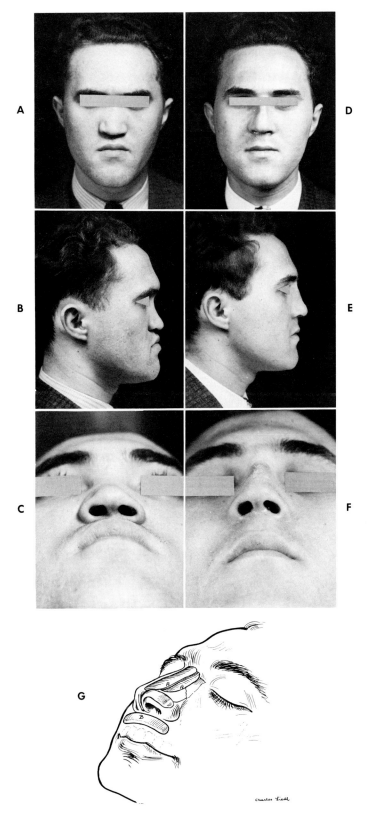

Fig. 11-4. A to **C,** Dish face before surgery. **D** to **F,** After corrective surgery. **G,** Technique of correction: *A,* cartilage graft to nose; *B,* retrolabial cartilage graft.

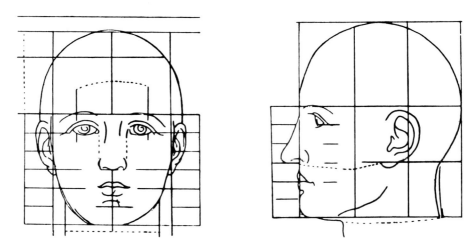

Fig. 11-5. Classic facial proportions according to Schadow's Canon. (From Joseph, J.: Nasenplastik und sonstige Gesichtsplastik nebst einem Anhang ueber Mammaplastik, Leipzig, Germany, 1931, Verlag von Curt Kabitzsch.)

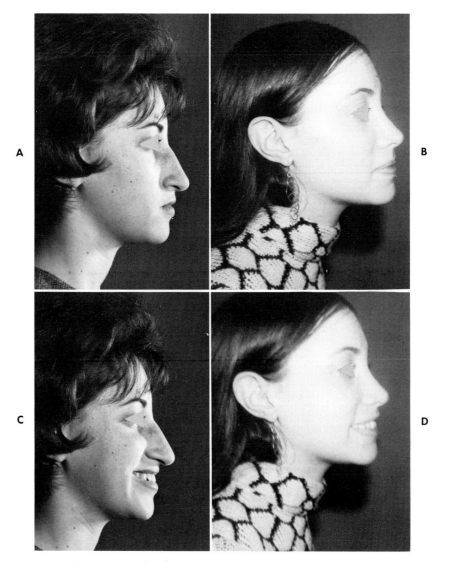

Fig. 11-6. Crowded upper lip, **A** and **C,** before correction, and **B** and **D,** after correction.

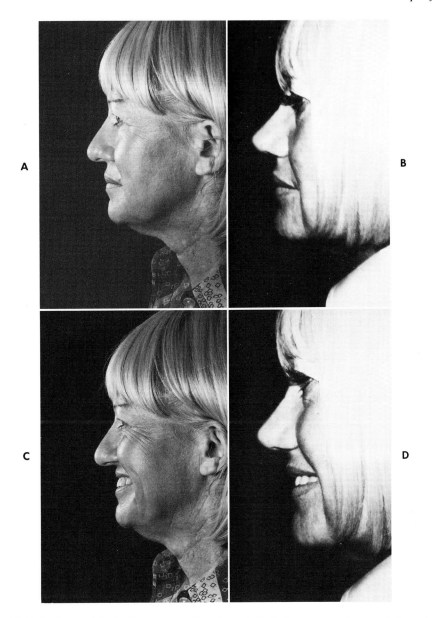

Fig. 11-7. Patient with shallow upper lip, **A** and **C,** before operation, and **B** and **D,** after operation.

The various objectionable configurations of the upper lip amenable to surgical correction include (1) a short or crowded upper lip, (2) a shallow upper lip, (3) an acute labiocolumellar angle, (4) an obtuse labiocolumellar angle, and (5) an overretracting upper lip.

The crowded upper lip is caused by a too-long nose, which appears to take up room at the expense of the upper lip (Fig. 11-6). The downward protruding septum presses the columella down or sometimes sideways (subluxation). The upper lip is visibly handicapped in motion. When a person

with this aesthetic defect smiles or laughs, the central portion of the mouth remains down, and the corners curl up. In other cases the lip may fold up in a sharp angle, often causing a permanent crease. Some self-conscious patients with this condition actually refrain from smiling or laughing.

The shallow upper lip and the acute labiocolumellar angle (with normal length nose) are due to an overly backward-slanting maxilla. It may be exaggerated by a prominent alveolar process and protruding teeth. This configuration, if objectionable, can be corrected with retrolabial grafts (Fig.

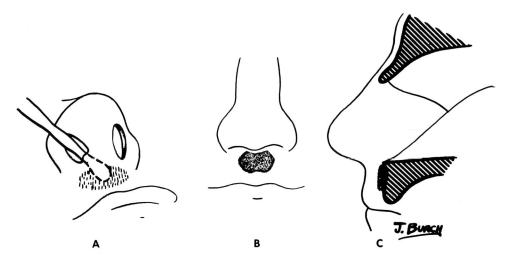

Fig. 11-8. Retrolabial graft. **A,** Retrolabial tunnel prepared with periosteal elevator. **B** and **C,** Graft in situ. (From Aufricht, G.: Plast. Reconstr. Surg. **43:**219, 1969.)

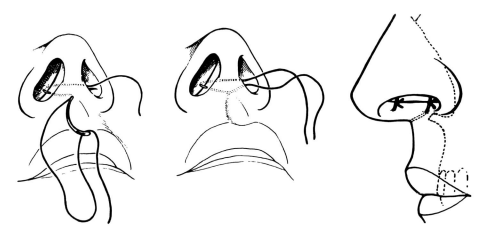

Fig. 11-9. Submerged suture. (From Aufricht, G.: Laryngoscope **53:**317, 1943.)

11-7). (Dental malocclusions require more radical treatment.) For these grafts a pocket is formed in front of the maxilla, the approach being through the base of the detached columella. The incision may be extended on one side toward the vestibulum.

The pocket is prepared with a periosteal elevator at bone level but not subperiosteally (Fig. 11-8). It should be symmetric and just large enough to accommodate the graft. There is no other fixation but the limits of the pocket. The septal cartilage is usually cut into uneven hexagonal pieces about 15 × 18 mm. A shallow indentation is made on the broad side to allow space for the inferior nasal spine. Several layers of cartilage can be used, as

can pieces from the lower lateral cartilage or bone from the nose. The incision is closed with interrupted plain catgut sutures.

An obtuse labiocolumellar angle is usually due to a partial, downward protrusion of the septum or to an overdeveloped inferior nasal spine or to both. In either case the excess cartilage and bone are resected. Often subcutaneous soft tissues, fat, and muscle are also removed at the base of the columella. The 90-degree labiocolumellar angle is formed then with heavy, submerged silk sutures, which are left in place for about 2 weeks (Fig. 11-9). They create scarry contraction in the angle without leaving visible marks on the skin.

Patients with a retrolabial graft often experi-

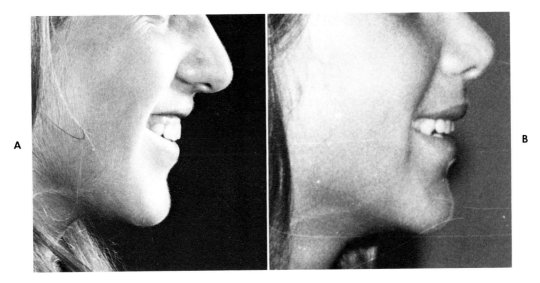

Fig. 11-10. Overretracting upper lip, producing so-called gummy smile. **A,** Before correction. **B,** After correction. (From Aufricht, G.: Plast. Reconstr. Surg. **43:**219, 1969.)

ence stiffness of the upper lip, which makes it difficult to retract the lip or show the teeth. This symptom is temporary; the lip limbers up in a few weeks, a process that can be speeded up by lip exercises. This phenomenon gave me the idea of using larger grafts on patients with an overretracting upper lip, which produces the so-called gummy smile (Fig. 11-10). With the idea of preventing this overretraction, I extended the postlabial pocket below the labial sulcus, transposing the sulcus to a lower level, and made it larger transversely (Fig. 11-11). The graft (approximately 20 to 22 mm wide and 30 mm long) lessens the retraction even if it does not completely eliminate it.

MARKINGS AND MEASUREMENTS

All preoperative markings are done before the infiltration of anesthetics. The purpose of marking and measuring is partly to review the existing condition and partly to outline the extent of the required corrections. The marks serve as a reminder of the operative plans and mensurations. The tissues become distorted once the anesthetic is administered, and the markings lose their projected values. The profile for all three features—nose, chin, and upper lip—should be planned simultaneously to visualize their aesthetic correlation.

Chin augmentation is planned and measured in the following manner. The soft tissues of the mentum are pinched between the thumb and fingers and pressed forward until the chin reaches a normal level in relation to the lower lip; this pro-

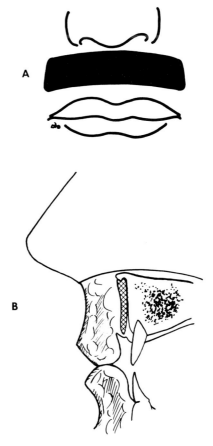

Fig. 11-11. A, Large retrolabial graft for correction of overretracted upper lip (gummy smile). **B,** Side view. (From Aufricht, G.: Plast. Reconstr. Surg. **43:**219, 1969.)

jection is marked on the skin of the lower lip. The distance between the chin and the mark usually measures 4 to 10 mm, or occasionally more with an extremely receding chin.

Here a minor but important detail is considered: the part of the chin that should be most prominent. For this purpose the vertical dimension of the chin is divided into three parts (upper, middle, and lower third), and the augmentation is made according to aesthetic judgment. In some cases, in addition to the receding chin, the mental fold is too deep. For such instances the augmentation is done on two levels, one under the fold and the other for the chin. In another patient the lower third of the chin may be flat, in which case lower-third augmentation is in order without changing the overall prominence.

THE NOSE

The surgeon establishes the new profile by manipulating the nose with his fingers. Its relation to the radix nasi and the lower lateral cartilages is noted and marked with a suitable dye. If the nose is to be shortened or the tip raised, the amount is marked on the cheek.

The procedure to lengthen a crowded upper lip proceeds in the following manner. The lower third of the face, from the base of the nose to the edge of the chin, is measured; it usually ranges from 6 to 7 cm, a third of which is normally occupied by the upper lip. A ruler or compass is now placed from the closed lip upward, and the proper distance is marked on the side of the columella. The distance between the edge of the columella and the mark is the amount the nose is raised or the lip lengthened.

The extent of the shallow upper lip can also be measured. A sterile applicator is placed inside the upper lip and raised to the desired level. Its projection is marked on the columella. The distance between the mark on the columella and the shallowest point of the upper lip is the extent of addition required (usually 2 to 7 mm).

After its profile is established, the width of the chin must be planned. This is determined in frontal view. (It can be done after the nose is infiltrated with the anesthetic, while anesthesia is being established.) First a vertical line is drawn from the middle of the upper lip downward, bisecting the chin into two equal parts. The line extends to the submental fold, which is marked with a transverse line; the lower border of the mandibular bone is also marked. The soft tissue of the chin is then pressed together between the thumb and fingers

to simulate the width, and it is decided whether the chin should be broad or narrow in relation to the mouth; again, this is a decision made according to the surgeon's aesthetic judgment. The implant or transplant should never extend to the cheek (unless there is a defect), lest the augmentation look or feel abnormal.

The width is marked with two vertical lines, the distance between the lines representing the length of the implant. This distance is usually 18 to 22 mm, and the vertical dimension of the graft is generally 8 to 12 mm.

TECHNICAL HINTS

Once on the operating table, the patient is draped so that the entire face from the forehead to the submental region is exposed. I do all rhinoplasties with the patient under local anesthesia to observe normal function and to avoid distortion by the anesthetist's paraphernalia. The same procedure applies to chin and upper lip surgery. With proper premedication and local infiltration anesthesia, the operation is painless, the patient is comfortable, and the field is dry.

When the nose is being straightened, the nasal hump is removed in one piece, since it is to be used as a graft. This is best accomplished by Joseph's saw technique. After the bony part of the hump is sawed through, resection of the cartilaginous part is completed using Joseph's button-end knife. The specimen is placed in a nonalcoholic antiseptic solution, such as hexylresorcinol (S.T. 37). After the bony work is done and the tip remodeled, the nose is shortened by resection from the lower border of the septum according to the preoperative plan.

To raise the tip of the nose, a triangular piece is resected with the base directed forward. The crowded upper lip is corrected by resecting a quadrangular piece from the cartilage and including part of or the entire inferior nasal spine, again according to Joseph.

When the crowding is combined with a shallow upper lip, I resect a quadrangular piece from the cartilage only and posteriorly leave a steplike cartilaginous prominence in front of the inferior nasal spine (Fig. 11-12). This advanced spine provides support for the elongated upper lip. Retrolabial grafts can be added if necessary. All the superfluous mucous membrane corresponding with the cartilage resection must be removed. To avoid scarry stenosis at the base of the vestibulum, I leave a small, posteriorly based V-Y flap on the side of the septum.

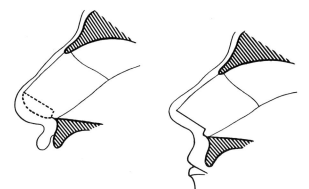

Fig. 11-12. Quadrangular resection from lower border of septal cartilage. Note steplike prominence in front of inferior nasal spine. (From Aufricht, G.: Plast. Reconstr. Surg. **43:**219, 1969.)

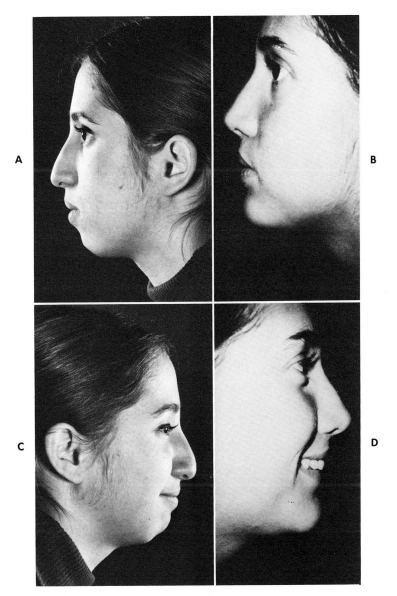

Fig. 11-13. Tri-feature aesthetic syndrome. **A** and **C,** Patient before correction. **B** and **D,** After correction. This combination of contours involves nose, upper lip, and chin.

If septal resection is required, it is performed after the rhinoplasty, including shortening the nose. (An exception is that the alar base excision is left until after the columella is resutured to the septum.) Thus the extent of septal window resection can be adjusted to the new proportions of the nose. The submucous resection can be done under direct overhead surgical light. The exposure is more than adequate, since the mobilized bony sides can be expanded, permitting a good view of the depth of the nasal cavity. The mucoperichondrial flap is raised at the freed lower border of

the septum. From here on, the resection proceeds in the usual manner.

For chin augmentation, gloves are changed after rhinoplasty, and a new set of instruments is used. The osteocartilaginous hump and other specimens are prepared on a wooden board. The mucous membrane is carefully removed from the inside of the hump. The sharp bone end is rounded, and the cartilaginous end is trimmed to proper length (usually 20 to 22 mm). The septal cartilage is cut into pieces of the same length and 6 to 7 mm wide. The vomer and all other skeletal

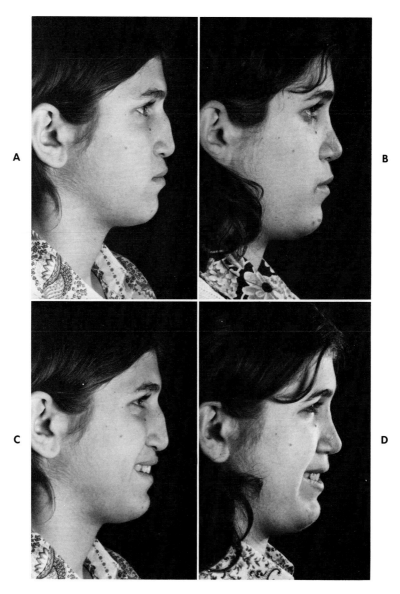

Fig. 11-14. Congenital absence of inferior nasal spine and a short columella (parakeet nose) before and after correction. This syndrome involves nose, upper lip, and chin. **A** and **C,** Before correction. **B** and **D,** After correction.

tissues may be used. The chin is injected with 1% procaine (Novocain) (usually at the time of the septal injection).

A 7 to 10 mm incision is made in the submental fold. A pocket is then prepared directly at the bone but not subperiosteally. It can be extended laterally using chin elevators. The pocket should be symmetric and just large enough to accommodate the graft. I try to place the bones closest to the mandible, but this is not important in this case. The incision is closed with a few sutures. There is no other fixation except the nest of gauze and adhesive dressing built around the chin.

If there is not sufficient live material available from the nose, I use Dow's Silastic silicone rubber implant. I make several perforations in the rubber block with a puncher. Eventually fibrous bands grow through these channels and firmly fix the implant to the bone. The implant is prepared in the operating room (while the local anesthetic takes effect). It takes only a few minutes and is carved according to the individual's need.

The implant is usually 20 to 22 mm long, 10 to 12 mm wide, and 5 to 10 mm thick. It should not extend to the side of or below the mandible; if it does, the patient may become overly conscious of its presence.

Due to repetition, certain stereotypes evolve in the plastic surgeon's mind during the process of studying facial configurations, especially in situations where the nose, chin, and upper lip are all involved. A common type is characterized by a hump nose, receding chin, and a disproportionate configuration of the upper lip. This could be called the *tri-feature aesthetic syndrome* (Fig. 11-13). The person often keeps his mouth open because forcing closure causes the chin to become even flatter. It sometimes lends an involuntary, disagreeable expression to the face. Correction in these cases often produces marked, favorable behavioral changes.

There is another typical deformity that deserves mention: congenital absence of the inferior nasal spine. This actually borders on defective or incomplete development and occasionally is caused by trauma or infection during early childhood. The condition is characterized by a short columella and therefore insufficient prominence of the tip of the nose; it can be said to resemble a parakeet's nose (Fig. 11-14). It is often also combined with and exaggerated by a receding chin. The labiocolumellar angle is acute, the nostrils practically facing the upper lip. Correction of this deformity requires use of a combination of surgical methods: bone work, radical advancement of the tip of the nose, and massive retrolabial graft. A detailed discussion of these techniques is not within the scope of this presentation, the purpose of which is to call attention to the often combined imperfections of the nose, upper lip, and chin and to the possibilities for their simultaneous surgical correction.

Patients often say that they want only a "little" change; they "want their friends to recognize them" or, more often, "not to know they have been operated on." In my experience, however, there is no purpose in performing partially corrective surgery when a maximum of improvement is possible. The surgeon's aim should be total harmony and balance of features. He should not leave imperfections that could have been safely corrected. I find that even with extreme alterations (including simultaneous correction of the nose, chin, and upper lip), if the face is well balanced and attractive, and even if it seems strange at first, the patient quickly becomes accustomed to the improved appearance and happily accepts all compliments.

SUMMARY

The purpose of rhinoplasty is not only to correct the objectionable contours and proportions of the nose but to improve the harmony and appearance of the entire face. For this effect, auxiliary correction of the chin, the upper lip, or both is often necessary and is advocated. Attention is called to an almost typical facial configuration, which may be called the tri-feature aesthetic syndrome.

Discussion

Musgrave: Is there some discussion from the audience or questions for Dr. Aufricht? Yes?

Participant: I wonder if Dr. Aufricht would consider putting a batten cartilage into the feet of the medial crura to lengthen the columella?

Aufricht: I mentioned somewhere that I don't use struts. Any strut would make the columella wide. But I have done it. Perhaps in an extreme case you might.

Participant: I would like to ask Dr. Aufricht if stripping the origin of the orbicularis oris or depressor septal muscle from the nasal spine when he plants that cartilage batten next to the bone might be part of the cause of lengthening the upper lip? When that patient smiled, it pulled the tip of her nose down, and I wonder if just stripping that muscle alone will help that?

Aufricht: I doubt it. Very often, with a thick columella, especially when the base of the columella is thick, I remove that muscle with some other soft tissue. It is not a frequent procedure, but I do it. You will find an extremely wide columella, and it interferes with the breathing also. Cosmetically if I want to narrow the alar base, I often remove those muscles and soft tissue, and I don't notice lengthening of the lip.

Participant: Could you amplify your discussion of what happens 30 years later to a nose that has been operated on? Does the alar cartilage continue to enlarge and the membranous septum stretch?

Aufricht: I have quite a number of patients whom I really should publish as they appear now 30, 35, or 40 years after surgery. I find their noses changed very little. There are some, who were 17 or 18 years old when I operated on them, who got married, pregnant, and had a few children. On these there might be some changes, as on other parts of the face and hands during pregnancy, especially broadening. However, the general contours are the same.

Chapter 12

Open-flap rhinoplasty

Rex A. Peterson, M.D.

Dieffenbach used external incisions in aesthetic rhinoplasty, and so did Jacques Joseph in his early years of rhinoplastic surgery (Chapter 4). Open-flap rhinoplasty is not, however, a rhinoplasty by an external incision, but rhinoplasty by intranasal techniques *plus* a flap lift of the nasal tip.

The primary indication for open-flap rhinoplasty is a long, hooked nose in an elderly person whose skin is loose and without turgor. The tip of the nose can be set at a satisfactory level and angle by lifting the tip on a soft tissue skin flap made by an upside-down, U-shaped incision in the thin skin just below the intercanthal level and extending downward in the nasofacial grooves (Fig. 12-1, A).

I have used the open-flap rhinoplasty regularly in specifically indicated cases for more than 10 years with good results except for one elderly man with a cleft lip nasal deformity. (The complication in this case was caused by lifting the nasal tip too high by an excessive excision of the upper edge of the flap.) It has also been used in correction of the postrhinoplasty dropped tip caused by excessive lowering of the dorsal edge of the quadrilateral cartilage at its caudal angle and to lift fallen nasal tips after overzealous submucous septal resection.

SALIENT POINTS IN OPEN-FLAP RHINOPLASTY

1. A rhinoplastic nasal reduction is accomplished according to the technique of the surgeon's choice.

2. The dorsal line of the quadrilateral cartilage must be reduced sufficiently because the lifting effect of the flap tends to elevate the tip and supratip skin (Fig. 12-1, D).

3. Thick, sebaceous skin is a contraindication, since a convexity of the supratip profile will probably result in patients having this type of skin.

4. At the conclusion of the intranasal reduction, the open-flap incision is marked and incised to include all the soft tissues between bone or cartilage and the skin surface. After reaching the bony level of the nose superiorly, the flap is elevated inferiorly by blunt dissection to join with the intranasal incisions (Fig. 12-2).

5. Approximately 6 mm of the superior edge of the flap and 2 to 3 mm of the lateral edges are excised. This is sufficient (Fig. 12-2).

6. A two-layer 6-0 clear and 6-0 black monofilament nylon repair of the skin is completed.

7. The nasal vestibule is inspected, and redundant mucosal lining, if any, at the intercartilaginous or intracartilaginous incision is excised. The nasal incisions are then repaired.

8. Alar wedge excisions are almost always required to set the bases of the nares into good position. These are accomplished by whatever pattern befits the situation (Fig. 12-1, B and C).

9. The nose is immobilized carefully with a nasal splint metallic or plaster of Paris placed over a Telfa dressing covering the suture lines.

The open-flap rhinoplasty has been satisfactorily used primarily in older patients. Many of these people have wanted a rhinoplasty all their lives but could not have one for some reason.

A more youthful appearance is always gained by shortening the nose, as the image of a long nose, in which the tip almost touches the upper lip, is connected with advanced age. Thus rhinoplasty, or open-flap rhinoplasty, if indicated, is an important adjunct to rhytidoplasty and blepharoplasty in creating a more youthful image.

In no case has any patient so treated been dissatisfied with the more youthful appearance of the newly lifted nose. Typical results obtained with the open-flap rhinoplasty are illustrated in Figs. 12-4 to 12-8.

Text continued on p. 98.

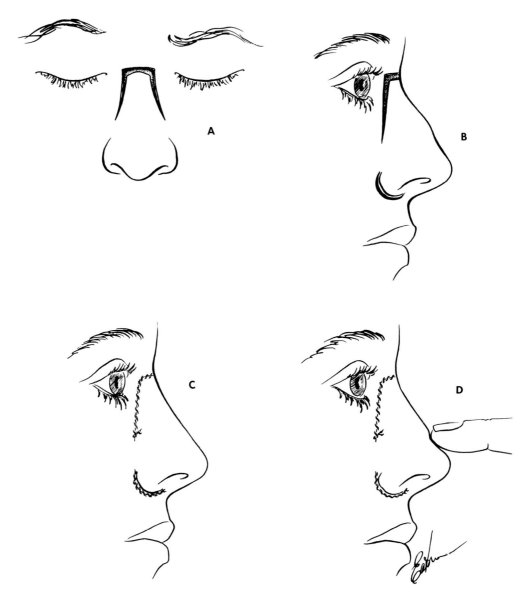

Fig. 12-1. Diagrams representing placement of skin incisions for open-flap rhinoplasty. **A** to **C,** Transverse limb of inverted-U incision is in thin skin at or just below canthal level. Elderly people may already have a transverse rhytid here, and postoperative scar is usually no more conspicuous than wrinkle. Eyeglasses frames also conceal it. Oblique limbs extend inferiorly where nasal planes meet cheeks for at least 2 cm. **B** and **C,** Alar wedges are almost always required to counteract forward thrust of nasal tip, which occurs as flap is lifted. **D,** Profile edge of quadrilateral cartilage must be reduced adequately to prevent supratip convexity. Lift of tip seems to increase this tendency.

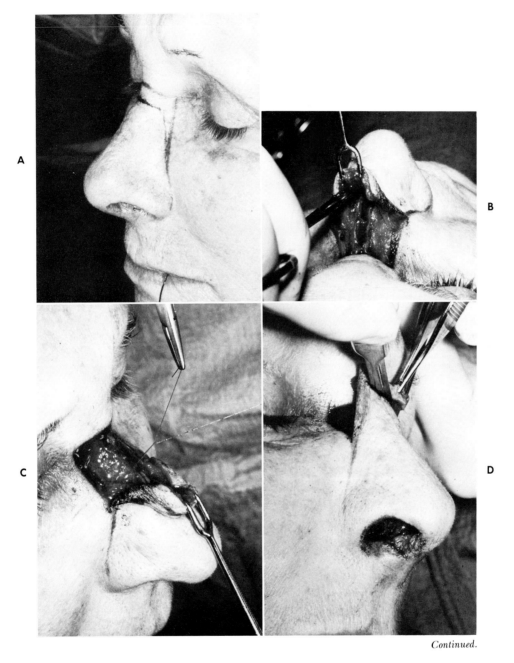

Continued.

Fig. 12-2. A, Incision marking. **B,** Flap elevated and dissected inferiorly at level of nasal bone to join intranasal incisions. **C,** Periosteum of nasal bones sutured together. **D,** About 6 mm of skin resected along superior transverse edge.

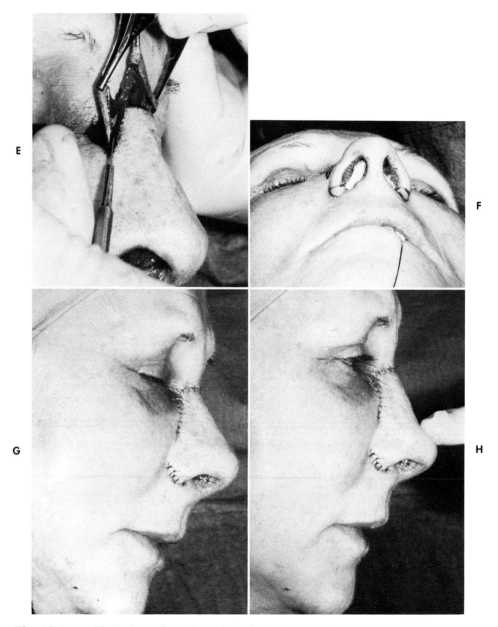

Fig. 12-2, cont'd. E, One of two lateral vertical triangles of skin is resected from flap. **F,** Alar wedges are almost always necessary to set nasal tip closer to face. **G,** Incisions are repaired. Note forward thrust of tip. **H,** Digital pressure reveals septum lowered to assist in preventing supratip convexity.

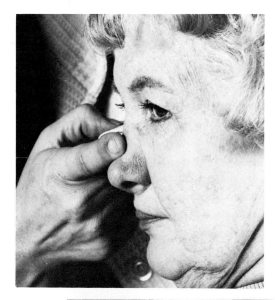

Fig. 12-3. Digital pressure applied to supratip midline skin several times daily helps prevent permanent supratip convexity.

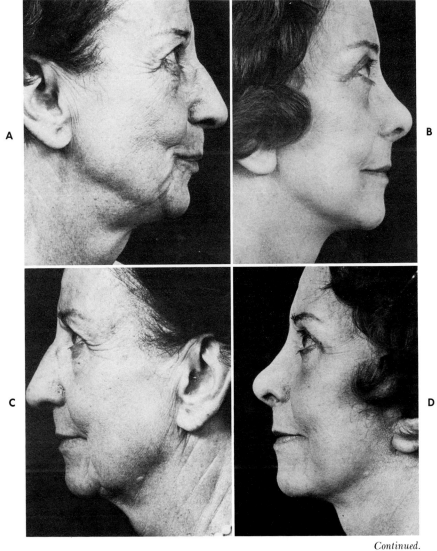

Continued.

Fig. 12-4. I. H., age 71. Patient had desired nasal reduction for many years. She was so pleased at more youthful appearance, she subsequently had a rhytidoplasty and blepharoplasty. Postoperative photographs were taken a year after surgery. **A, C, E,** and **G,** Before surgery. **B, D, F,** and **H,** After surgery.

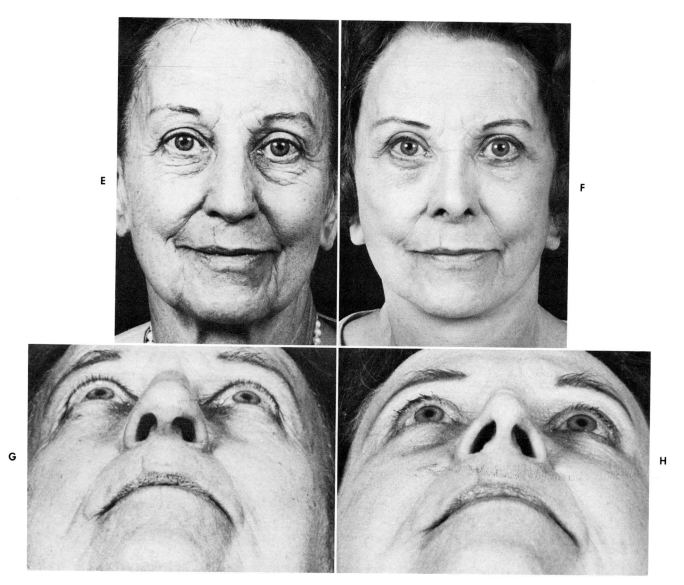

Fig. 12-4, cont'd. For legend see p. 87.

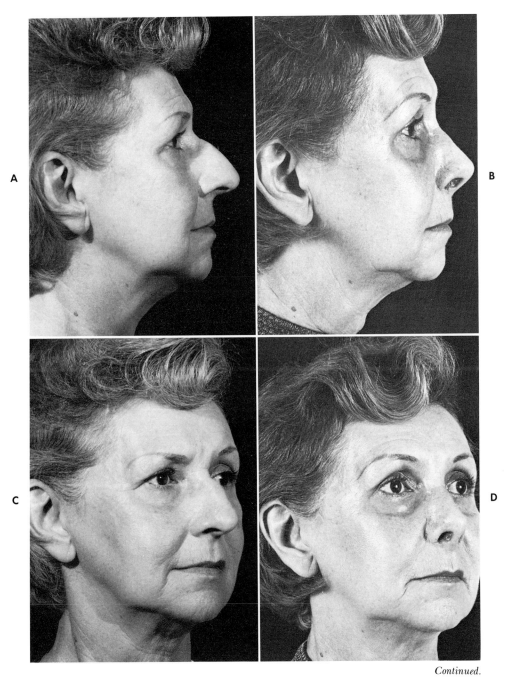

Continued.

Fig. 12-5. B. W., age 60. Large hook nose with inelastic skin. Additional bone and cartilage could have been removed from profile line. Operative photographs are shown in Fig. 12-2. Postoperative photographs were taken 3 months after surgery. Tip will drop later. **A, C, E,** and **G,** Before surgery. **B, D, F,** and **H,** After surgery.

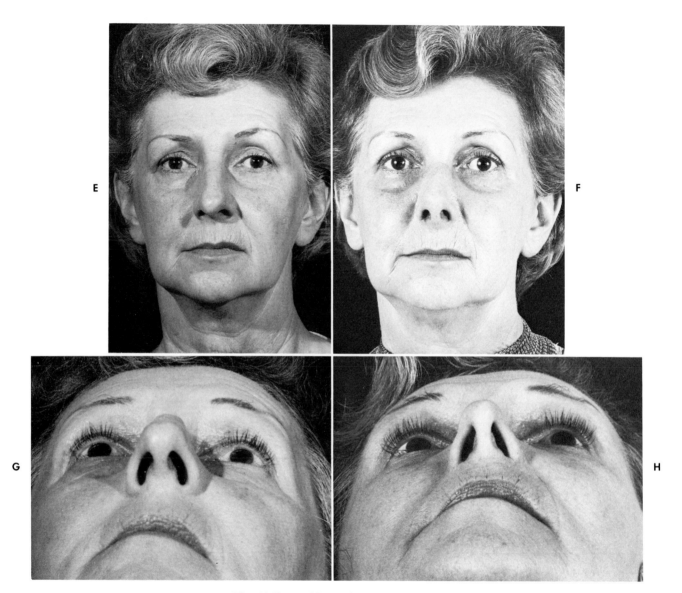

Fig. 12-5, cont'd. For legend see p. 89.

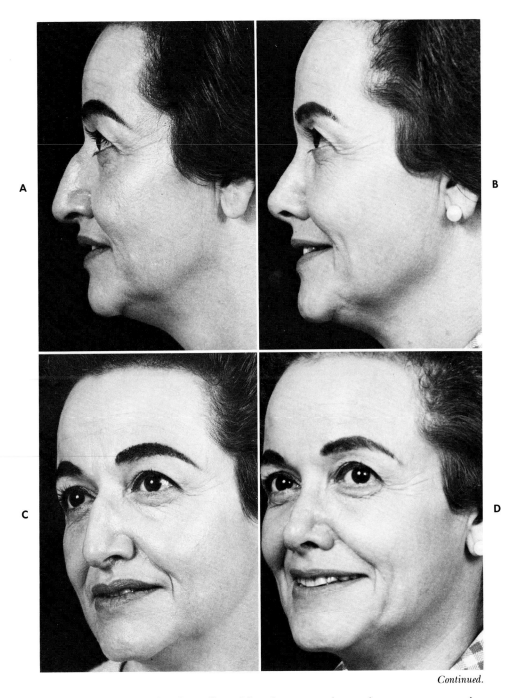

Continued.

Fig. 12-6. B. H., age 51. Open-flap rhinoplasty was chosen because nose was long and hooked, and skin was elastic. Extensive submucous septal resection of deviated quadrilateral cartilage, vomer, and vertical plate of ethmoid was accomplished at same operation. Postoperative photographs were taken a year after surgery. **A, C, E,** and **G,** Before surgery. **B, D, F,** and **H,** After surgery.

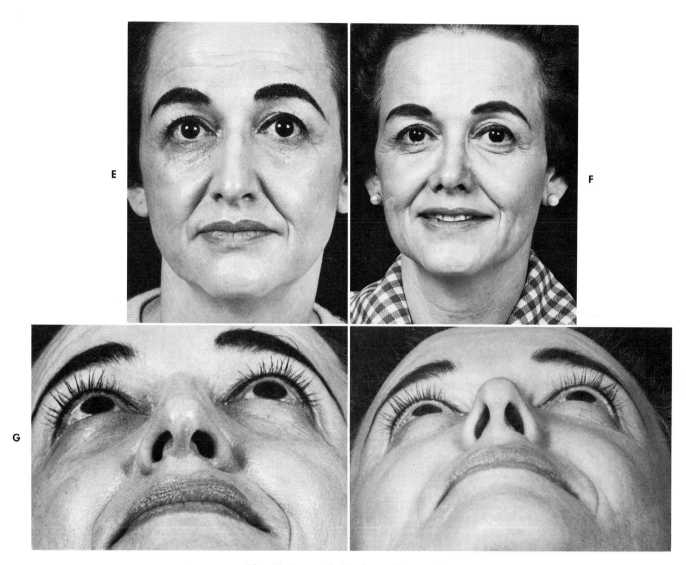

Fig. 12-6, cont'd. For legend see p. 91.

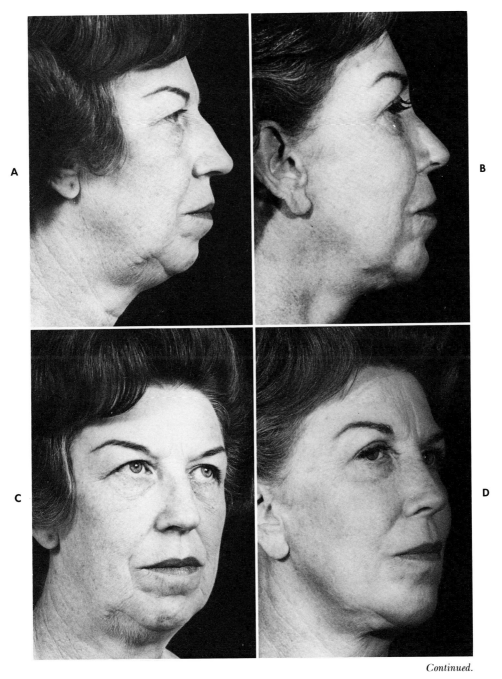

Continued.

Fig. 12-7. D. C., age 51. Open-flap rhinoplasty. Transverse incision line became infected and required revision. Subsequent rhytidoplasty, blepharoplasties, submental lipectomies, and chin implant were performed. Postoperative photographs were taken 16 months after surgery. **A, C, E,** and **G,** Before surgery. **B, D, F,** and **H,** After surgery.

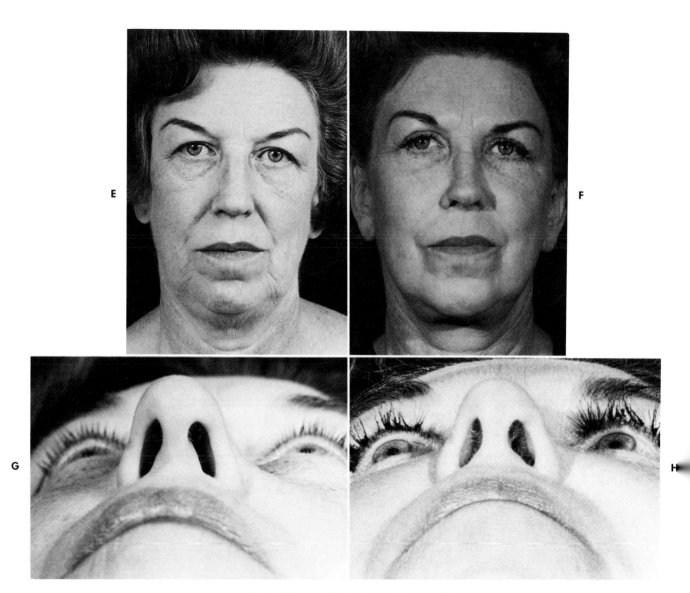

Fig. 12-7, cont'd. For legend see p. 93.

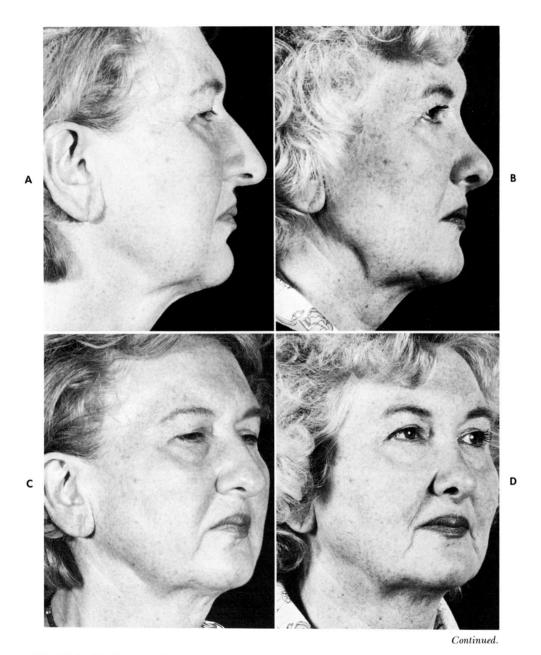

Continued.

Fig. 12-8. M. H., age 57. Open-flap rhinoplasty. Note tendency to supratip convexity associated here with upward projection of tip. This is same patient illustrated to have adequate resection of profile edge of quadrilateral cartilage in Fig. 12-3. Postoperative photographs were taken a year after surgery. **A, C, E,** and **G,** Before surgery. **B, D, F,** and **H,** After surgery.

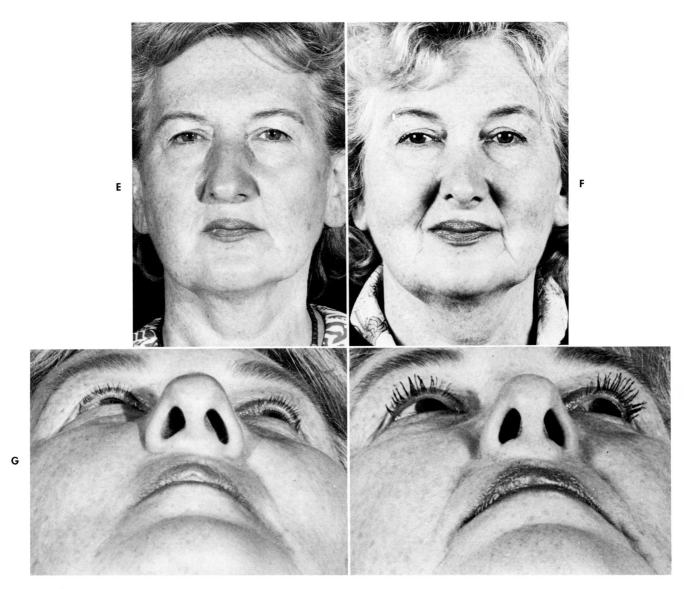

Fig. 12-8, cont'd. For legend see p. 95.

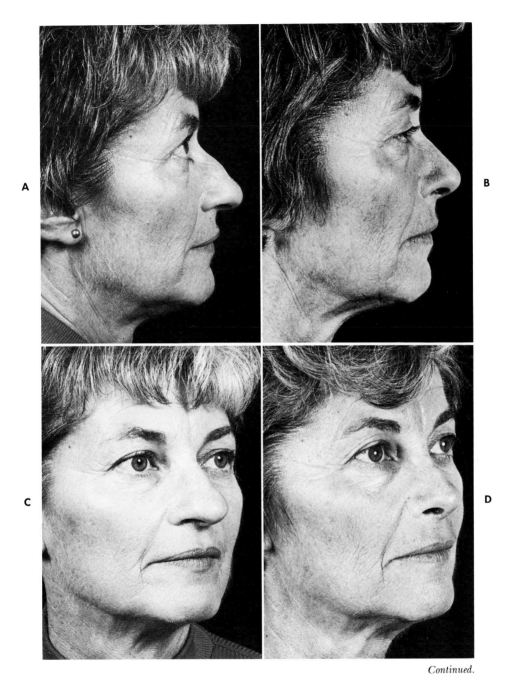

Continued.

Fig. 12-9. D. B., age 51. Large nose in all proportions. Open-flap rhinoplasty was performed. Postoperative photographs were taken 3 years after surgery. **A, C, E,** and **G,** Before surgery. **B, D, F,** and **H,** After surgery.

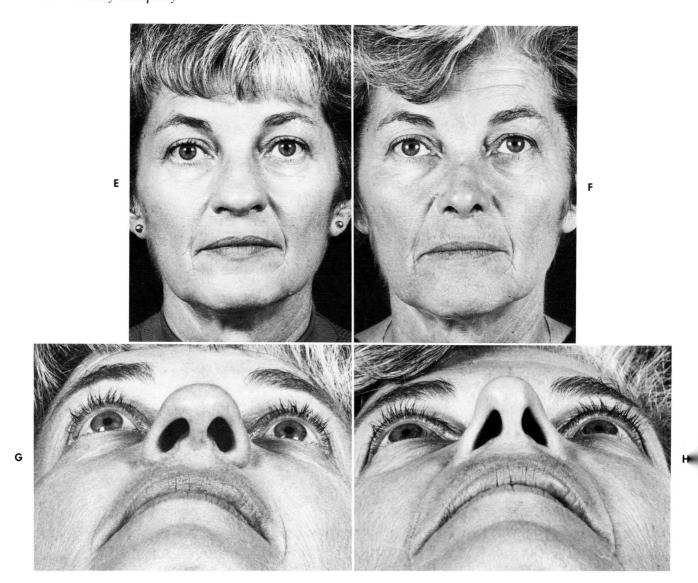

Fig. 12-9, cont'd. For legend see p. 97.

SUMMARY

Open-flap rhinoplasty (rhinoplasty plus flap lift of the nasal tip) is indicated when rhinoplasty is desired by an elderly patient with a long hooked nose, where the skin is loose and inelastic to a degree that the nose cannot be shortened by rhinoplasty alone. The flap lift of the tip produces an upward and forward thrust, which increases the tendency to supratip convexity in long noses (Fig. 12-3), but the aesthetic results are nevertheless worthwhile. It may also be helpful for certain postrhinoplasty or postseptoplasty deformities in which the nasal tip has fallen.

Discussion

Musgrave: Are there questions to be directed to Dr. Peterson?

Millard: Ross, I've been over here afraid I might have to put a straitjacket on Dr. Safian. This presentation tends to stray from the conservative, and Dr. Safian feels pretty strongly about this. Shall I call on him?

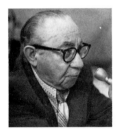

Dr. Safian

Peterson: Please don't!

Musgrave: Questions out there, somebody?

Participant: Dr. Peterson, if you're really worried about excessive skin in the older rhinoplasty, why not combine the routine rhinoplasty with the forehead lift rather than the flap?

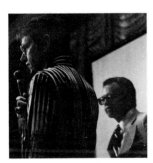

Dr. Peterson and Dr. Millard

Peterson: Well, I also happen to be an advocate of brow lifts, and I have considered extending brow lifts right across at the brow margin. I have done forehead lifts at the scalp margin. I have never done a coronal lift. I have seen the brow on coronal lifts, and they look like a high arched surprised look to me, and sometimes they are not necessarily symmetrical. Therefore to me this is less of a procedure even though it looks extremely radical in these operative photos. These patients do not have any great problem after this open-flap procedure. They are grateful, the scar is minimal, and we frequently operate on this very area for basal cell carcinoma. You get a fine scar, and, even at my elderly age, I have a transverse crease exactly where that scar is. Also, almost all these people wear glasses.

Musgrave: Spectacles would hide that scar. Blair, did you have something?

Rogers: Rex, I just want to know why you believe you have to go through such an extensive operation to accomplish what I think many of us accomplish in people in this age group through a routine rhinoplasty?

Peterson: As I said, the only indication in this age, Blair, is the very large hooked nose with very loose skin. The other patients I use it for are pinched noses, for people who have dropped tips that touch the upper lip combining it with a Dingman type of intranasal composite graft of the ear as a reconstructive sequence. I got into it on a reconstructive case and it worked for that, and I decided to extend it to the other type. Now, I don't necessarily advocate this, but I thought it an interesting procedure to see the inside of the nose on a living person!

Musgrave: You did!

Peterson: As I said, I've done it about twenty-seven times in 7 years.

Participant: Were there any bad emotional changes to such a radical change in the patient's features?

Peterson: No. As a matter of fact, this patient who was shown in the operative series has not had a face lift, which would make her look extremely youthful if I combined the two. She wanted the nose operated on, and she wanted it up. The emotional responses are all very good.

Weybright: I have a similar number of these, and I started doing them to help in the thinning of the primary rhinoplasty. In defense of myself, I must say not all cases were mine. Some were from you all. I was able to take up three quarters of the skin on the upper portion of the dorsum of the nose without dropping the incision vertically down the face. The excess skin falls rather well in the inner canthal area.

Peterson: That's true. A simple elliptical excision may do just as well as the pattern that I've shown here.

Musgrave: You certainly see that in basal cells in this area where you get a real nice result. Ralph?

Millard: Rex, the shortest exit is right over there to the left behind that screen. I say this because there are still so many questions waiting, and we don't want to wear you out, yet!

Chapter 13

Simplifying the corrective rhinoplasty

John R. Lewis, Jr., M.D.

The three fundamental principles for simplifying most surgical procedures (this particularly applies to the corrective rhinoplasty) are the following:

1. Proper evaluation of the problem
2. Proper planning for the correction (this is almost automatic for the experienced surgeon if the evaluation has been properly made)
3. An orderly procedure or group of procedures for carrying out the surgical correction

Proper evaluation of the nose consists of, first, consideration of the appearance of the nose as a whole as it sits on the particular face involved. This means the surgeon should evaluate the nose in proportion to the other features and particularly in proportion to the forehead, lips, and chin, both in the front and in both profile views. The full-face examination also involves the observation of the width of the nasal bridge, base, and tip along with the relative proportions of forehead, nose, lips, and chin. A long nose does not fit properly on a short face, nor does a wide nose suit a narrow or slender face. Wide alae obviously do not fit the narrow face or the patient with a small mouth and narrow eyes, and a wide nasal bridge and base further accentuate close-set eyes. Narrowing of the nasal base and bridge tend to give the illusion of wider eyes.

This brief oversimplification touches on most of the principles involved in evaluation of the nose as a whole, but the size and the height of the patient also play a part in the evaluation and determination of what changes will be most appropriate.

EVALUATION AND PLANNING

Proper evaluation and planning involve a judgment of the patient and the patient's desires. One should always know exactly what the patient wishes to achieve for the nose and for the appearance in general by the surgery anticipated. If the patient wishes something that cannot be achieved or that would not be appropriate for the other features, then it is best that the surgeon know this beforehand. If the surgeon believes he can achieve a desirable result for the particular patient, he should attempt to give the patient what he or she desires so long as it is consistent with his own judgment of an appropriate correction. Minor variations often mean the difference between a happy patient and a dissatisfied one, so it is most important that the surgeon know the desires of the patient.

I have found that a measuring instrument such as the Straith profilometer (Fig. 13-1) can be of great help in demonstrating the changes desired to the patient and in actually achieving these changes in the operating room. Certainly the surgeon can benefit from such a guide, or else he should have photographs of the patient in the operating room.

Proper planning and the achievement of the desired nose involve a decision as to what portions of the nose are to be corrected and to what degree. It is well to have an orderly arrangement of recorded thoughts in regard to any surgical procedure. The simplest method for me has been to list the stages generally involved in the corrective rhinoplasty and to specify these steps with a "slight," "moderate," or "marked" change in that particular step. I use step 1 to indicate the lowering and contouring of the nasal bridge (Fig. 13-3); step 2 indicates the tilt-up or shortening in the end of the nose, including the septum and sidewalls (Fig. 13-4); step 3 is the narrowing or adjusting of the nasal tip with or without raising or lowering of the tip on the end of the septum (Fig. 13-4, *B*); step 4 is the freeing of the nasal bones from the

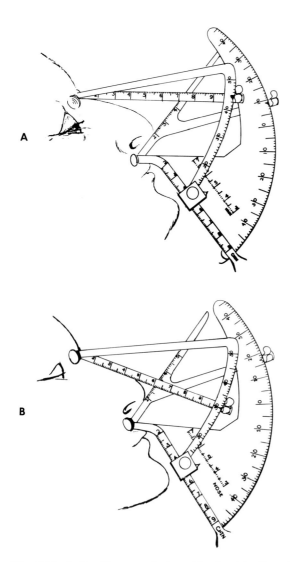

Fig. 13-1. A, Profilometer designed by Straith allows for measuring of nasal bridge angle, tip angle, length of base of nose from glabella to base of columella, relative lengths of nose, and nose-to-point-of-chin distance. Measurement in this nose shows angle of 45 degrees in bridge and about 9 degrees at tip, and length at about 5.2. **B,** Setting of profilometer to aid in determining amount of tissue to be removed in rhinoplasty shows bridge setting at 30 degrees, which is about right for male or female nose, leaving male nose with full bridge and female nose with slight swoop to bridge. Setting of tip angle is 17 degrees, which is what I usually use for female nose. Length setting is now at 5 cm, which is right for petite girl. For male nose, length should be in cm approximately that of patient's height in feet and inches, that is, 6 ft male should have nose about 6 cm long, allowing of course for measurements of face. A long face should have a longer nose than a short face. Note also Figs. 18-1 and 18-2. (From Lewis, J. R.: Atlas of aesthetic plastic surgery, Boston, 1974, Little, Brown & Co.)

septum and from the frontal process at the nasal root (Fig. 13-5, *A*); step 5 is the separation of the nasal bones from the maxillae bilaterally, with repositioning of the nasal bones and narrowing of the base and bridge in most instances (Fig. 13-5, *A* and *B*). Step 6 usually is the submucous resection and/or reconstruction of the septum with or without a cartilage or bone graft to the columella and/or anterior maxillary spine. Step 7 allows for any additional special steps such as the Z-plasty inside one ala, a small rotation flap in an ala base or, most commonly, the bilateral ala base resection. The orderly planning of these various steps along with the appropriate documentation of the patient's nose and of the face from the front, side, inferior, and oblique aspects, as indicated, facilitate carrying out the operative procedure when that time arrives.

The orderly procession of steps in the corrective rhinoplasty has been considered in the planning stage, during the first consultation, subsequent consultations, or both, and is further solidified in the surgeon's mind when he rechecks a nose on the admission day or on the morning of surgery. This also gives the surgeon a chance to reevaluate the patient's desires in regard to the type of nose and the changes desired. Then a procession of the surgical steps, repeated regularly and orderly, allows the surgeon to proceed almost automatically from one step to the next.

One may be deceptive in calling anything automatic or semiautomatic because each nose is different, and the steps for any one single nose vary from the steps of surgery on a preceding case or a subsequent one. This keeps rhinoplastic surgery from becoming monotonous, since each nose is different in enough details to make each one a separate and distinct problem, and this ordinarily keeps up the surgeon's interest in this most artistic of all operative procedures. When one follows the principles of adequate examination with an adequate consultation with the patient, adequate planning, and an orderly procession of steps in the correction, one is most likely to achieve a reasonably happy result.

SURGICAL PROCEDURE

The steps of surgery are as follows:
1. Incision or incisions (Fig. 13-2, *A*)
   Undermining (Fig. 13-2, *B* and *C*)
   Freeing of special attachments (columella from end of septum) (Fig. 13-2, *D* and *E*)
   Correction of nasal bridge (osteotomy with dorsal removal of bone from nose) (Fig. 13-3, *A* to *E*)

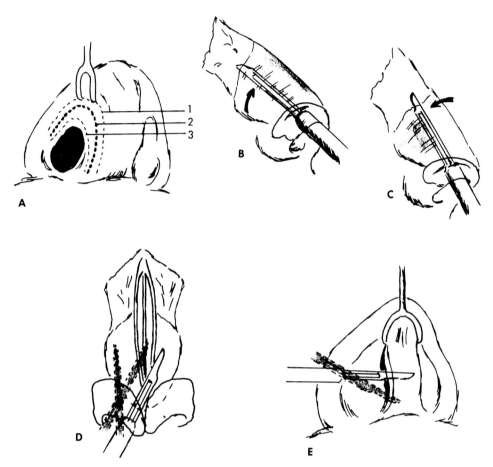

Fig. 13-2. A, Incisions may be made as, *1,* marginal or rim incision, *2,* transcartilaginous incision, or, *3,* intercartilaginous incision. **B,** Undermining is carried out in subcutaneous plane with knife beveled slightly toward upper lateral cartilage and toward nasal bone. It is carried upward over nasal bridge where undermining is met from other side. **C,** Undermining is carried toward cheek by reversing knife blade, still keeping it beveled slightly toward nasal bone and upper lateral cartilage to avoid any danger of penetrating skin. Undermining toward cheek is carried only so far toward cheek as is required for adjustment of nasal skin and must be carried wider for large bony hump, or somewhat wider in the older patient, to allow for shrinking. It is left attached to upper lateral cartilage and nasal bone at base to help accomplish stability of structures after base osteotomy in later stage of procedure. **D,** Undermining is carried across top of nasal bridge. **E,** Blade is carried to membranous septum separating columella from end of septum. (From Lewis, J. R.: Atlas of aesthetic plastic surgery, Boston, 1974, Little, Brown & Co.)

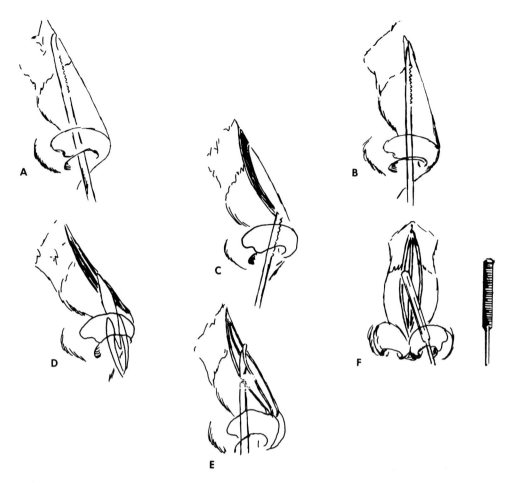

Fig. 13-3. A, Nasal bony hump and dorsum are lowered with nasal saw. Chisel may also be used for this stage. **B,** Nasal saw continues on through nasal bone. **C,** Saw continues, usually cutting through nasal bone, and then knife is inserted to sever remainder of upper lateral cartilage and to sever septum in central area, but nasal saw may be carried to remove whole hump as is done here. **D,** Hump is removed with forceps. **E,** Rasping of sides of nasal bones to smooth off sharp edges and to lower nasal bones slightly below level of septum in midline. **F,** Trimming of dorsum of septum to contour nasal bridge. (From Lewis, J. R.: Atlas of aesthetic plastic surgery, Boston, 1974, Little, Brown & Co.)

Trim top of septum (Fig. 13-3, *F*)
Trim top of upper lateral cartilages (Fig. 13-4, *A*)
2. Tilt-up of nose (Fig. 13-4, *D* and *E*)
Trim excess (lower areas of upper lateral cartilages, shortening of upper lateral cartilages, shortening of end of septum with rounding of tip)
3. Correction of alar cartilages in tip (Figs. 13-4, *B* and *C*)
4. Dorsal osteotomy with separation of nasal bones from septum and frontal process (Fig. 13-5, *A*)
5. Lateral osteotomy, separating nasal bones from maxillae (Fig. 13-5, *A*)

Pressing nasal bones medially, with or without outfracture (Fig. 13-5, *B*)
6. Submucous resection of septum with straightening of septum
Reduction of lower turbinates as needed
7. Alar base resection, as indicated, and repair
8. Suture of incisions; reapproximate upper and lower lateral cartilages and columella to end of septum
9. Packs and splinting
I usually make the incision in a transcartilaginous fashion (Fig. 13-2, *A*), penetrating the lower lateral cartilage between its midpoint and its junction with the upper lateral cartilage. The un-

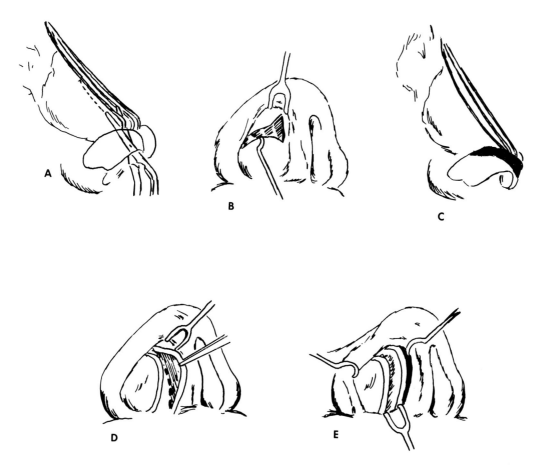

Fig. 13-4. A, Trim of nasal septum in lower portion accomplishes beveling of end of septum and rounding of tip to avoid prominence in supratip area as healing and settling of tip occur. Then upper lateral cartilages are lowered slightly below level of septum and are beveled at tip, as is done with tip of septum. **B,** Trim of lower lateral cartilage is varied depending on need. However, usually a triangle of cartilage is resected adjacent to midline, and second cartilage based toward first triangle goes along upper edge of lower lateral cartilage as seen in **C. C,** Long ellipse composed of two triangles as described in **B** accomplishes narrowing of tip and some degree of lowering of tip. **D,** Trim of lower end of septum and similar trim of upper lateral cartilages accomplishes shortening of nose. **E,** End of septum is left long enough that columella will be more prominent than lower margin of alae. End of septum is rounded and is not trimmed in straight fashion. (From Lewis, J. R.: Atlas of aesthetic plastic surgery, Boston, 1974, Little, Brown & Co.)

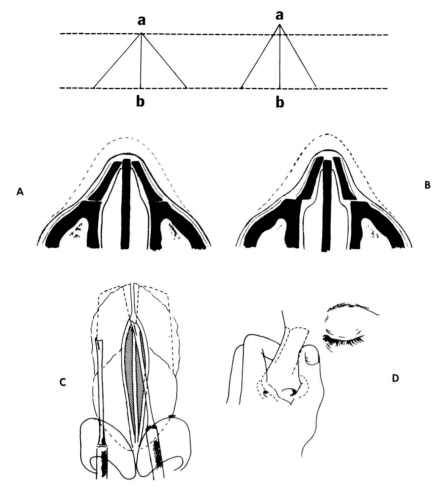

Fig. 13-5. A, Use of saw or chisel to accomplish dorsal osteotomy separates nasal bones from septum and from each other in midline and if followed by base osteotomy separating nasal bones from maxillae. Nasal bones have usually been lowered slightly below level of septum at this point, and upper lateral cartilages also have been lowered slightly below septal level. **B,** Narrowing of nasal base and bridge by moving nasal bones together is like moving base of two tent poles together, which raises top of tent (see insert *A* and *B*). Nasal bones have now been raised up to level of septum or a little above in this instance. This then requires trim of top of upper lateral cartilages and rasping or trim with osteotome of dorsal edge of nasal bones to keep from having flat-top appearance to bridge of nose. Nasal bones and upper lateral cartilages are again lowered slightly below level of septum to allow rounded bridge in cross-section view. If skin is freed completely from nasal bone exteriorly and if mucosa is cut through in base osteotomy, it is natural for nasal bones to slip inward and fall internally inside base of nasal bones and maxillae, lowering nasal bone height on each side. This is undesirable, since it is difficult to control, and, further, it decreases blood supply to nasal bones by separating skin and subcutaneous tissue more widely than required and cutting through mucosa more than necessary. It is much more desirable to leave skin intact and attached to nasal bones laterally, undermining no more than is required to shrink and adapt itself on nasal bridge after removal of dorsal hump. It is undesirable to cut through mucosa, and it is much better to preserve it intact. This can usually be checked easily by inspection in nose after lateral or base osteotomy. **C,** Chisel or saw is carried along base of nasal bones, freeing nasal bones from maxillae bilaterally, and chisel is carried along adjacent to septum, separating nasal bones from each other and from septum in midline dorsally. This allows nasal bones to be mobilized for narrowing, straightening, and repositioning as it requires. A 4 mm or 3 mm chisel may be pushed in without incision, making its own incision, or through a narrow incision with little or no undermining of tissues and causes minimal trauma in osteotomy. **D,** Nasal bones are simply pressed together at base after dorsal and lateral osteotomies, narrowing bridge and base of nasal bones. (From Lewis, J. R.: Atlas of aesthetic plastic surgery, Boston, 1974, Little, Brown & Co.)

dermining is carried out in a subcutaneous plane, and no particular effort is made to raise the periosteum from the nasal bones (Fig. 13-2, *B* and *C*). Freeing of special attachments includes freeing the columella from the septum by penetrating the membranous septum (Fig. 13-2, *E*). This allows for removal of the bony hump (Fig. 13-3, *A* to *E*), trimming of the dorsum of the septum (Fig. 13-3, *F*), and shortening of the end of the septum (Fig. 13-4), as well as beveling the lower portion of the septal bridge.

The correction of the deeper tissues includes the osteotomy with removal of the excess bone of the nasal bridge and rasping the top of the nasal bones (Figs. 13-3 and 13-4), followed by trimming the dorsum of the septum and dorsum of the upper lateral cartilages. Repositioning of the framework includes the separation of the nasal bones from the septum on each side in the bridge, using a saw or chisel (dorsal osteotomy), freeing the nasal bones from the maxillae bilaterally, using either a saw or chisel (lateral or base osteotomy),

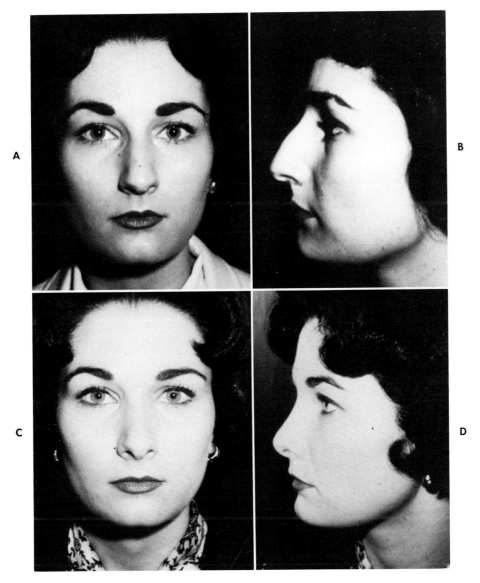

Fig. 13-6. A, Preoperative appearance of somewhat long nose, showing wide nasal bridge, base, and tip. **B,** Tip of nose is pulling upper lip at base of columella upward. **C** and **D,** Postoperative appearance showing narrowing in base, bridge, and tip, shortening of nose, and relaxation at base of columella as tip has been lowered. Effort by surgeon should be to give nose that seems natural for face and not exaggerated change.

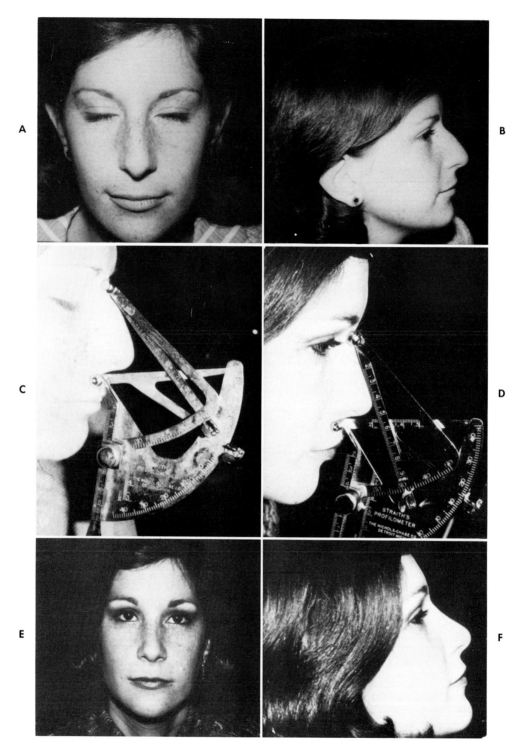

Fig. 13-7. A and **B,** Preoperative appearance showing nose with broad tip, base, and bridge, a nose that is too long and has prominent hump. **C,** Measurement with profilometer reveals bridge angle of about 45 degrees, tip angle of about 15 degrees, and length of about 6 cm. **D,** Postoperative measurement of nose showing bridge angle of 30 degrees, tip angle of about 16 degrees, and length of about 4.8 cm. For a short face this is a satisfactory measurement. **E** and **F,** Postoperative appearance of nose in front and side views.

A   B   C

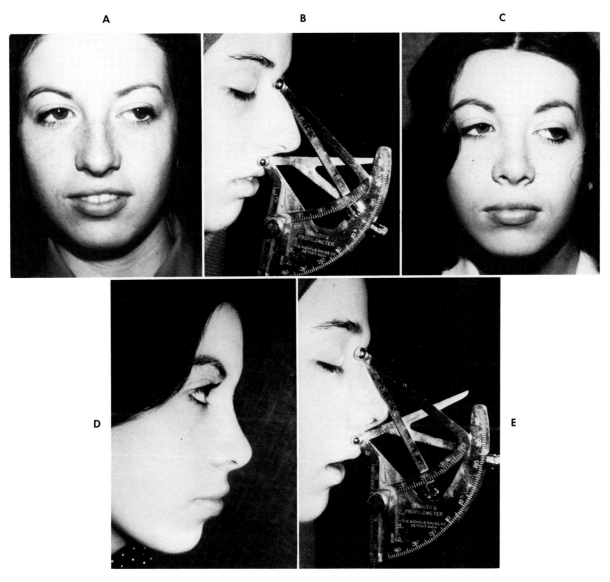

D   E

Fig. 13-8. A, Front view of nose before surgery, showing heavy look to bridge tip base. **B,** Measurement of nose with profilometer, indicating high bridge angle, high tip, and increased length of nose, which does not give adequate length to upper lip, particularly in profile view. **C,** Immediately at end of rhinoplasty showing exaggerated tilt-up of tip because of swelling at base of columella, with tip angle at this point of 24 degrees and slight swoop of bridge below straight line of bridge measurement. **D** and **E,** Postoperative view of nose, still with some swelling in bridge and tip. Note in postoperative profile view that tip is beginning to come down and does not have exaggerated tilt-up. However, for this patient we intended to have relatively nice tilt-up of about 17 or 18 degrees, and patient has about 19- or 20-degree angle in this view.

and then moving the nasal bones together to narrow the nasal base and bridge (Fig. 13-5). Trim of the excess includes trimming the dorsum of the septum and rasping of the nasal bones if there are high points (Figs. 13-3, *E* and *F*, and 13-4, *A*). It also includes a trim of the dorsum of the upper lateral cartilages to a level slightly below that of the septum in the midline (Figs. 13-3, *E* and *F*).

The upper lateral cartilages are often trimmed at their lower edges toward the lower lateral cartilages (Fig. 13-4, *D*), and usually the necessary amount of cartilage is excised without any trim of the mucosa.

Correction of the tip is usually done by the inversion technique, turning the tip cartilages downward into the nostrils and trimming from the

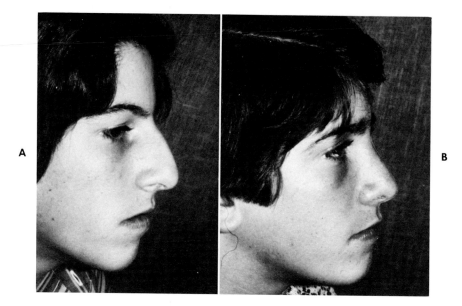

Fig. 13-9. A, Teen-age boy with high nasal bridge and increased length of base of nose. Note that nose comes almost off forehead with practically no glabellar notch. **B,** After rhinoplasty, showing shallow glabellar notch and relatively full nasal bridge. Nose has not been tilted up to the degree of female nose, and bridge has not been given swoop. This patient would have benefited from small augmentation to chin, but his family preferred to delay chin correction until later if needed.

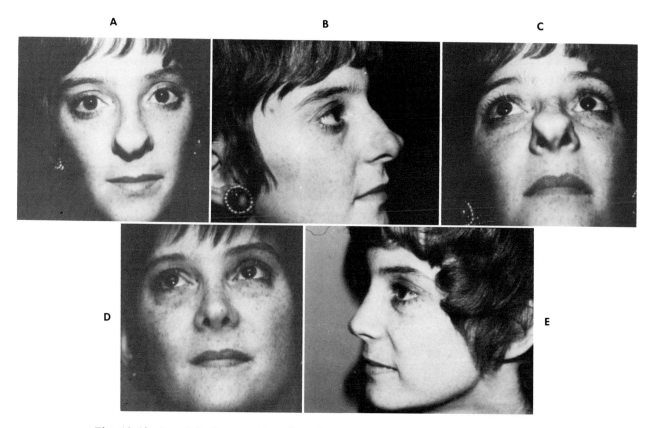

Fig. 13-10. A and **B,** Preoperative view of nose reveals that major corrections will be of nasal tip. Front view reveals somewhat wide nasal base and bridge about distorted wide asymmetric nasal tip and prominent long alae from cheek to tip. **C,** Underneath view reveals extreme width of alar cartilages and some increased width of alar base itself. **D** and **E,** Postoperative views showing correction in nasal bridge and base, alar base resection, and heavy reduction of alar cartilages.

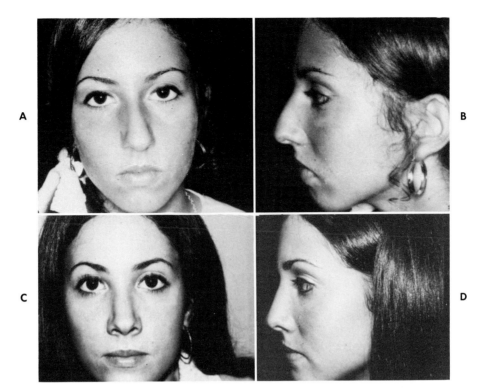

Fig. 13-11. A and **B,** Preoperative view revealing overly large nose for face of girl of medium height and medium facial features. Nose is heavy in base and tip, and side view reveals high nasal bridge with bony hump. Upper lip appears short, and chin is receding. Hypogenia should be corrected along with nose at same stage as preliminary to rhinoplasty. **C** and **D,** Postoperative view revealing nose that is consistent with other facial features. **D,** Chin has not been made overly large, and some undercorrection has been carried out to keep chin looking more normal. Chin is usually made a little more full in men than in women.

upper edge, taking a triangle adjacent to the midline and a narrower triangle based toward the first triangle and tapering sharply toward the alar base (Fig. 13-4, *B* and *C*). Little trim is carried out toward the base of the lower lateral cartilages. As a rule only cartilage is excised, leaving the mucosa intact. Repair by absorbable sutures is usually carried out, reapproximating the columella to the end of the septum, reapproximating upper and lower lateral cartilages, and fixating cartilage placed in the columella by a through-and-through penetrating suture if this is required. A suture of the mucosa at the point of septal resection may also be carried out.

The submucous resection of the septum is usually carried out by carefully elevating the mucosa on each side through an incision on only one side. An attempt is made not to penetrate the opposite mucosa and to remove only that cartilage and bone which are obstructing breathing or contributing to curvature of the bridge or tip. Often the septum can be straightened into the columella

when it deviates to the side without actual resection in the end portion. A substantially wide segment of septum is left dorsally for support and in the columella for tip support. The lower turbinates are frequently fractured laterally, flattened against the sidewall, and then injected with corticosteroid with or without sclerosing solution added. Packs are inserted to keep the sidewalls separated from the septum and to splint the septum, and these packs are not tight. A nasal splint is then applied, usually well padded with sponge rubber. Often sterile strips are applied to the skin to minimize the immediate postoperative edema, but it is advisable to look under the splint at 48 to 72 hours and to trim the tape strips away from the dorsum of the tip, particularly in patients who have acne.

Illustrative cases (Figs. 13-6 to 13-11) show the results obtained by these relatively straightforward steps of the corrective rhinoplasty. I have made notes of the special attention given to some areas of the corrections.

SUMMARY

The surgical steps are, basically, (1) lowering the bridge, (2) shortening the tip by shortening the end of the septum and shortening the lower end of the upper lateral cartilages, (3) narrowing of the tip, (4) separation of the nasal bones from the septum in the midline, (5) narrowing of the nasal base, (6) management of the septum, and (7) management of the alar bases.

A measuring instrument, such as the Straith profilometer, can be of aid in planning and in execution of the rhinoplasty. Photographs of the patient may be useful to refer to in the operating room.

The average rhinoplasty need not be complicated, but each step must be carried out meticulously and studiously so that the ultimate result will be a satisfactory blend of all the steps into one proportioned nose that appears natural and pleasing for that particular face.

REFERENCES

1. Aufricht, G.: Combined plastic surgery of nose and chin, Am. J. Surg. **95**:231, 1958.
2. Broadbent, T. R.: Anatomy of a rhinoplasty—saw technique. In Masters, F. W., and Lewis, J. R., Jr., editors: Symposium on aesthetic surgery of the nose, ears, and chin, St. Louis, 1973, The C. V. Mosby Co.
3. Crosby, J. F.: Aesthetics: the ideas and ideals of beauty. In Masters, F. W., and Lewis, J. R., Jr., editors: Symposium on aesthetic surgery of the nose, ears, and chin, St. Louis, 1973, The C. V. Mosby Co.
4. Horton, C. E.: Osteoplastic rhinoplasty—osteotome technique. In Masters, F. W., and Lewis, J. R., Jr., editors: Symposium on aesthetic surgery of the nose, ears, and chin, St. Louis, 1973, The C. V. Mosby Co.
5. Lewis, J. R.: Atlas of aesthetic plastic surgery, Boston, 1974, Little, Brown & Co.
6. Millard, D. R.: Twenty-five helpful hints in corrective rhinoplasty. In Masters, F. W., and Lewis, J. R., Jr., editors: Symposium on aesthetic surgery of the nose, ears, and chin, St. Louis, 1973, The C. V. Mosby Co.
7. Peck, G. C.: Surgery of the nasal tip. In Masters, F. W., and Lewis, J. R., Jr., editors: Symposium on aesthetic surgery of the nose, ears, and chin, St. Louis, 1973, The C. V. Mosby Co.
8. Safian, J.: Fact and fallacy in rhinoplastic surgery, Br. J. Plast. Surg. **11**:45, 1958.
9. Straith, C. L.: Personal communication, 1946.
10. Straith, C. L.: Reconstruction about the nasal tip, Am. J. Surg. **43**:223, 1939.
11. Straith, R. E., Teasley, J. L., Linde, M. G., and Moore, L. T.: The treatment of lateral deviations of the nose by pin fixation, Plast. Reconstr. Surg. **15**:346, 1955.

Chapter 14

Sculpturing the nasal tip

George C. Peck, M.D.

The rhinoplastic surgeon is constantly searching for a technique that will produce an anatomically normal and aesthetically pleasing nose. This technique must be technically simple and allow the surgeon to predict his results. It is the purpose of this chapter to demonstrate a technique for nasal tip sculpturing that will be both predictable and reproducible.

Before beginning surgery, the surgeon must examine the nasal tip and feel the borders of the alar cartilage (Plate 1, *A*). He then marks on the skin the outline of the lower margin of the alar cartilage (Plate 1, *B*). The surgeon must now examine the *projection* of the nasal tip as shown by the blue arrow (Plate 1, *C*). He must now determine if the tip height is too high, about right, or too low. If the tip height is too high, he must position his incision so that he leaves a minimum of alar cartilage in continuity in the alar rim. This diagram shows the position of the sculpturing incision placed about 3 mm above the lower line (Plate 1, *D*). These lines are drawn on the skin of the nose before surgery. Here we see the position of the sculpturing incision in the large, projecting tip (Plate 1, *E*). If the nasal tip projection is good, he then places the intracartilaginous or sculpturing incision higher and leaves 5 or 6 mm of alar cartilage in continuity in the alar rim (Plate 1, *F*). If a surgeon has doubts about positioning of the sculpturing incision, he should use moderation and leave 5 or 6 mm of cartilage for a slightly larger nose with good aesthetic lines.

Surgery begins with elevation and sculpturing of the nasal tip followed by reduction of the nasal bridge. It was found that more consistently good profiles would result, since the surgeon can control the reduction of the nasal bridge better than that of the tip. Initially the surgeon must not infiltrate local anesthesia in the nasal tip or bridge. The area

that must not receive infiltration, so that there will be no distortion of the tip or bridge, is marked in red (Plate 1, *G*). The infiltration (approximately 8 to 12 ml) is confined to the area of the inner canthus, the infraorbital nerve, the alar base, and the nasal spine. Next, infiltration is confined to the area of the intercartilaginous incision. The intercartilaginous line is the red-white line created by the junction of the white vestibulum skin and the red nasal mucosa.

Surgery begins with the intercartilaginous incision between the upper lateral and the alar cartilages, extending around the spetal columella in one sweep of the scalpel (Plate 1, *H*). The nasal tip is shortened when necessary. The columella is always shortened with a resulting obtuse angle, which produces an elevation of the tip without a subsequent elevation of the columella (Plate 1, *I*). This eliminates the retracted columella or piglike appearance. The shaded area represents the area of excision. Good nasal aesthetics should have the columella slightly lower in profile than the alar rims. The nasolabial angle in a woman should always be 100 to 110 degrees. Plate 2, *A*, shows the straight-line excision of the columella septum as shown in Joseph's textbook, which tends to produce a retracted columella with the piglike look.

The sculpturing of the alar cartilages is the next step in our surgery. The suction tip is placed intranasally into the concavity made by the dome of the alar cartilage (Plate 2, *B*). By pressing with the index finger, an impression can be made intranasally, which represents the dome. This marking must be made at the sculpturing line that was drawn on the nasal skin before surgery. Now the stage is set for the sculpturing incision, which begins in the dome area and extends medially for 2 to 4 mm and laterally in the lateral crus (Plate 2, *C*). The incision is made through and through the nasal lining and cartilage, leaving an intact segment of alar cartilage in the alar rim (Plate 2, *D*). The alar cartilage above the incision is now removed. This is accomplished by first undermining the skin from the underlying fat and alar cartilage with a blunt scissors (Plate 2, *E*). It is important to remove all fat lying in the **V** between the two medial crura and the two domes. A hemostat has grasped the nasal lining and, by pulling inferiorly, the cartilage with the overlying fat is exposed (Plate 2, *F*). By sharp dissection, the alar cartilage that is to be removed is separated from the nasal lining (Fig. 14-1). The lining is now a bipedicle flap attached medially and laterally. The cartilage is then removed. Notice that the fat is removed in continuity with the cartilage (Fig. 14-2). At this point in the surgery the nasal tip has been sculptured according to predetermined lines. Above the sculpturing incision the alar cartilage and fat have been removed, leaving skin externally and nasal lining internally. Below the sculpturing incision are skin externally, fat, cartilage, and nasal lining. This sculpturing line has produced a level discrepancy, which light will hit and which will make a shadow. In essence, this is no different than a scar having a level discrepancy between the two sides. Even in the thick, sebaceous skin, the slightest level discrepancy will produce a shadow that will impart the good aesthetic lines of the sculpturing incision. The tail of the lateral crus is preserved if the nasal tip shows an external depression in this area. It is removed if the nose is bulbous in this area (Plate 2, *I*).

It is important to note that the domes have not been transected by removal of wedges. It is not necessary to do dome-wedge resections. The box-like nasal tip is eliminated, as are the sharp bumps of protruding edges of alar cartilage. The normal anatomy and lines of the nasal tip have been preserved. One must remember that it is not the size of the nose that is important but the aesthetic lines that are achieved. Certainly a slightly larger nose with excellent lines and anatomic symmetry is more to be desired. It is important to preserve normal anatomic lines to prevent the possibility of bumps or irregularities.

An analytic evaluation of the geometry involved reveals that the alars are not flat structures shaped as an inverted **U**. Many anatomic diagrams would lead us to believe that this is true. It can be seen, however, that the resected cartilage is a three-dimensional structure, and, after excision, as shown, there is a reduction of the nasal tip in all planes (Fig. 14-1). On removal of the cartilage, the

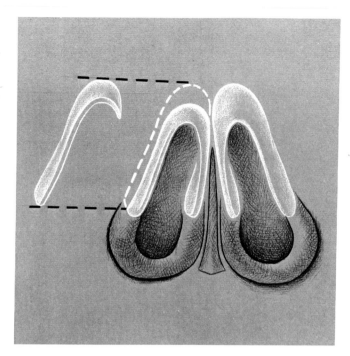

Fig. 14-1. Resected cartilage is three-dimensional structure. After excision, there is reduction of nasal tip in all planes. (From Masters, F. W., and Lewis, J. R., Jr.: Symposium on aesthetic surgery of the nose, ears, and chin, vol. 6, St. Louis, 1973, The C. V. Mosby Co.)

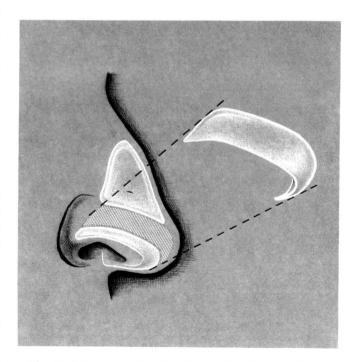

Fig. 14-2. Because of loss in volume of resilient cartilage, tip has reduced size in its entire pyramid. (From Masters, F. W., and Lewis, J. R., Jr.: Symposium on aesthetic surgery of the nose, ears, and chin, vol. 6, St. Louis, 1973, The C. V. Mosby Co.)

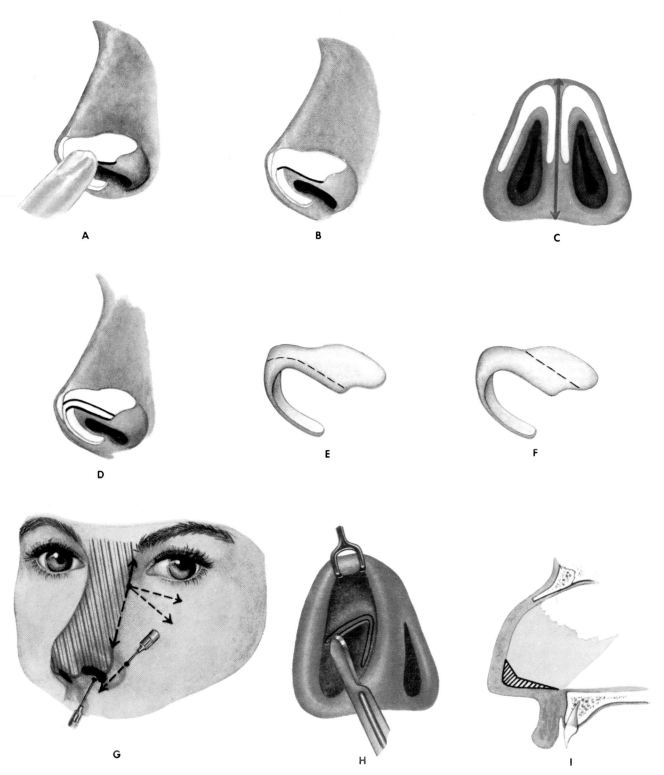

Plate 1. A, Surgeon feels borders of alar cartilage. **B,** He outlines lower margin of alar cartilage. **C,** Projection of nasal tip is examined. **D,** Sculpturing incision is placed 3 mm above lower line in high projection tip. **E,** Position of sculpturing incision is drawn on skin before surgery. **F,** Sculpturing or intracartilaginous incision leaves 5 or 6 mm of alar cartilage in tip with good projection. **G,** Tip and bridge marked in red will not be injected, to prevent distortion. **H,** Intercartilaginous incision is made between upper lateral and alar cartilages, extending around septal columella. **I,** To produce elevation of tip but not of columella, columella is shortened with a resulting obtuse angle. (**G** and **I** from Masters, F. W., and Lewis, J. R., Jr.: Symposium on aesthetic surgery of the nose, ears, and chin, vol. 6, St. Louis, 1973, The C. V. Mosby Co.)

Plate 2. A, Straight-line excision of columella septum is to be avoided. Note that there is less cartilage taken in obtuse angle illustration. **B,** Suction tip is used to mark position of sculpturing incision in dome of alar cartilage. **C,** Sculpturing of alar cartilages is done with curved incision made at beginning of dome (in suction tip imprint) and extending medially across medial crus for about 2 to 4 mm and laterally across lateral crus, always remaining parallel to rim margin. **D,** Position of incision together with preserved cartilage below and cartilage to be removed. **E,** To remove alar cartilage above sculpturing incision, first skin from underlying fat and alar cartilage is undermined with a blunt scissors. **F,** Cartilage with overlying fat is exposed when hemostat is used to grasp nasal lining and pull it inferiorly. **G,** Alar cartilage that is to be removed is separated from nasal lining. **H,** Cartilage is then removed. Fat is removed in continuity with cartilage. **I,** Tail of lateral crus is preserved if nasal tip shows external depression in this area. It is removed if nose is bulbous in this area. (**A** and **E** from Masters, F. W., and Lewis, J. R., Jr.: Symposium on aesthetic surgery of the nose, ears, and chin, vol. 6, St. Louis, 1973, the C. V. Mosby Co.)

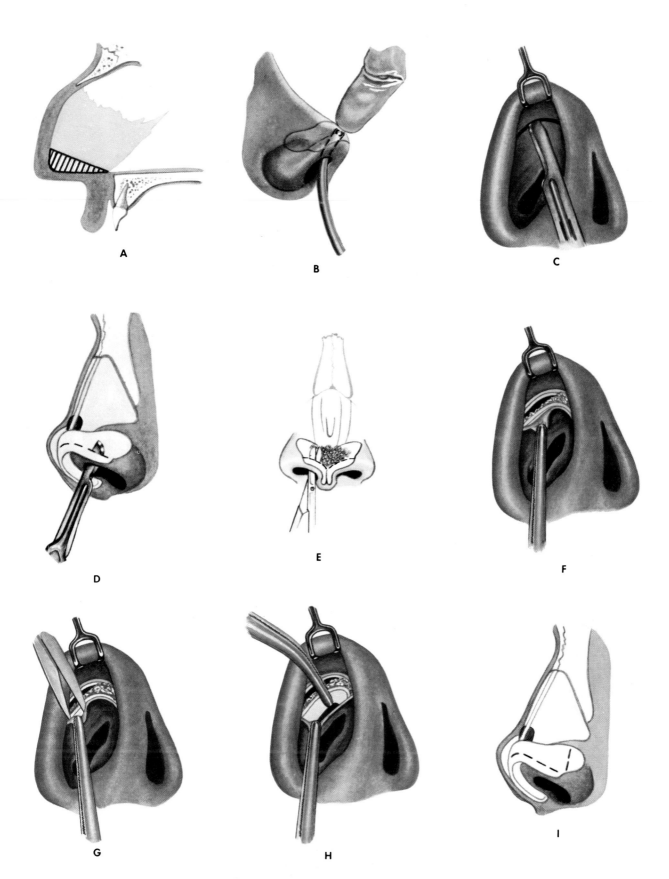

Plate 2. For legend see opposite page.

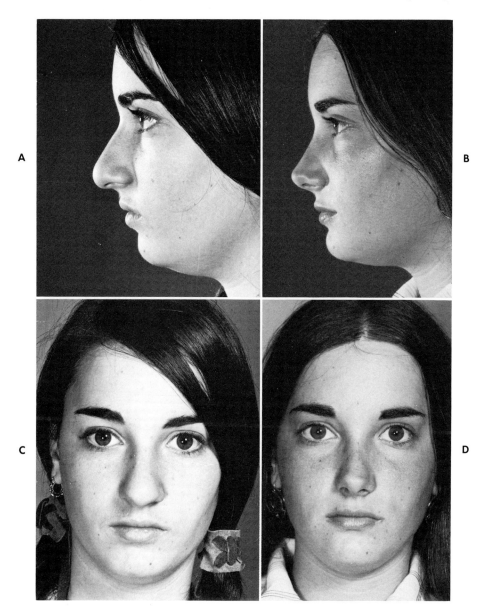

Fig. 14-3. A, Preoperative appearance of 16-year-old girl. **B,** Her postoperative appearance 2 years later. Notice improvement in chin lines by Silastic chin implant. **C,** Preoperative front view. **D,** Postoperative front view.

tip has reduced size in its entire pyramid. This is directly related to a loss in volume of resilient cartilage. A reduction in entire nasal tip size has been achieved without sacrifice of anatomic symmetry, and there is an obvious reduction in tip height (Fig. 14-2). Fig. 14-3 shows preoperative and postoperative results in a 16-year-old girl, with the postoperative photographs taken 2 years later. Note the definition and normal anatomic appearance of the alar cartilage. The patient had a receding chin that was corrected by a Silastic implant. Fig. 14-4

shows a 32-year-old woman and her postoperative results 18 months later. Again note the alar definition. Fig. 14-5 shows a 14-year-old girl and her results 2 years postoperatively.

The sculpturing technique as described has been used successfully in 90% of my patients. The remaining 10% represent the abnormally high tip projection or wide, bulbous tip. In these cases I must resort to transection of the nasal dome, to lateral rotation of the alar cartilage, or to crosscutting of the alar domes. Also in this 10% is the short

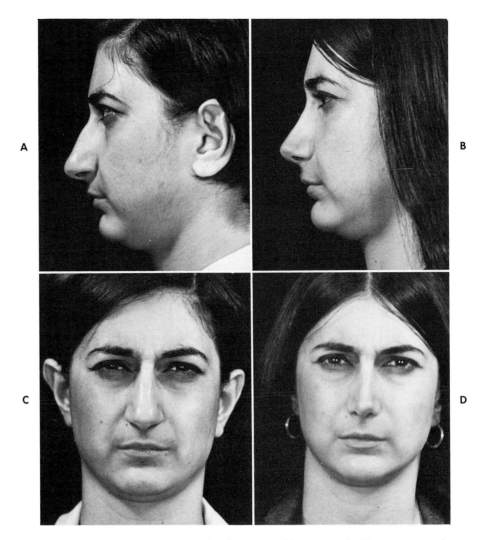

Fig. 14-4. A, Preoperative photograph of 32-year-old woman. B, Her postoperative appearance 18 months later. C, Preoperative front view. D, Postoperative front view.

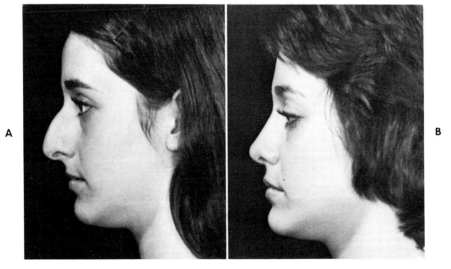

Fig. 14-5. A, Preoperative photograph of 14-year-old girl. B, Her postoperative appearance 2 years later.

tip projection, which can represent a real trap if not diagnosed before surgery. Such a nose may have a high hump with a low tip projection. The usual rhinoplasty as described, accompanied by a tip cartilage graft or strut, will usually give satisfactory results. However, one word of caution:

When in doubt, use moderation, and utilize the sculpturing technique as described. One can always come back for a minor revision, and it is amazing how often one will be pleasantly surprised.

Chapter 15

Adjuncts in primary rhinoplasty

D. Ralph Millard, Jr., M.D., F.A.C.S.

The moment a prospective rhinoplasty patient enters the consultation room, a generalized scrutiny begins, taking in height, weight, hair style, *nose,* facial bone structure, chin prominence, *nose,* personality, style of dress, overall effect, and *nose.* By the time full attention has focused on the nose the third time, *most of us have made a decision as to what this specific patient needs and how close we can come to our goal.* A tall, glacial lady will usually require a higher bridge with less tip turn-up than a tiny, vivacious one. Then comes the second stage of the campaign, discovering *what the patient wants.* Achievement of this should be obtained along two levels: (1) *direct* questioning and listening to the patient's expressed desires and (2) counterintelligence maneuvers to uncover the patient's ideal hopes and hidden fears.

The third stage of the campaign is probably the most difficult—*the meeting of the minds,* explaining to the patient not only what is ideal but what is possible and giving an educated guess how close one can approach the other in reality. If the surgeon and the patient do not agree on the ideal, then that should conclude the consultation. If the patient is not satisfied with the frank prediction of the probable final result, then the patient will conclude the consultation and should be allowed to do so. If the surgeon understands the patient's desires and thinks he has a reasonably good chance of achieving them and if the patient understands what the surgeon has in mind and realizes the possible degree of deviation from perfection, then the surgery has its best chance of psychologic success.

The chance of aesthetic success depends on the condition and degree of difficulty of the nasal deformity itself, the artistry, training, and skill of the surgeon, the postoperative healing phase, and an unknown and hopefully minor quantity of luck.

PHOTOGRAPHIC RECORDS

It is essential that standard, accurate photographic records be kept. The preoperative condition must be recorded not only for postsurgical reference but also for legal protection. These photographs should be printed soon enough before surgery not only to ensure their success but also to enable their presence in the operating room during the surgery.

Of course the photographs can be taped to the wall, but there is a far better way. Three sheets of transparent plastic can be stitched into a two-sided compartmental holder. A slit at the top of each separate pocket enables the nurse to insert or withdraw each photograph. A second case can be similarly presented on the opposite side. If this composite photographic holder is hung from an intravenous stand, it can be maneuvered to within easy view of even a myopic surgeon (Fig. 15-1).

From the moment the administration of the local anesthetic is begun and through all the stages of a rhinoplasty, the original nose is continually changing its shape. Infiltration in the columella base lifts the tip temporarily, and reduction of the alar cartilages gives the effect of shortening the nose. Thus a long nose, without being actually reduced in length, can appear, during surgery, to be short enough. *Only a preoperative photographic record can make available at all times a baseline reference and counteract transient false effects to encourage the surgeon to do what had to be done from the beginning.*

PREPARATION FOR SURGERY

Approximately 45 minutes after sedation with pentobarbital (Nembutal) and meperidine (Demerol), my special nurse clips the vibrissae of the nostrils and cleans the nasal airways. About 20

118

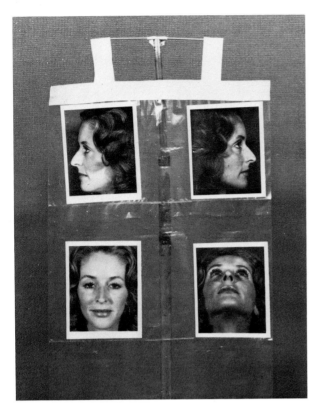

Fig. 15-1. Simple photograph holder for on-the-spot referral to original deformity at any time during surgery.

minutes before surgery, she packs the nostrils with half-and-half 10% cocaine and epinephrine (Adrenalin), 1:100,000. Injection with a no. 27 needle of 1% lidocaine (Xylocaine) with epinephrine, 1:200,000, is carried out with gloves before scrubbing. The injection starts at the root of the nose continuing along the sides subperiosteally when possible, with special focus on blocking the infraorbital nerve medial to its exit. The needle continues down under the alar bases, is withdrawn, and is again inserted just back of the columella base. A slight amount of local anesthetic is inserted along the bridge line and immediately massaged flat. In a test series, Maisels and I[6] found that the most common complaint from the rhinoplasty patient under local anesthesia occurred during the lateral osteotomies when the saw or chisel was working against the lateral vestibular mucosa. Thus a final generous injection is made in this area bilaterally within the nose near the inferior edge of the nasal bones where the stab incisions will be made later in the operation.

The nasal airways are then packed with Vaseline gauze to seal off blood passing into the nasopharynx. If much blood is swallowed during sur-

gery, there often follows the syndrome of feeling of warmth, nausea, and vomiting, which is most disturbing to both the patient and the surgeon.

SURGICAL PROCEDURE
Vestibular incisions

The membranous septal incision is placed according to the plan of reduction. If the columella shows minimal retraction or if the tip suggests the need for strut support, then the membranous septal incision is placed back flush with the septal cartilage to leave ample tissue in front for the insertion of cartilage struts.

Extending bilaterally from the membranous septal incision are the anterior vestibular incisions, which are made approximately 0.75 cm from the margin and leave approximately 4 mm of the alar cartilage distal. These single anterior vestibular incisions give direct access to the entire alar cartilages without various chondromucosal flaps being cut and turned out of the nostril. It leaves the valvelike structure at the intercartilaginous junction intact, and it avoids the necessity of a true marginal soft tissue incision. Then, of course, it simply reduces the amount of intranasal scarring.

The alar cartilages proximal to this incision are resected after being freed by sharp subperichondrial dissection inferiorly and by scissor snipping to remove any excess fatty tissue over the tip superiorly. Distal to this incision, the alar cartilage can be reduced as required. Every effort is made to retain at least a 2 mm intact distal rim of alar cartilage as emphasized by Peck.[13] Under specific circumstances such as an extremely projecting tip, a wedge resection medial to the angle can be carried out without great concern (Fig. 15-2).

These incisions also give access to the lateral crus, angle, and medial crus of each preserved distal intact rim of alar cartilage. In certain broad-tipped noses where there is soft tissue separating the alar cartilage, this tissue can be excised and its two cartilages sutured together for extra refinement of the tip.

If the medial crura of the alar cartilages are wide in depth, they can be reduced; if the nasal tip is long, the feet of the medial crura may be amputated; if the feet splay to create a wide columella base, they can be reduced, or the tissue between them can be excised and the feet shackled with a suture.

Sidewalls not divided

In 1958, Anderson[1] described retrograde intramucosal hump removal, which involved subperi-

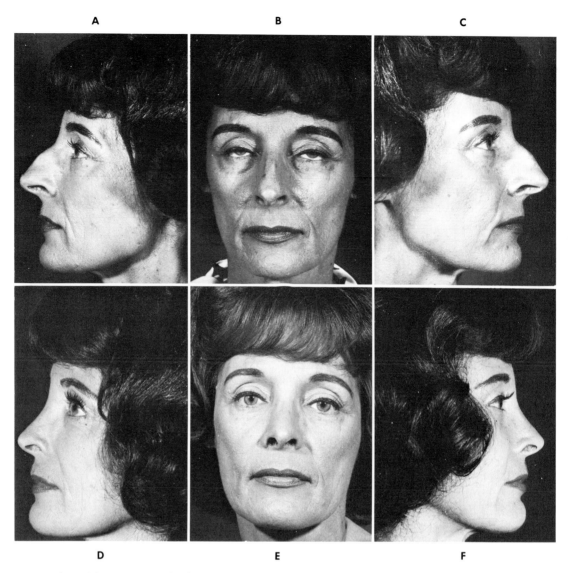

Fig. 15-2. A to **C,** This 47-year-old woman had high-bridged, humped nose that projected severely from her face with exceptional length from tip to lip. Her nostrils were long and slightly retracted. **D** to **F,** Through usual anterior vestibular cartilage-splitting incisions, superior three quarters of lower lateral cartilages were removed, and *wedges were excised from medial portion of each crural angle.* Bridge was lowered, and rectangle was resected from anterior septum, including nasal spine. Bilateral osteotomy and resection of wide alar base wedges completed this rather radical reduction.

chondrial and subperiosteal freeing of the entire length of the cartilaginous and bony nasal dorsum to facilitate scissor-and-gouge hump removal. Although the results he published suggested possible insufficient bridge lowering, there is an aspect of this approach that has appeal. Not dividing the mucosal continuity of the sidewalls to the septum may increase the technical difficulty slightly but is overcompensated by the reduction of scars with easier healing and fewer secondary deformities. Over the past few years, I have not divided the

sidewalls from the septum but do not follow Anderson's extensive subperichondrial and subperiosteal dissections. Rather, after the skin has been freed from the dorsum of the nose and the full-thickness bony hump lowered, the mucoperichondrium of the septum is peeled down from above enough on either side along the bridge to allow shaving down the cartilage septal bridge. In the bony hump area, the sidewalls are divided from the septum, if not during hump removal, then with an osteotome during bilateral osteoto-

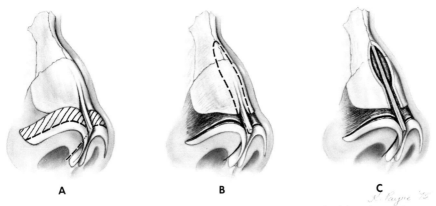

Fig. 15-3. A, Broken line indicates position of anterior vestibular incision through mucosa and lower lateral alar cartilages and extending down membranous septum. Cross-hatched areas indicate usual removal of lower lateral cartilage. **B,** Marking hump and upper lateral cartilage reduction. **C,** Note after all reductions, vestibular mucosal lining is still attached to septum distal to nasal bones.

mies. The important point is that the mucosal attachments of the sidewalls to the septum are respected in the distal half of the nose and tip, which reduces scarring and the incidence of supratip swelling (Figs. 15-3 and 15-4).

Hump and bridge

I still prefer the controlled reduction of the hump with saws and the cartilaginous bridge with the scalpel. A sharp chisel and an Echoff rongeur under direct vision help to chip away toward a smooth, natural bridge line. The rasp is being used more and more for minor to moderate lowering of the bony hump (Fig. 15-5).

Septal shortening

It is important that nasal shortening be conservative and that the nose not be uptilted too much. I have no qualms about reducing the nasal spine when it is excessive or when it causes the columella to protrude into the lip.

Submucous resection

When there is a deviation of the septum that is obstructing the airway, a submucous resection is carried out but only after the bridge has been lowered and the anterior septum has been shortened. Once the septum has been tailored around its periphery to its final form, then it is safer to resect its central portion, of course always maintaining an intact L-shaped septal support. The septal cartilage removed is available for use as strut grafts and, when necessary, may have to be obtained even when no septal obstruction is present.

When the septal deviation is seen externally, either in a curve of the external nose or presenting in one nostril, then in addition to a submucous resection, the residual cartilage is scored on the concave side, and the anterior strut is freed from its dislocated position, reset, and fixed in the midline (Figs. 15-6 and 15-7).

Osteotomy

Bilateral osteotomy is postponed until the tip, bridge, and septum have been completed, since the bleeding after this maneuver is greatly responsible for much of the swelling and ecchymosis in the area of the eyelids. Through lateral vestibular stab incisions, the frontal process of the maxilla is divided as close to the maxilla as possible with a button-guarded 6 mm chisel. Further freeing of the bone along this line is carried out with a 4 mm chisel. This is done without periosteal dissection to maintain some control of the bones. Then an osteotome inserted between each nasal bone and the septum high up is tapped gently through the intact mucosa and used to outfracture the bony component on each side. When free, they are then moved medially and set neatly in narrowed position. The outfracture is not always necessary, and simple infracture may be sufficient.

Septal cartilage grafts

In 1965 I stated:

Routine reduction rhinoplasty is limited in its potential for in principle it is *all take and no give.* Occasionally, the mere removal of tissue may produce an improvement but still fall short of ideal. A subtle addition in

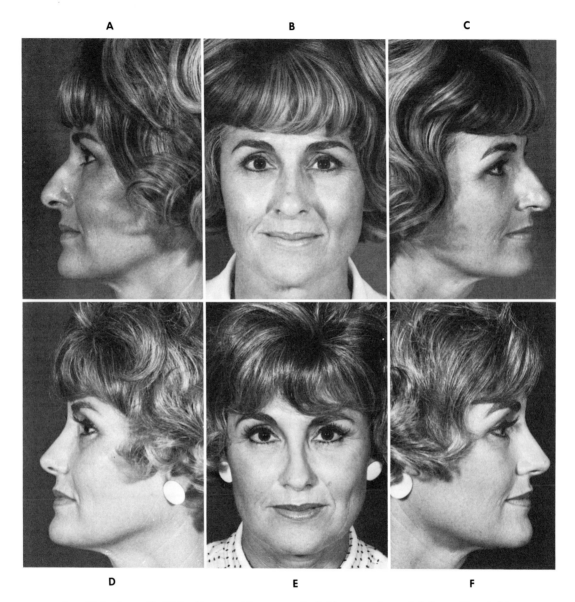

Fig. 15-4. A to **C,** This 44-year-old woman had history of nasal injury. Her bridge was elevated; tip was slightly bulbous and hooked when she smiled. **D** to **F,** Through anterior vestibular incisions, maintaining lateral wall attachments to septum, superior three quarters of lower lateral cartilages were removed and medial foot was amputated on left, bridge was lowered, and septum was shortened by rhomboid resection, bilateral osteotomy, alar wedge resections, and submucous resection of left obstruction.

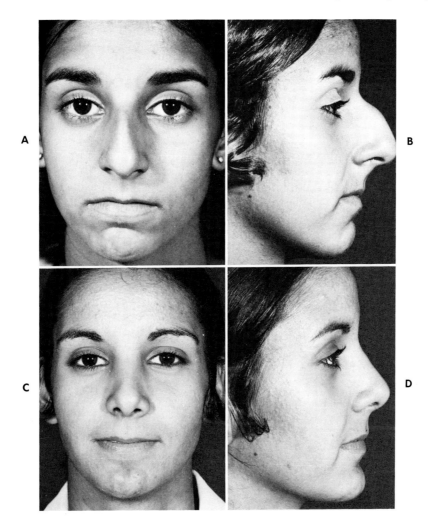

Fig. 15-5. A and **B,** Thirteen-year-old girl 5 feet 11 inches tall with overpoweringly high bridge, hooked nose, and slightly receding chin. **C** and **D,** At 15 years, corrective surgery included removal of superior three quarters of lower lateral cartilages, bridge lowering with saw, anterior septal resection as a square including nasal spine, bilateral osteotomy, alar base resections, and Silastic sponge implant to chin through lower sulcus incisions. Seventeen months after operation, slight supratip swelling was excised.

the right place along with the reduction can tip this gain into a full-fledged success.

Autogenous septal cartilages taken by the usual submucous resection is by far the material of choice for the adjunct of the columella strut. It is close at hand, usually available in sufficient amounts, thin enough to avoid bulk, but of a structure and strength suitable to render support as well as contour.*

An intact pocket in the columella can be made whatever length is required; it should be made slightly less in dimension than the cartilage strut so that the oomph of a little spring is maintained

after insertion. It is important that the strut not be too long or the pocket carried so close to the tip that its point shows white even with smiling.

It seems that this approach is becoming more and more popular. When the tip is flat and the columella sagging, one or two septal cartilage struts, using the nasal spine as the push-off, can get a rise out of a moderately flat nose. A true flat nose deserves a costal osteochondral graft as modified from Gillies.[4] Tessier[14] has added a little trick by splitting one end of the cartilage strut so that it splays like a fleur-de-lis in the tip. When septal cartilage is not available, Gorney's gull-wing auricular graft[3] gives a similar, if not as stiff, lift.

---

*From Millard, D. R., Jr.: Adjuncts in augmentation mentoplasty and corrective rhinoplasty, Plast. Reconstr. Surg. **36:**48, 1965.

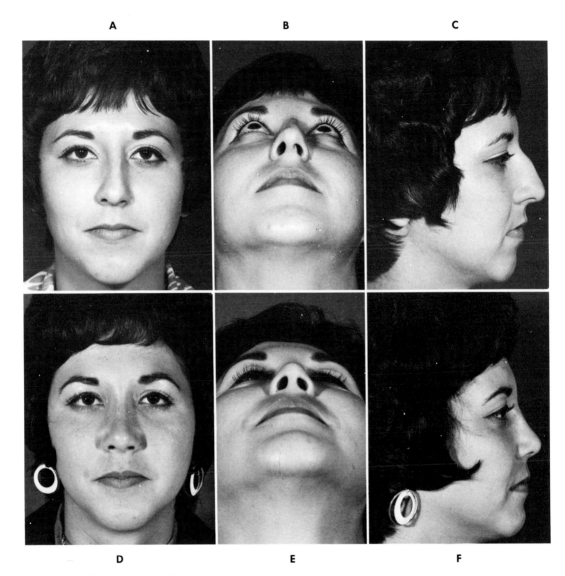

A   B   C

D   E   F

Fig. 15-6. A to **C,** This 26-year-old woman with history of nasal trauma revealed humped nasal bridge with deviated septum presenting in left nostril and receding chin. **D** to **F,** Corrective surgery included removal of superior three quarters of lower lateral cartilage, hump reduction, anterior septal shortening including nasal spine, submucous resection of obstruction, bilateral osteotomy, alar wedge resections, and Silastic sponge implant inserted on chin through lower sulcus incision.

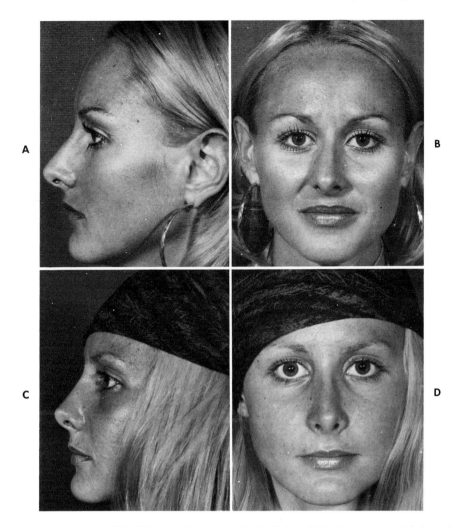

Fig. 15-7. A and **B,** This 25-year-old woman had slightly high, long nose with hanging columella and deviation of her septum with definite slant of nose to right. **C** and **D,** Corrective rhinoplasty through anterior vestibular incisions maintaining lateral wall attachments to septum included removal of superior three fourths of lower lateral cartilages, slight lowering of bridge, minimal anterior septal resection involving nasal spine, bilateral osteotomy, and submucous dissection of septum with scoring of cartilage of residual bridge on concave right side high up in bend to bring nose into straight line.

When the tip itself needs only definition, then shorter struts are effective.

Recently, Sheen[15] has been advocating small pieces of bone for tip definition. His work is artistic, but he has not followed this technique more than a few years, and, since free-floating bone does not always maintain its total presence, later results will be of interest.

Alar bases

As noted by Joseph[5] and elaborated by Aufricht,[2] wedge resections of the alar bases are of value. The need for this refinement is often not obvious preoperatively, but during the process of alar cartilage reduction and septal lowering, the main lift of the anterior tip is reduced, resulting in sag of the sidewalls and degrees of flaring of the nostrils. In 1960, I[8] was using alar base wedge resections in 65% of reduction rhinoplasties, and, by 1965, I[9] had increased it to 98%, which is about my percentage today. If the nostril flares with a long, horizontal limb, the wedge resection is obvious. In certain cases where the nostrils are wide but there is little horizontal limb, it is important to leave a slight nostril sill on the columella side, as noted by Sheen.[15] Do not excise so much of the wing of the ala that it is forced to run straight into the cheek. There must be a gentle curve into

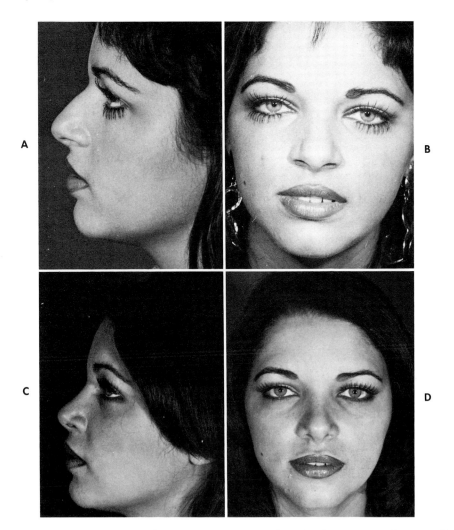

Fig. 15-8. A and **B,** Twenty-five-year old woman with vivacious personality revealing broad nose with wide tip, flaring alae, slight hump, and prominent columella base in profile. **C** and **D,** Reduction rhinoplasty included removal of superior three quarters of lower lateral cartilages leaving intact 2 mm rim and suture of crura together in tip, slight lowering of bridge, reverse triangle excision of anterior septum with greatest amount at nasal spine area, and wide alar base excisions.

the sill for naturalness. All cases shown here have had alar base resections of some degree, but it played a major role in the transformation in Fig. 15-8.

Alar margins

When the original nose is long but has sidewalls that challenge the columella and tend to hide it in profile, producing a relative retraction, there is a dilemma. First, the septum must be shortened. Then the sidewalls will need to be shortened even more. This can be achieved indirectly by reduction of the vestibular lining, but if this is insufficient, alar marginal excisions can be used to reduce di-

rectly the length and thickness of the sidewalls[10] (Fig. 15-9).

Chin

One out of four patients requesting nasal reduction deserves augmentation mentoplasty, and three out of the seven patients presented here had chin implants. For 24 years, I have used the lower labial sulcus route for insertion of chin implants. Beginning in 1951,[7] homologous costal cartilage was used, but after about 10 years, it became evident that these grafts were being absorbed. It was then that the fine Silastic sponge was first used, and except for a shrinkage of about a third its orig-

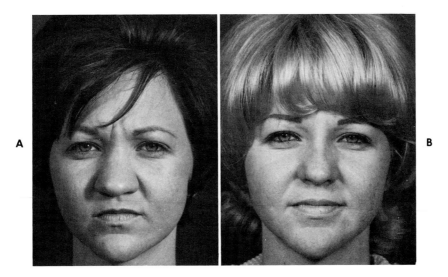

Fig. 15-9. A, This 24-year-old woman with thick, broad, flat nose without definition was first presented in *Plastic and Reconstructive Surgery* **40:**337, 1967. **B,** Improvement was obtained by radical reduction of lower lateral alar cartilages, anterior septal resection, alar marginal and alar base wedge resections twice, and insertion of Silastic implant to bridge to give effect of refinement and definition.

inal size, this implant was free of problems. Unfortunately, its manufacture was discontinued. More recently, a slightly firmer sponge (Heyer-Schulte) has been made available. It is as easily shaped for the specific case, and, although it is too soon to make a final decision, it promises to show less shrinkage.

The technique of its insertion is the same.[11] A 1 cm midline stab incision is made with a no. 15 B.D. blade in the mucosa of the lower lip 0.75 cm above its mucosal attachment to the mandible in the labial sulcus. Leaving soft tissue over the mandible for 1 cm, a no. 10 B.P. blade is directed down to the periosteum of the mandible, and a pocket averaging 7 or 8 cm is dissected parallel and in front of the mentum. The dissection is not carried beneath the periosteum to avoid bone resorption but is kept close to the periosteum to avoid injury to the mandibular and marginal branch of the cervical nerve to the depressor muscles of the lower lip. The sponge implant is shaped with tapering ends that are fashioned extremely thin at the extremities to facilitate their hugging the mandible and avoiding projection. The implant is folded, and its center is marked with a methylene blue stab mark, after which it is soaked in a solution of neomycin-bacitracin. The implant is then taken at the very tip of one of its ends by a smooth forceps and is inserted all the way to the end of the pocket on one side. Then the other end is similarly inserted completely into the other side. The blue mark on the implant should be seen dead center in the 1 cm stab incision, indicating that the implant is in perfect position. A 4-0 chromic catgut suture takes a bit of subcutaneous tissue of the lip inside the pocket, then a small nip of the implant at the blue point, and finally picks up the subcutaneous tissue over the mandible. After this suture is tied, the implant is fixed, and a further two-layer subcutaneous closure is carried out to seal off the implant. Finally, the labial sulcus mucosa is closed with 4-0 chromic mattress sutures, and a gentle pressure dressing with transverse compression between lip and chin is applied. Antibiotics are used for 5 days as prophylaxis. Except for early temporary swelling, complications have been minimal, and the improvement in the overall effect is important (Fig. 15-10).

Postoperative nasal dressing

The operative packs are removed and the nasal airways suctioned. Then new Vaseline gauze is packed on both sides gently but fully enough to ensure apposition of all lining to outer structures and closure of dead spaces, the temptresses of hematomas. The skin is molded with 3M tape to the skeletal structures of the bridge and tip with special pressure in the supratip area. A split piece of Telfa is fitted over the dorsum of the nose, and nine layers of plaster of Paris are molded as a cast to hold the bones in their new position. Once this cast has set, eyepads and folded cotton are placed

A   B   C   D

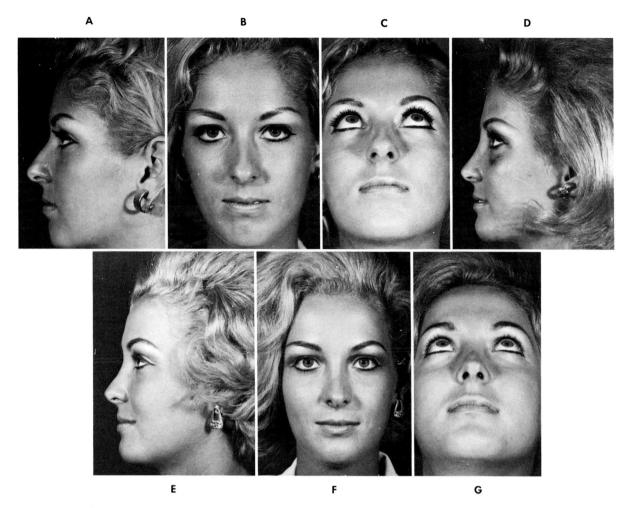

E   F   G

Fig. 15-10. A to **C,** This 23-year-old woman had slightly more nasal projection and tip fullness than ideal, deviation of anterior septum, slightly protruding lower lip, and receding chin. **D** to **G,** Corrective surgery included removal of superior three quarters of upper lateral cartilages, slight bridge reduction, narrow rectangle resection of anterior septum with subperichondrial scoring on concave side, bilateral osteotomy, small alar base excisions, and small Silastic chin implant inserted through 1 cm lower sulcus incision. **D,** Note minimal swelling and ecchymosis after splint removal at eighth postoperative day.

over the eyes, and a gentle pressure dressing is applied over the splint and eyes for several hours. Care is taken to make certain that this bandage does not shift the splint, causing upward telescoping or down-sliding of the dorsal skin of the nose. A gauze sling is laid across the nostrils, being tucked under the eye bandages on each side. This additional gentle pressure has reduced postoperative edema and ecchymosis to a minimum.

REFERENCES

1. Anderson, J. R., and Rubin, W.: Retrograde intramucosal hump removal in rhinoplasty, Arch. Otolaryngol. **68:**346, 1958.

2. Aufricht, G.: A few hints and surgical details in rhinoplasty, Laryngoscope **53:**317, 1943.
3. Falces, E., and Gorney, M.: Use of ear cartilage grafts for nasal tip reconstruction, Plast. Reconstr. Surg. **50:**147, 1972.
4. Gillies, H., and Millard, D. R., Jr.: Principles and art of plastic surgery, Boston, 1957, Little, Brown & Co., pp. 575-576.
5. Joseph, J.: Nasenplastik und sonstige Gesichtsplastik, Leipzig, Germany, 1931, Curt Kabitzsch.
6. Maisels, D. L., and Millard, D. R., Jr.: Local anesthesia in cosmetic surgery, Br. J. Plast. Surg. **19:**187, 1966.
7. Millard, D. R., Jr.: Chin implants, Plast. Reconstr. Surg. **13:**70, 1954.
8. Millard, D. R., Jr.: External excisions in rhinoplasty, Br. J. Plast. Surg. **12:**340, 1960.

9. Millard, D. R., Jr.: Adjuncts in augmentation mentoplasty and corrective rhinoplasty, Plast. Reconstr. Surg. **36:**48, 1965.

10. Millard, D. R., Jr.: Alar margin sculpturing, Plast. Reconstr. Surg. **40:**337, 1967.

11. Millard, D. R., Jr.: Augmentation mentoplasty, Surg. Clin. North Am. **51:**333, 1971.

12. Millard, D. R., Jr.: Aesthetic rhinoplasty. In Saad, M. N., and Lichtveld, P., editors: Reviews in plastic surgery: general plastic and reconstructive surgery, Amsterdam, 1974, Excerpta Medica Foundation, pp. 371-386.

13. Peck, G. C.: Tip rhinoplasty. In Masters, F. W., and Lewis, J. R., Jr.: Symposium on asthetic surgery of the nose, ears, and chin, vol. 6, St. Louis, 1973, The C. V. Mosby Co.

14. Pollet, J.: Utilisation des exérèses ostéo-cartilagineuses au cours de la rhinoseptoplastie, Ann. Chir. Plast. **17:**90, 1972.

15. Sheen, J.: Achieving more nasal tip projection by the use of autogenous vomer or septal cartilage graft. (In press.)

Secondary rhinoplasty

Chapter 16

Secondary rhinoplasty surgery

Jack H. Sheen, M.D.

Sheen: This 27-year-old patient had a primary rhinoplasty done approximately 11 years ago. Fig. 16-2 is her preoperative photograph, which I would like to briefly go over. There is a very slight nasal hump; the tip is a little rounded with poor differentiation. The nasolabial angle is excellent; the subnasion has an appropriate fullness. On frontal view, I would consider the nasal configuration to be excellent. The lower lateral cartilages are a little broad; the nasal bridge, however, is what I would consider to be excellent.

In the postoperative photograph, one is immediately struck by the different look through the middle third of her face. I have frequently mentioned the separation of eyes in white people (Fig. 16-3). In the preoperative photograph, the dorsum does in fact separate the eyes as an anatomic structure that is not present in the postoperative photographs. Frequently, when the bridge has been resected too low, patients will complain, "Something funny has happened to my eyes!" The effect of this can be seen very well in the postoperative photograph. Furthermore, with a reduction of the dorsum or an overreduction of the dorsum, the supratip area becomes a separate anatomic part as you can see here. So, you have a flat, nondifferentiated area,

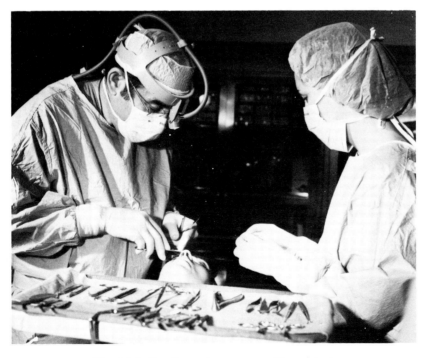

Fig. 16-1. Dr. Sheen in surgery with assistant.

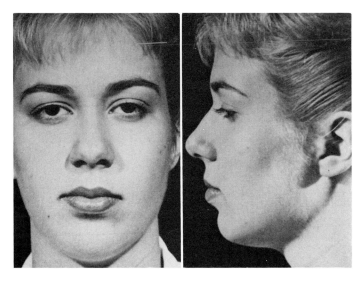

Fig. 16-2. Preoperative photographs of patient.

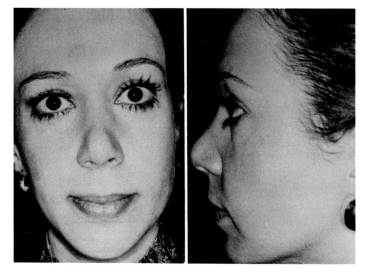

Fig. 16-3. Patient after first surgery.

which is your low dorsum, and a bulbous, poorly differentiated tip without facets and with visible nares. The apparent length of her lip has increased significantly because of the resection of the caudal septum.

Now, back to the preoperative lateral view. I would never have touched the caudal septum on this patient, since all elements of the base of the nose are near perfect. In the postoperative picture, the subnasion is full, but there is no cartilage there. I can push it up almost 3 or 4 mm. A point of nomenclature I would like to make: The subnasion is that point at the base of the columella overlying the anterior

nasal spine. The lobule is that area of the tip that is above the nares and columella, so when I refer to the columellar-lobular junction, you will know that it is precisely this point.

I would next like to illustrate some relationships on this three-quarter profile to show what I'm going to try to achieve on this patient. The dorsum begins high or in line with the superior tarsal fold. It is relatively straight, ending in a tip, which is the highest point in the nasal profile. The tip is well differentiated from the dorsum. The thing that gives your nose the look of length is an uninterrupted line from the root to the base. This nose appears shortened because it begins at the point of the rise of the supratip area. The subnasion is very important in giving you proper aesthetic nasal-labial relationships. It can be neither too full nor too sharp. On the lateral preoperative view, the nasal-labial angle is wider than it is on the postoperative picture, yet the tip has a *down* look preoperatively. Now the down look (of the tip) is by virtue of the relationship of the nasal parts, obviously, but the deepening of the nasal-labial angle (recessing subnasion by resection of inferior caudal septum or spine) is very important. The relationship of the columella to the alae is also important, and it should be lower than and parallel to it.

So, on this patient, the thing that we're going to try to do is to first do something to elevate her dorsum. The tip is flat and nonprojecting, exaggerated by virtue of the high supratip area. So what I'd like to do are these three things: raise the dorsum, lower the supratip, and do something to elevate that tip area. The nasal-labial angle is wide open, so obviously nothing should be done to touch that. I will not do a transfixing incision; my incision will stop just below the angle of the septum. So, just to repeat one more time, the thing that we're going to try to do is elevate the dorsum, reduce the supratip, and do something to project the tip.

Now, if I can, I'm just going to very briefly go through the technique I use for anesthesia. I use a total of 5 to 6 ml of 1% lidocaine (Xylocaine) mixed with epinephrine (0.75 ml of 1:1000 Adrenalin to 30 ml of 1% Xylocaine).

While we're waiting for a needle, please come back to the pictures, and let me go through a couple more things. In this view, there is one thing that worries me. If you'll notice in the preoperative photograph, her nasal bones look perfect. In the postoperative photograph, the caudal border of the nasal bridge appears distracted and wide. The roof is obviously open, the septum forms the middle part, and so you have a triangular deformity. I'm concerned about the width of these nasal bones, and I'm sure they've been fractured because I can feel some knots close to the root of the nose. But when I do a septum, I hate to do an osteotomy too. But there is a possibility that if I can't get a proper pyramid reconstructed with my septal cartilage, I may have to do an osteotomy on both nasal bones to bring the caudal edges in.

Musgrave: How late after a primary do you think you can do that (move the bones in) without having to do an osteotomy?

Sheen: As you know, nasal bones do not heal by callous but by fibrous union, so I feel you can move them in with an appliance or digital pressure up to perhaps 6 months. After that, you have to do something to sever the union.

Musgrave: What preoperative medicine did the patient receive?

Sheen: She has been given 20 mg of diazepam (Valium) and 50 mg of meperidine (Demerol) intravenously. I also keep a 500 ml bottle of Ringer's lactate with 100 mg of meperidine added. I can then titrate the patient during the procedure.

Now then, to anesthetize the nose, I begin with less than 1 ml at the radix. Following that, I place the needle along the malar groove to the root, and drawing the needle out, lay in approximately 0.5 ml on each side. Next, the columella and area over the spine is injected, followed by a small amount over both lower lateral cartilages. The needle is then placed over the angle of the septum to the root of the nose with solution injected as the needle is again withdrawn.

Before I do anything else, I'm going to pack the nose with cocaine. I use 5%.

Musgrave: Any epinephrine?

Sheen: No. Cocaine is one of the most effective vasoconstrictors we have.

Musgrave: I'm just going to ask for a show of hands from the audience. How many of you use epinephrine along with your cocaine? We have about 40%.

Sheen: Well, perhaps we can change their minds. One of the main reasons for using cocaine or any topical anesthetic is to anesthetize the mucosa overlying the area where you plan to do your osteotomies. The patients frequently complain of pain because you're hurting them on the mucosal side, not the cutaneous side.

A lot of people feel that a secondary rhinoplasty should be approached through the normal tissues, entering into the area of distortion. I feel strongly that the area of distortion should be entered directly and that no incisions be made in areas not directly involved with the correction. I make an incision much like George Peck uses for his cartilage-splitting incision: it is gull-wing shaped, and I carry it through the scar tissue in an effort to develop a plane (to thin out the supratip area) and then go right over the angle of the septum.

Musgrave: Have you run into any cartilage at this point in your dissection?

Sheen: I have not encountered any so far. Now, at this point, I take a sharp Joseph scissors and dissect right under the skin cephalad, trying to get into some kind of a plane, which is difficult to do in scarred tissue such as this is. This is actually a thinning maneuver. I do no more skeletonizing than I absolutely have to. I use my Joseph elevator and try to get under the caudal part of the bony vault and try to preserve as much tissue of the dorsum as I can, especially if it is a secondary.

Musgrave: How far down on the maxilla are you?

Sheen: I'm just at the edge of the nasal bone. In my dissection, I'm trying to get under the periosteum. I then use a hockey-stick knife and place it across the radix and draw it caudally against the nasal framework, preserving as much tissue as possible. Finally, I use a Cottle periosteal elevator to make certain that the soft tissue is freed away from the entire dorsal surface of the nose.

This having been done, I can explore the nasal structure with an Aufricht retractor. I can see that the nasal bones are intact at the root, then approximately 1 cm caudally they separate. Caudally, I can now see it is not cartilage causing the supratip swelling, because the cartilage of the distal superior septum has been overcorrected by trimming it down 3 or 4 mm. Now you can see that whoever did the primary did an overresection of this part of the septum to avoid supratip swelling, but it did not work.

Next, I would like to do the septal part. In doing the septum, the first thing I like to do is to infiltrate with 1% lidocaine (no epinephrine), which is actually a dissecting aid. If you elevate the perichondrium, it is enormously helpful. I feel that if you are doing septal surgery in order to obtain cartilage for reconstruction, the Ballinger knife will not provide you with the superb piece of cartilage that lies at the osseochondral junction or in the vomerian groove. Whenever I take septal cartilage for reconstruction, I like to leave at least 1 cm and preferably 1.5 cm for support. An incision is made 15 mm cephalad to the caudal border of the septum and carried through the mucoperichondrium. The perichondrium is carefully elevated; if you get under the perichondrium, it really is a simple procedure. This is carried past the osseochondral junction. After having completed the dissection on one side, the septum is transected and the dissection continued on the opposite side. After this has been done, I use a Jackson turbinatome to cut across the cartilage

into the perpendicular plate, placing a finger on the frontal junction to make certain I have not fractured the attachment at that point. After that has been done, another parallel cut is made 12 to 15 mm below the first, the specimen is carefully extricated, and this, then, will be used for the dorsal graft.

Musgrave: What do you do if it's not straight?

Sheen: If it is not usable, I will try going after the vomer, which also makes an excellent dorsal graft. I would prefer using material that is not in any way modified by fracturing or attenuating. In the event that nothing else can be found, tight crosshatching or morselizing is done to prevent curling.

I am going to resect this small tag of the cephalic border of the right lower lateral cartilage because it has been annoying me, and it serves no real purpose. Even in a patient such as this with a large supratip swelling, I think it is important to retain as much tissue as you possibly can, because these patients are really tissue deficient.

Musgrave: What do you do if the tissues cannot accommodate to the bony framework?

Sheen: The important thing to remember is that no matter what you do to the bony skeleton, if you reduce it beyond the point of nasal tissue contractility, you're going to get a supratip hump. It would then follow that if the supratip hump is caused by tissue inability to contract down to the skeletal framework, no matter how many times you thin it out, the hump will in fact remain. So to answer your question, if the tissues cannot accommodate to the bony framework, you simply raise the bony framework with suitable material, which is what we are doing here.

Musgrave: Couldn't the low, wide, bony dorsum be raised and narrowed by means of lateral osteotomies and infractures?

Sheen: That's probably one of the greatest misconceptions in plastic surgery. How can you take nasal bones based on the maxilla, fracture them inward so they are in the pyriform aperture, and expect them to rise above the level of the dorsum? This might be true if they were on a platform, but they are not.

Musgrave: What difference does the position of the little piece of bone at the edge of the graft make? In other words, should it be up toward the radix, or can it be down toward the tip?

Sheen: It doesn't make any difference. The only important thing is where you want the thickness. If the largest defect is near the root, the thickest portion of the graft (i.e., the bony junction) is placed at the root.

Musgrave: What happens if there is no septum—if it was all taken out in a previous surgery? What type of material would you use?

Sheen: I have always been able to find some material between the nasal bones, or very often, I have utilized the vomer. If the primary surgeon was using a Ballinger-type knife, there is always sufficient material to be found. This at least has been true of my last 300 or so secondaries.

Musgrave: Did you use anything else prior to those 300?

Sheen: I used silicone three times, and two of those came out.

It is at this point that I am going to place a tip graft to obtain some finesse or projection of the tip. To be effective, a tip graft must be free floating or not be dependent on support from the maxilla. That is important because with a strut based on the maxilla, the action of the zygomatic and facial muscles pulls the tip down and could cause a tent-pole effect or even perforate the tip. Autogenous cartilage is ideally suited to the type of graft that I plan. The shape is designed to reduplicate the normal domes of the lower lateral cartilages. It tapers down to a narrow base with a notch to avoid slippage and to give lateral stability.

Musgrave: Where is this graft in relation to the medial crus?

Sheen: In front of it. Now, after the graft has been placed, the profile view shows excellent tip differentiation. In fact, incredible as it may seem, I am going to place another graft under the caudal part of the dorsal graft to shore it up even further. This in the area of the supratip fullness. Following the insertion of the small $11 \times 5 \times 2$ mm piece of cartilage, the relationships of the nose appear to be excellent. All of the preoperative objectives are now compared with the photos, and it is felt that no more can be obtained at this time.

Musgrave: Are you happy at this stage with the left nasal bone?

Sheen: Not entirely, but whenever anything is minimally displaced or distorted after this much surgery, I wait to see how it looks after some of the swelling is down. Then, if it still seems out too far, without skeletonizing, I simply do the osteotomy and bring the caudal borders in more medially.

Safian: I feel that what you see in the secondary nose is due to the result of undifferentiated scar-ring from a lack of dissection in the proper tissue planes.

Peterson: Dr. Sheen, you said the vomer was very important to the integrity of the nose and to nasal function, and then you stated later that you would frequently take a portion of the vomer as graft material if septum is not available.

Sheen: That is correct. I feel that the status of the vomer in nasal physiology is in a state of limbo at this time. Some people feel it is very important, especially to provide a structure for the turbinates to abut against. I feel that you can take the vomer (or part of it) out as long as you do not violate the bony part of the turbinate, and I am careful about this phase of turbinate surgery when I do a partial vomerectomy. I have spoken to men who do radical septal surgery as I do, and over a 20-year period they report they have had no nasal problems, which confirms my clinical impression.

Peterson: One very significant point of yours is that you always get supratip swelling if you take too much dorsum. Would you expand on that?

Sheen: Any time you remove too much dorsum, or lower the skeleton past the point of tissue contractility, then the skin just can't respond, and a supratip hump will result. The skin of the nasal tip is much thicker than it is at the root, so its contractility is much less.

Peterson: In reference to the last 300 secondary rhinoplasties that you have done, if the bridge had been so badly lowered at the first procedure that there was not enough material, would you then go to bone graft, rib, or homograft?

Sheen: With rib or iliac bone graft there is a problem of resorption unless there is good host bone contact. If I were forced to go to something other than the patient's own material, I would elect to try an alloplastic graft rather than subject the patient to the trauma and morbidity and uncertainty of the grafts you have mentioned.

Operation notes

Hospital: Victoria Hospital, Inc., Miami, Florida
Date: January 17, 1975
Operation: Major septoplasty—nasal reconstruction
Surgeon: Jack H. Sheen, M.D.
Assistant: Mrs. Anitra Sheen, R.N.
Preoperative diagnosis (Fig. 16-4, *A* to *C*): The patient presents with a moderate saddle deformity of the nose. The roof is open with the septum visible in the midline. There is a moderate supratip hump ending in an ill-defined, poorly differentiated tip. The nasolabial angle is open. The subnasion is modestly retracted, and the columellar insertion is higher than

A   B   C

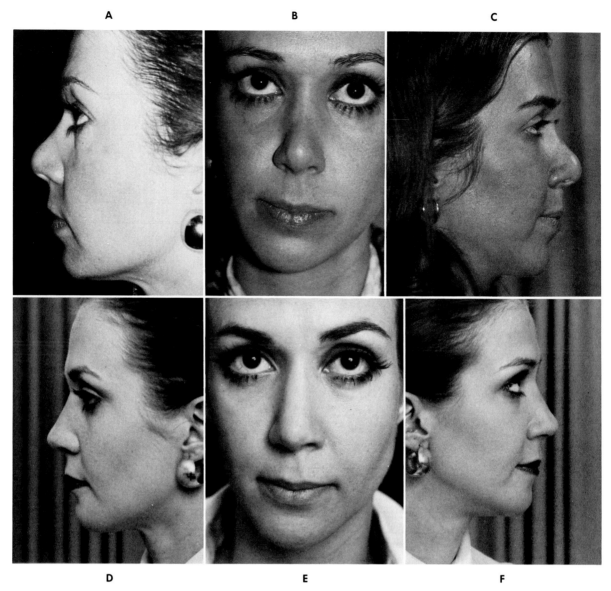

D   E   F

Fig. 16-4. A to **C,** Preoperative photographs of patient. **D** to **F,** Postoperative photographs of patient after correction of first surgery.

the insertion of the lateral alar lobules. The inferior caudal septum has been partially resected. On internal examination, the cartilage is found to be intact, and, on palpation, it is found to be moderately thin. The vomerian ridge is over to the left. All internal structures appear to be normal in size and location; the mucosa is of normal color. There are no discharges.

With the patient in the dorsal supine position, a thorough preparation and drape of the face and neck was done. The nasal airways were packed with pledgets of cotton dipped in 5% cocaine, carefully dried before insertion. The nose was infiltrated with approximately 6 ml of 1% lidocaine (Xylocaine) with epinephrine. After this, gull-wing

incisions were made approximately 5 mm cephalad to the border of the alar rim. This was carried through the scar tissue just below the surface of the skin. Using a sharp Joseph scissors, the dissection was carried cephalad to the caudal border of the bony vault, where a Joseph periosteal elevator was used to elevate the tissues from the dorsal edge of both nasal bones. This was continued across the radix, at which point a hockey-stick knife was inserted, and the separation of soft tissues from the skeleton was completed across the angle of the septum.

The septum was next infiltrated with 1% lidocaine without epinephrine. The perichondrium was elevated away from both sides. A Jackson tur-binatome was used to make two parallel cuts to obtain a specimen approximately 14 mm wide and 3 cm long. Further dissection of portions of the septum in the vomer was done to obtain more material.

The single cartilage graft was shaped to approximately 9 mm wide with both sides beveled to recreate the normal dorsum, and this was secured in place with a percutaneous mattress suture of 6-0 nylon. After this, a pocket was dissected in the tip, and a tip graft was fashioned to produce a more projecting tip. This was secured by suturing the wound with interrupted 5-0 plain catgut. Because of the new projection of the tip, another piece of cartilage, which was approximately 2 mm

thick, 1.5 × 1 cm rectangular, was slipped under the caudal edge of the dorsal graft.

The contour of the nose was felt to be appropriate at this time, so Adaptic gauze packing and a routine nasal split and dressing were applied.

Blood loss during the procedure was minimal. The patient withstood the procedure well and was returned to the recovery room in good condition. (See Fig. 16-4, *D* to *F*.)

Postscript: You may notice that I did a chin augmentation on her (the first week after surgery) and at the same time did an osteotomy on both sides (lateral only) without undermining as I had discussed, because it seemed that I would eventually have to bring in the caudal part of that left nasal bone.

Chapter 17

Secondary rhinoplasty surgery

D. Ralph Millard, Jr., M.D., F.A.C.S.

Musgrave: Let's have a look at the photographs (Fig. 17-2).

Millard: Right profile. There is a depression of the bridge as you can see. I feel a small amount of cartilage, but there is little to no septum beyond a small piece, as the previous surgeon must have resected the anterior portion, producing retraction of the columella along with the depression of the bridge.

Musgrave: How tall is she?

Millard: What is your height, dear?

Barrett: She's about 5 feet 7 inches.

Millard: She's about average, so we'll work on that basis.

The important thing to notice also is that the sidewalls are long. Here is the front view. Can you see how the alar wings sort of overlap the columella slightly? The tip is bulbous and spongy. She has had Weir wedges excised so the scars go around into the cheek, but the nostrils seem a little bit wide, even so. We may have to revise that slightly. But the main points are the depression of the bridge, the bulbous, spongy tip, the flaring and overhang of the alar rims medially, the retraction of the columella without any definition, and the hanging sidewalls. The nose is too short, and the lip is too long relatively. So we have to lengthen the nose a bit.

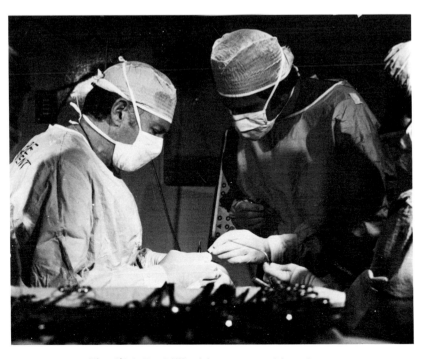

Fig. 17-1. Dr. Millard in surgery with assistant.

Are there any questions? If anyone would like to come and help me with this, I'd appreciate it!

Musgrave: Are you asking for someone to step forward?

Millard: Anybody!

Musgrave: What are you putting in there, Ralph?

Millard: Lidocaine (Xylocaine), 2% and epinephrine: 1:200,000. We've had epinephrine half and half with the cocaine in the packing, and she's being very good.

Take flaps of the vestibular sidewalls as chondromucosal flaps to swing into the releasing incision in the membranous septum to lengthen the nose, particularly at the tip, and to lift the alar rims slightly. At the same time, I hope to put in a bridge support. As I've not done the two together, it may be a little difficult transposing two flaps within the vestibule and still get a watertight closure to protect the cartilage that I've taken from her rib. I much prefer septal cartilage, of course; it's thinner, more dependable, and it's much easier to get. Unfortunately, there is no septal cartilage left. There is shortness of lining in the membranous septum region. Can you see? When I take hold of it and pull, it has no give at all; it's tight. So there is no point in trying to shove pieces of cartilage in it to bring it down. New tissue is needed. The important thing in the chondromucosal flap technique is to cross from your membranous septal incision into the lateral vestibule, estimating approximately what you need, and extend it taking cartilage as well as mucosa where you can. Then the second incision will be up forward more, parallel, and taking these long, thin flaps with carti-

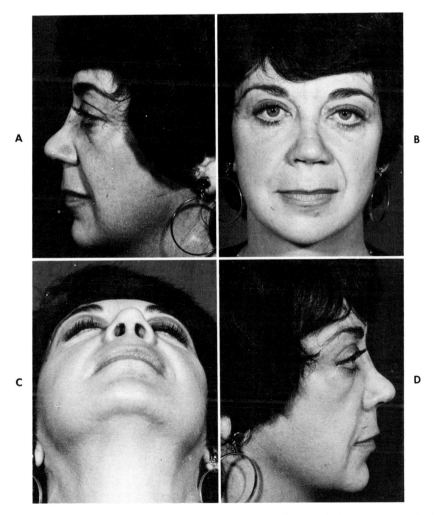

Fig. 17-2. Preoperative photographs of patient. **A,** Left lateral view. **B,** Frontal view. **C,** Basal view. **D,** Right lateral view.

lage to splint them. I've done quite a few without mishap, but of course this could be the first one to give up the ghost.

Patient: You shouldn't say that!

Musgrave: You need a little more diazepam (Valium) there, buddy.

Millard: She's happy about the whole thing.

Patient: I only care about the results.

Millard: I'm with you, dear.

The reason for her original rhinoplasty was a bulbous tip. She still has much of this quality, so taking these flaps may benefit this problem.

Musgrave: You have a pedicle there about three to one or two and a half to one?

Millard: No, it will be four to one, I imagine. It is important to base these flaps on the tip in front and on the columella so that when this component moves forward, the flap goes with it. If you leave it behind, you're in trouble.

Musgrave: Ralph, what is that you're using?

Millard: It's a thimble with a forceps on one side and a double hook on the other so you can rotate it forward to pick up the suture, and spin it back for retraction.

Musgrave: You looked like the drum major of the Hurricane band there the way you were twirling that!

Millard: Storz, I think, made this one for us.

I guess I've done thirty of these flaps and they have all done well. It's amazing because they have been taken with scars across their base and across their body. The blood supply in the tip lobule of the nose is so abundant that flaps in this vicinity are winners.

Musgrave: Does it bother you to have so much epinephrine in it?

Millard: I avoid putting any in the base of the flaps.

Musgrave: What you're doing is a three-dimensional Z-plasty.

Millard: You won't get an argument from me on that! Understand one point. The proximal incision for the flap must be continuous with the membranous septal incision. The distal incision runs parallel to create the flap.

Musgrave: You can feel that against your index finger?

Millard: Yes. That's the point of the thimble hook. So I have two or three fingers free for palpation. Incidentally, I sit down to work.

Musgrave: Are you sitting on your embroidered stool?

Millard: I've got a new one now that you haven't seen yet, Ross. It has a Viking on horseback.

Musgrave: I hope he doesn't have the horns!

Millard: I haven't noticed them yet; the spear occasionally.

All right. Now it's hard scar in the membranous septum. I can feel it fighting me.

Musgrave: That's a no. 11 blade now?

Millard: Yes, a no. 11 blade, and I'm going to keep cutting until I get no more resistance. See how the right-angle scissors work under the flaps at the tip to get them free now with the membranous septal incision releasing the retracted columella? You can see the two flaps whirl down in the nostrils, anxious to swing into the septal defect.

Musgrave: Do your two pedicles go back to back?

Millard: That's right. Cartilage to cartilage, just like in the medial crura of the normal. I picked this difficult case because it presents the most common use I've found for this flap. If someone finds it helpful, then I guess it was worth it. Try not to take too big a bite with each suture in the flap because after two big bites, one on each side, you've tied off the whole blood supply. All right now, it's sewn in on the anterior side of the membranous septal incision. Now, we'll go behind and stitch the mucosa to the mucosa behind and pick up cartilage whenever it is available. This is just sewing the flap into the membranous septal incision. I don't make up my mind what I'm going to do until I'm in the operating room.

Musgrave: You're calling audibles at the line of scrimmage!

Millard: That's about right. You see, you have to in all of plastic surgery.

Musgrave: Can you talk?

Millard: I'm choking a little, but . . . I'm a little worried about the closure of the right side. Just because I'm suturing doesn't mean I'm a blank. I'm trying to figure out how I'm going to get that other side closed. I'm probably going to have to rotate the lining.

Musgrave: You're photographing well.

Millard: See, this has got to be watertight and trustworthy if I'm going to insert a rib cartilage strut to the depressed bridge. Now the left side is loose and coming nicely. There's a terrific shortness of tissue on the right with scarring, but I think I see a savior. There is excess soft tissue inferiorly and laterally.

Musgrave: I hate to throw a curve, but somebody asked would you please get a speculum and demonstrate the size of the nostril so we can get an idea of possible stenosis. Can you put a speculum in your sutured side? That leads to another question: Doesn't the juncture of the donor site incision and the insert suture line ever web?

Millard: I've never seen a web here. There is no reason it should with a transposed, full-thickness composite flap breaking the scar line at the potential position of the web.

Musgrave: Your left nostril looks better.

Millard: That's right. There is a tightness of tissue on the right. Let's see with the stitch out how well it looks. Yes, it's better. Shall we put the implant in and then go from there?

Musgrave: Yes, it shows. Is that fresh cartilage?

Millard: Yes, it was taken about 40 minutes ago. Can you see that, Ross, at all?

Musgrave: Yes, it's showing.

Millard: Now, she's a little too high in the bridge. At least the columella is no longer retracted.

Musgrave: Gustie is saying on my left that the cartilage graft is not too large.

Millard: I'm afraid that it will stand up just a little too much here at the root of the nose if I leave it.

Musgrave: Gustie is saying, "Shave it down but don't shorten it."

Millard: Okay. Thank you, Gustie.

Musgrave: Can the camera come in on that? Gustie says, "Tell him a little bit shorter."

Millard: Okay, that's what I want. How's that?

Musgrave: How is that, Gustie?

Millard: One thing, this pocket is only the size of the cartilage, so it's not going to slip around anywhere.

Musgrave: One of the people in the audience wants to know: Can you put another graft under the anterior portion to give it a little extra lift?

Millard: No, I can't afford to push it up any more in front, which is already absolutely what I want.

Musgrave: We want to see what you're talking about before you take it out, because it looks good on the screen. Tell us what it is you're concerned about.

Millard: It's too high at the root of the nose.

Musgrave: The plebeians in the stands have thumbs up.

Millard: What does that mean—they want me to take it out?

Musgrave: No, they want you to leave it in.

Millard: All right. I think they want to get back to their coffee!

From deep in the vestibule laterally where it can be spared, a transposed mucosal flap is being turned up to close the defect on the right.

Can you see that? Yes, it's coming nicely, and now it will no longer pull.

Musgrave: You just called another audible.

Millard: Now there is enough, and the donor area of the chondromucosal flap can be closed without pulling on the right.

Musgrave: You're breathing easier. Please show us the side view before you put that little piece in. Is it possible to turn her head or turn the camera?

Millard: Now the retraction is corrected.

Musgrave: If the rib graft had already been obtained, why not use a sliver of it for a columella implant instead of the flap?

Millard: Because there was not enough lining. You can't just shove a piece of cartilage into a contracted compartment; that's a mistake I think is made too often. There was not enough lining which required a release.

Musgrave: Why not elevate that slight angulation on the dorsum by sandwiching more cartilage below your graft?

Millard: That's the obvious thing, to tip the cantilever. But when you drop one end down, you push the other up and get a supratip prominence, which I don't want. I have gotten the definition I want, and I'm very encouraged.

Musgrave: Can we go back and look at the profile?

Millard: Yes, let's try. Now, I want to think a minute about these alar bases.

Musgrave: They look pretty good.

Millard: They don't look too bad on the preoperative pictures. I'm just thinking about a little more delicacy. I believe I'll do it. No. 11 blade.

Musgrave: They were kind of grumbling when you said that.

Millard: Yes, well, the only way we can tell for sure is to do it. When I first looked at her, I thought that even though the nostrils weren't noticeably wide, they gave a grossness that when refined, would improve the total effect.

Musgrave: Questions: The chondromucosal flap seems to have been rotated approximately 105 degrees, and they are bilaterally concave to each other. Is that correct?

Millard: That's right. The raw surface is in and the epithelial surface is out.

Musgrave: Ralph, we thank you very much. The photography's been great!

Operation notes (*Fig. 17-3*)

Hospital: Victoria Hospital, Inc., Miami, Florida
Date: January 17, 1975

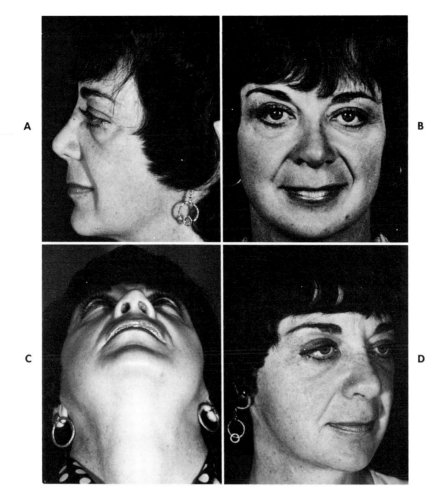

Fig. 17-3. Postoperative photographs of patient. **A,** Left lateral view. **B,** Frontal view. **C,** Basal view. **D,** Right three-quarters view.

Preoperative diagnosis: Deformity of nose and septum, including retracted columella, collapsed nasal bridge, and bulbous tip

Operation: Chondromucosal flaps to membranous septum and rib cartilage graft to bridge and tip

Surgeon: D. Ralph Millard, Jr., M.D.

Assistant: Bernard Barrett, Jr., M.D.

Rib graft: The right chest was prepared and draped, and under local anesthesia through a 2-inch inframammary incision, the sixth rib was exposed, and a 5 cm section of costal cartilage was resected. The cartilage specimen was soaked in bacitracin solution, and the wound was closed in layers. Surgeons were Gary Burget, M.D., and Bernard Barrett, Jr., M.D., residents.

Nasal preparation: Thirty minutes before surgery, vestibular vibrissae were trimmed and nasal airways were cleaned thoroughly before packing with gauze soaked lightly with 10% cocaine and epinephrine (Adrenalin), 1:100,000, half and half. The entire face was then prepared and draped, leaving both forehead and chin exposed. Before scrubbing, gloves are used to give the local anesthetic. An injection of 2% lidocaine (Xylocaine) with epinephrine, 1:100,000, is given with a

no. 27 needle. The local anesthetic is given a chance to take full effect while the surgical team is scrubbing. Then the nurse removes cocaine packing and replaces it with Vaseline gauze packing to seal off the nasal airway from the pharynx.

The obstruction on the left was far back and included a large adhesion of the sidewall to the septum. Under satisfactory local anesthetic, a mucosal flap was elevated, obstructing cartilage was removed, and the flap was replaced and later packed into position.

Then with a two-prong hook eversion of the alar rim, the chondromucosal flaps were marked with methylene blue on the lateral vestibular wall. The superior incision of the parallel incision of each flap was marked in continuity with the membranous septal incision. Then the chondromucosal flaps were incised full thickness with a no. 15 B.P. blade and dissected from the dorsal skin with a right-angled scissors. These flaps included not only mucosa and alar cartilage but also scars from the previous operation. These flaps were freed from the nasal tip skin. The upper incisions were then joined at the lower tip of the septum as a membranous septal incision with a no. 11 B.P. blade. This incision was carried well down to the nasal spine, releasing the columella. When the retracted columella and shortened nasal tip were pulled forward, producing a large membranous septal defect, the chondromucosal flaps automatically whirled about and practically fell into the defect with cartilage to cartilage and mucosa turned outward. They were sutured into their new position with 4-0 chromic catgut without tension. In spite of their length-to-width proportion of 4 to 1 and the cross scarring, they retained their pink color at all times.

A narrow pocket was then dissected over the depressed bridge, and into this was inserted the autogenous rib graft shaved on all sides and shaped to extend from its root to just short of the tip. It was evident that the upper end of the rib strut was standing too high, but, since the rest of the profile was satisfactory, it was left.

Closure of the chondromucosal flap lateral donor area offered no difficulty on the left and lifted the long sidewall perfectly. On the right, the scarring had been more marked, and closure of this donor area caused retraction of the alar rim. Undermining the lateral mucosa provided insufficient lining for closure, so an inferior mucosal flap based laterally was transposed up and out to fill the defect without tension, and its donor area was easily closed along another axis. This achieved a watertight closure to protect the rib graft.

The slight flare of the alar bases and the presence of previous Weir wedge resections prompted minor alar wedge resections. A stab incision halfway up the side of the columella allowed a superficial pocket to be dissected into the tip. Into this was inserted a sliver of costal cartilage, which not only gave definition to the tip but, by compensation of columella contour, corrected the overhang of the alar rims. All lining incisions were carefully closed with 4-0 chromic catgut, and the alar base incisions were closed with 6-0 silk.

Old packs were removed, and new Vaseline packs were inserted to gently press all flaps into their new position. The bridge was fixed with 3M taping. Antibiotics were started as prophylactic protection of the cartilage implant, and a gauze sling was taped under the nostrils.

Progress report: As soon as Dr. Aufricht and Dr. Courtiss had left town, I brought the patient back to Miami and, through a tiny stab in the right vestibule, removed the rib cartilage graft. It was *shortened* and shaped slightly thinner, dipped in bacitracin solution, and reinserted with a 6-0 silk pull-out suture. The dorsal skin was fixed over the graft with 3M taping.

Had this not been a symposium case from out of state, the bridge graft would have been inserted separately into its own pocket at a second stage, bypassing the hazard of not having its own sealed compartment. Thus, if it eventually requires a further revision, little has been lost.

Chapter 18
The nasal profile

John R. Lewis, Jr., M.D.

The nose, to be pleasing and natural, should be proportioned to the rest of the face, both in the front and profile views. It also should be consistent with the general build of the patient. The profile is only one aspect of nasal correction, but it is an important consideration to the patient and therefore to the surgeon.

The nasal profile is a continuation of and a reflection of the remainder of the facial profile. It may vary considerably and still be pleasant in appearance, but its acceptable variations are limited by the length of the face and to a degree by the height of the patient, the length of the neck, and the general body type.

Those who have studied the profile at great length in the past and present, such as Joseph, Straith, Aufricht, Safian, and Ulloa, have generally agreed on the nasal proportions. Although nasal fashions change, and each surgeon must vary these proportions to suit himself and his patient, the general principles remain consistent. The nasal profile angle from the forehead should be about 30 degrees (Figs. 18-1, 18-2, 18-6, 18-9, and 18-13). It is surprising how close to this angle the pleasing nose will fall, whether male or female, tall or short, and no matter the length or width of the nose. Nearly always this angle will vary between 28 and 35 degrees, and variations beyond this will indicate room for improvement by a corrective rhinoplasty. The tip angle of the nose will vary more considerably, depending on the various other facial contour factors, but in general it should be 5 to 15 degrees in men (Figs. 18-1, 18-13, and 18-14) and 10 to 25 degrees in women. This angle which the columella makes with the upper lip may be varied to some degree, being tilted up a bit more for the petite nose in women, but it should seldom drop below these measurements (Figs. 18-1 to 18-3, 18-5, and 18-6).

THE NASAL BRIDGE

The contour of the nasal bridge should nearly always be straight or, if not, slightly above a straight line in men (Figs. 18-1 and 18-12 to 18-14) and below a straight line in women (Figs. 18-1 to 18-6 and 18-9). The female nose may be contoured to give a definite swoop, but most profiles will look more pleasant with a gentle and subtle swoop. The pug nose is seldom indicated.

The forehead contour is of great importance in limiting the contour of the nose. The straight forehead (the chin being within normal limits) allows for a distinct turn-up of the nasal tip (the tip angle) and allows for a swoop in the nasal bridge (to or approaching the Hollywood nose). The receding forehead, which slopes back from the brow, indicates a firmer nasal bridge and less tilt-up of the tip. The overly full or rounded forehead may indicate a firmer nasal bridge to keep the profile contour from appearing to be dished out in the center of the face (Fig. 18-4).

Likewise, the chin is a firm factor in determining the nasal contour. The chin that forms a relatively straight line with the forehead and lips allows for great variation in the tip angle and in the bridge contour. One may use considerable judgment and allow for the smaller petite nose with more swoop with the small face and the short patient or a more subtle swoop and a less sharp tip angle in the taller patient and the patient with the longer face. The long neck tends to accentuate the heightened tip angle and lower bridge profile in a similar fashion.

The firmer-than-usual chin (the forehead being within normal limits) allows for great variation of the bridge and tip angles. Frequently the nose looks nice with a fairly high tip angle and a distinct swoop in the nasal bridge contour (Figs. 18-4 and 18-5).

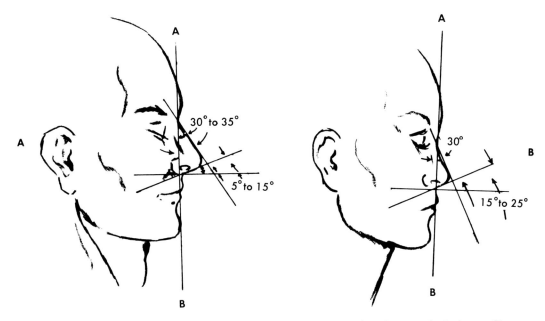

Fig. 18-1. A, Generally considered ideal measurements of male nose include profile angle of 30 to 35 degrees to vertical facial plane (*A-B*) and tip angle of 5 to 15 degrees above horizontal facial plane (which is at right angles to vertical facial plane). Thus male nose has bridge angle of about 30 degrees, with slight fullness or at least straight bridge, and tip angle usually not to exceed 15 degrees above right angle with upper lip. **B,** Ideal female profile includes profile angle of 30 degrees, or slightly under, to vertical facial plane (*A-B*) and a tip angle of 15 to 25 degrees above horizontal facial plane. In other words, nasal bridge should be at about 30 degrees to facial plane with slight swoop beneath straight line of 30 degrees in female nose, and tip angle should tilt up further than male nose and be about 18 degrees above right angle for most faces.

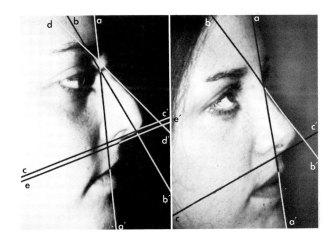

Fig. 18-2. Measurements of profile before surgical correction and after correction by rhinoplasty. *a-a'* represents line of base of nasal pyramid and extends through nasion and pogonion, or in general through root of nose below glabella and base of nose at anterior maxillary spine (the facial plane). *b-b'* represents angle of nasal bridge and should make angle of about 30 degrees with *a-a'*. *b-b'* then is profile line of bridge. *c-c'* is tip angle and should make angle of about 12 degrees in men and 18 degrees in women with base line *a-a'*. *d-d'* and *e-e'* are actual profile and tip angles in preoperative photograph.

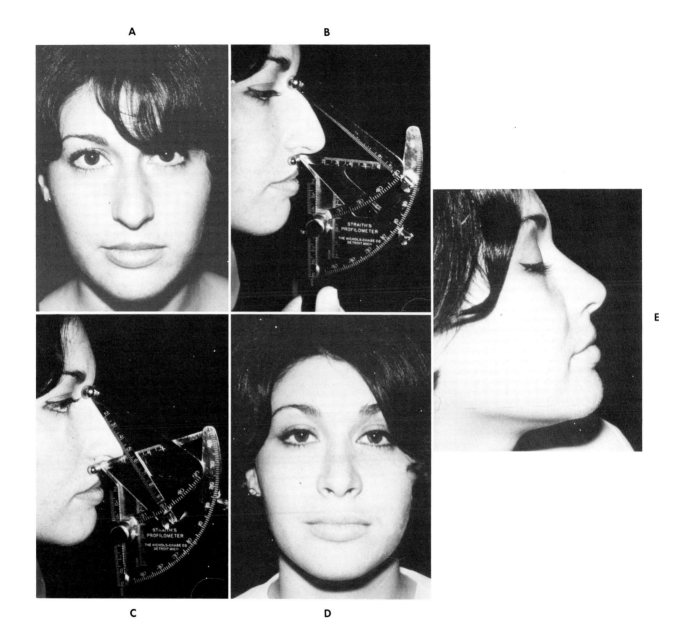

Fig. 18-3. A, Front view of patient with wide base and tip, long nose, and bony hump.
B, Profilometer in position measuring angles of nasal bridge and tip. **C,** Measurement
of nose at desired angles so that profilometer actually cuts off that portion of nose
one wishes to remove. Profilometer deals only in straight lines, and surgeon must use
his own best judgment as to degree of swoop in nasal bridge, rounding in columella,
and narrowing of tip. **D** and **E,** Postoperative view of patient after corrective rhinoplasty
utilizing profilometer in preoperative planning and in operating room.

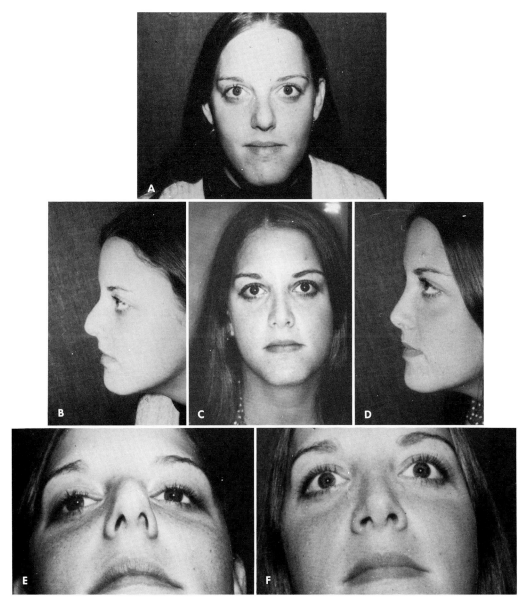

Fig. 18-4. Same patient as in Fig. 18-2. **A** and **B,** Wide nasal base, bridge, and tip and high nasal bridge, particularly in midportion and lower portion. **C** and **D,** Postoperative views of rhinoplasty proportioned to patient's other features and her general build. Note that nasal bridge and base have been narrowed, and tip has been narrowed. In side views profile has been contoured to give slight suggestion of swoop in nasal bridge and rounding of columella into tip. **E** and **F,** Inferior view shows reduction of alar width in tip and in base of columella.

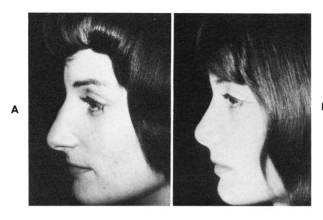

Fig. 18-5 A, High nasal bridge and long nose in small patient. Length of nose in its lower portion tends to accentuate shortness of upper lip from vermilion border to base of columella. **B,** Postoperative rhinoplasty showing contouring of nasal bridge and tip. Note longer appearance of upper lip, giving better proportion to facial features.

The receding chin poses a real problem in contouring the nasal bridge and tip. The receding chin should be corrected at the same operative procedure as the corrective rhinoplasty if it is considered abnormally recessive (Figs. 18-11 and 18-12). If it falls within normal limits but is somewhat small or recessive, then the nasal bridge should be left less distinctly swooped and the tip less tilted.

In general, then, the relatively straight forehead-lip-chin line in women allows for a swoop in the bridge and a distinct tilt-up in the tip, whereas the recessive forehead or chin or both indicate a more firm contour of the nasal bridge and less tilt-up of the tip.

In men the nasal bridge should be relatively straight under all circumstances. The depth of the glabellar groove should be less deep when the forehead or the chin or both are receding, and the nasal bridge should be firmer and the nose a little

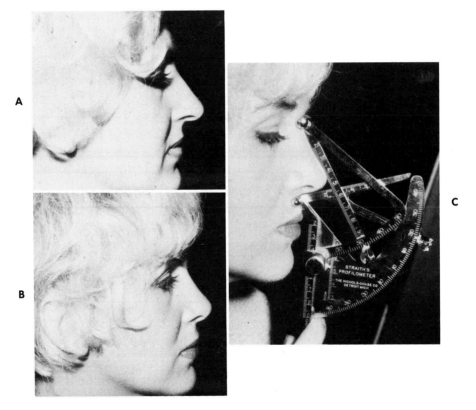

Fig. 18-6. A, Generalized enlargement of nose with increase in whole nasal bridge height, increase in length of nose, and slight overhang of tip and columella in older patient. **B,** Contouring of nasal bridge and tip from side with shortening of nose and slight swoop to nasal bridge. Deepest portion of nasal bridge is at top of bridge in subglabellar area. **C,** Measurement of nose with profilometer in postoperative period approximately 6 months after her surgery. Contouring of nose with shortening gives more youthful appearance to patient's face.

longer, with less tilt-up at the tip, when the forehead and chin are recessive (Fig. 18-11). The chin should be relatively firm, especially in men, for the most desirable profile, and a mentoplasty should be considered at the same operative stage as the rhinoplasty if the chin does not fulfill the normal qualifications (Figs. 18-11 and 18-12). Augmentation of the forehead can also be carried out using molded plastics, plastic sponge materials, injectable plastic materials, or cartilage or bone if it is definitely abnormal.

The point at which the depth of the swoop in the female nose occurs may be varied but must not be too deep. The lowest point is usually best at the top of the nasal bridge below the glabella or only slightly lower along the bridge (Figs. 18-2 to 18-6 and 18-9). One should definitely avoid a saddle nose appearance. The swoop should be a gentle one, not reaching a great depth at any point but coming upward gently into the tip without giving a full or high-tip appearance. The tip should be gently rounded rather than pointed and sharp, and the columella and alae should conform pleasantly so as to have the columella more prominent than the alae and the alae neither overly short nor overly long (Figs. 18-3 to 18-5, 18-7, 18-13, and 18-14).

The recessive columella in particular is to be avoided, and a cartilage graft (from the septum) may be used to make this more firm at the time of the corrective rhinoplasty, if indicated (Figs. 18-7 to 18-9 and 18-12 to 18-14). The recessive maxilla that allows for depression of the alar bases and base of the columella may be corrected by a cartilage or bone graft across the maxilla beneath the alae and base of the columella or at any one point where indicated. This gives a higher base from which to start the contouring and may help considerably in the general contour of the nose in the profile and full-face views.

THE NASAL TIP

A prominence of the dorsum of the nasal tip, where the alar cartilages create a fullness just to either side of the septum and into the midline, may spoil an otherwise perfectly effective rhinoplasty (Figs. 18-3, 18-4, and 18-9). The reasonable reduction of the alar cartilages, allowing for narrowing of the tip and blending into the nasal bridge line from the front, may not appear to blend into the bridge from the side unless the septal cartilage has been lowered somewhat below the level of the bridge higher up. Some have recommended a slight scooping out of the septum oppo-

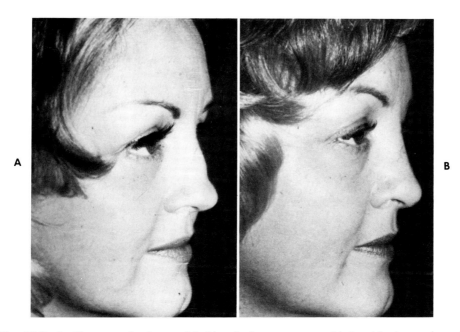

Fig. 18-7. A, Hypertrophy in nasal bridge in its upper two thirds with depression of nasal bridge in its lower third. Patient has wide nose and depression in lower portion due to traumatic fracture of nasal bones and septum. **B,** After lowering of upper portion of nasal bridge and augmentation with small cartilage graft from septum to lower portion of bridge. Columella strut was inserted for support of columella and tip as part of reconstruction of lower end of septum, which was deficient.

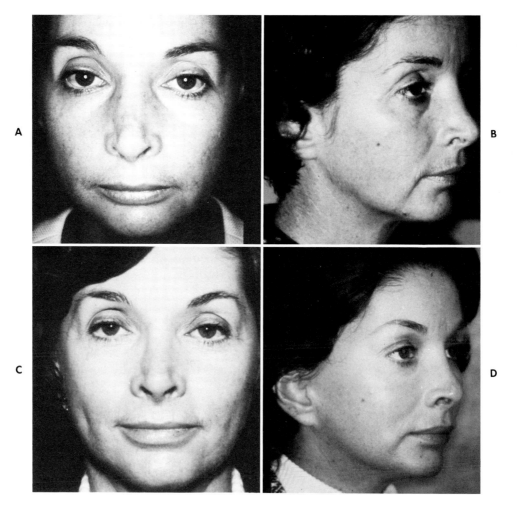

Fig. 18-8. A and **B,** Note flat, wide appearance of nose, including nasal bones and cartilages. Straight blow from front fractured nasal bones and septum, widening whole nasal complex. **C** and **D,** Postoperative views showing narrowing of nasal bones, including base and bridge, and of nasal tip. Columella strut has been inserted for support of tip. Nasal bridge has actually been heightened by moving nasal bones together, and it was necessary to reduce height of nasal bones by trim in bridge to maintain approximately same profile contour.

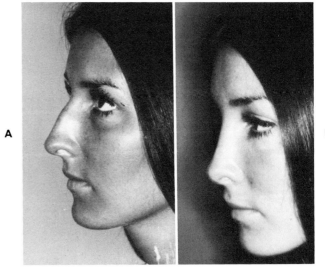

Fig. 18-9. A, Contour of profile is controlled in part also by lower lateral (alar) cartilages. Reduction in width of cartilages may also reduce height. Occasionally reduction at base of columella, resecting medial crurae at that point, may be required. Through-and-through resection of medial crurae at tip may also be carried out to reduce height of tip and to narrow tip (Fig. 13-4, *C*). **B,** After routine tip rhinoplasty, which accompanied relatively routine general corrective rhinoplasty with reduction of bridge.

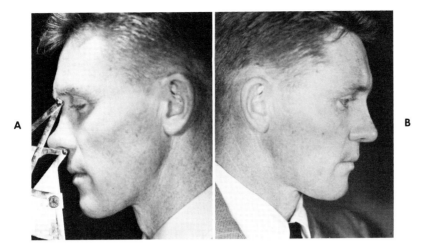

Fig. 18-10. A, Saddle nose with measurement by profilometer to determine amount of buildup in bridge. **B,** After cartilage graft to nasal bridge and to columella.

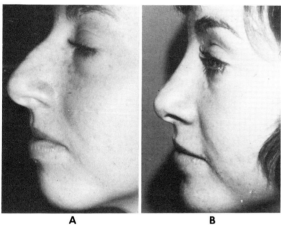

Fig. 18-11. A, Profile is also determined by contour of chin. Here corrective rhinoplasty has been carried out, reducing height of nasal bridge and augmentation of chin for recorrection of hypogenia. **B,** After heavy reduction of nasal bridge and shortening of whole length of end of septum to eradicate tendency to pull upper lip upward toward tip of nose, which gives longer appearance to upper lip. Chin has been augmented through small submental incision. It is usually important to undercorrect chin in augmentation mentoplasty.

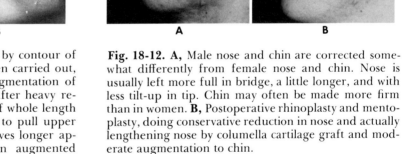

Fig. 18-12. A, Male nose and chin are corrected somewhat differently from female nose and chin. Nose is usually left more full in bridge, a little longer, and with less tilt-up in tip. Chin may often be made more firm than in women. **B,** Postoperative rhinoplasty and mentoplasty, doing conservative reduction in nose and actually lengthening nose by columella cartilage graft and moderate augmentation to chin.

site the top of the alar cartilages when the nasal bridge is being reduced. This may be effective, but it may also allow for a dip in the nasal bridge below that which is desired when all of the tissues have relaxed and the tip has dropped, after a period of months or as the patient grows older.

In my opinion a more effective and a safer method for routine use is a slight beveling down of the top of the septal cartilage when the nasal bridge is reduced. The tip of the septal cartilage

opposite the tip of the nose should be rounded off and not left pointed or prominent.

The excess fat in some nasal tips may delay or prevent the achievement of the desired contour in some instances. At the time of the reduction of the alar cartilages, a conservative and symmetric reduction of the fat in the tip may be carried out (Fig. 18-4), but overzealous reduction of the fat may be harmful.

The profile angle of the nasal tip should slant

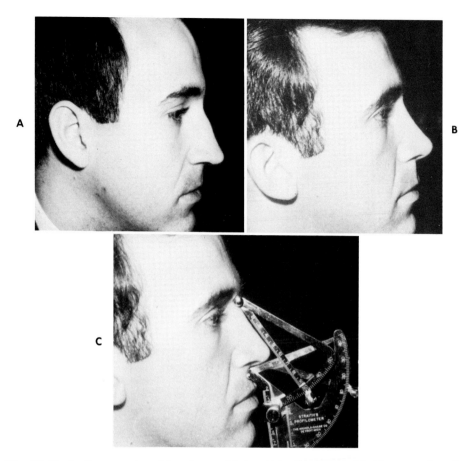

Fig. 18-13. A, Preoperative rhinoplasty with hypertrophy in nasal bridge, overhanging tip, and lack of columella support. Alae are longer than columella so that columella is lost in side view. It is not seen in front view unless head is tilted backward. **B,** After corrective rhinoplasty with reduction of bridge, narrowing of base, bridge and tip, and shortening in tip combined with columella implant to increase prominence of columella, which gives appearance of better proportioned width of nose, lip, forehead, and chin. **C,** Measurement with profilometer indicated acceptable measurement, although final judgment must be made by surgeon's eye.

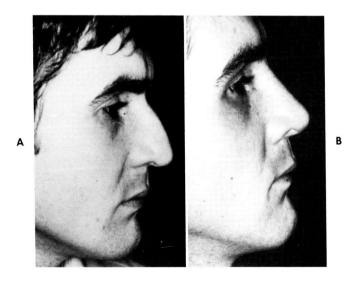

Fig. 18-14. A, Preoperative view of male nose showing adequate depth of columella, which perhaps is even too deep, hypertrophy of nasal bridge, and overhanging tip but with short base of columella. **B,** Corrective rhinoplasty including lowering of nasal bridge and tip, small augmentation to very top of nasal bridge in subglabellar notch, and cartilage graft at base of columella to give more prominence at base of columella. This increases appearance of tilt-up of tip and gives appearance of decreased length of upper lip from columella to vermilion border. Base of columella could be augmented more with improved result.

up from the upper lip at an angle of 5 to 15 degrees in men, or from 10 to 25 degrees in women, depending on the other aspects of facial contour. The shortening of the columella itself may be carried out by a simple elliptical through-and-through excision, then reapproximating the columella to the lower edge of the septum. The method most commonly employed is the trim of the lower end of the septum, reducing that part which is too prominent and slanting it upward to give the desired angle of the nasal tip, the columella-lip angle (Figs. 18-2, 18-3, 18-5, 18-6, and 18-11). Rounding of the lower end of the septum is preferred to a straight trim to give a more pleasing and a more natural look (Figs. 18-2 to 18-6, 18-9, 18-11, and 18-12).

The addition of cartilage from the septum into the columella may be required to give more prominence to the columella when this is deficient in support or when it is retracted (Figs. 18-7, 18-8, 18-10, 18-13, and 18-14). Often a small graft to the base of the columella will give a desirable result and make the nose appear to tilt up at the tip without actual shortening of the septum. A strut for the whole length of the columella, including the anterior maxillary spine, may be required, however.

The placement of the columella against the end of the septum may be varied without using forceful or strangulating sutures. If the columella is short, or if there is a groove or retrusion at the junction of columella and upper lip, the columella is advanced forward on the end of the septum. This will require enough dissection to free up the columella and will require free incisions between the base of the columella and the septum, and at times even into the floor of the nostrils to allow for more give. The addition of a small bone or cartilage graft in the area of the anterior maxillary spine will help. When the nasal tip is high or the septum has been lowered considerably, or when the alar cartilages themselves are long, the columella is brought downward on the end of the septum (Figs. 18-2, 18-3, 18-5, and 18-11). Whenever there is a large nasal hump, there is usually a need for this reverse advancement of the columella on the end of the septum. This is usually easy, but the incisions need extension to the base of the columella or even into the nostril floor bilaterally to allow for further give to bring the columella down on the end of the septum without tension and to assure its remaining in position. The use of small chromic catgut sutures will usually suffice, but nonabsorbable sutures may be used for longer support. I depend on the nasal splint to maintain the position for a week. If the alar cartilages themselves are long and have much spring, they keep pushing upward. The reduction of the alar cartilages at the tip reduces this tendency considerably, but complete section of the medial crurae may be required at the base of the columella or at the tip for the Pinocchio-type tip (Fig. 18-11).

MEASURING THE NOSE

The corrective rhinoplasty should always be performed to keep the nose consistent with the other facial features. Careful appraisal of the face should include the forehead, lips, chin, and cheeks, but the nose should fall within certain normal limits. The nose in both men and women should have approximately a 30-degree angle of the nasal bridge from the facial plane (the line extending from the pogonion through the nasion). It may be 35 degrees for a large man or one with large features (Figs. 18-1 and 18-13), or it may be 25 degrees for a small woman, especially if the face is petite as well (Figs. 18-1 to 18-3 and 18-6).

The tip angle (the angle of the columella at the upper lip) should be approximately 10 degrees (5 to 15 degrees) in the male nose and 17 degrees (10 to 25 degrees) in the female nose. However, it may be pleasing if it is varied somewhat from these measurements in individual cases. The teenage patient should have a higher tip angle than the adult, and treatment of the nose of the older patient should be the most conservative.

A rhinometer may be of great help to the surgeon, not only in planning the corrective rhinoplasty in the operating room, but also in showing the patient in the office at the consultation visit the measurements that are present and those which are desired. This is helpful during the office consultation in demonstrating to the patient those changes which are to be made, and it is also helpful to the surgeon in the operating room. It aids in determining the amount of hump to be removed and indicates the amount of buildup of the bridge for the saddle nose (Figs. 18-3, 18-6, 18-10, and 18-13).

For the past 20 years I have used the profilometer designed by Straith (Figs. 18-3, 18-6, 18-10, and 18-13). It is not a guide to be used without question or without utilizing one's sense of the aesthetic, for one must keep features of the face in mind as well as one's idea of proportion and symmetry, but it can be a considerable aid. It facilitates the planning of the rhinoplasty and checks on the surgeon's work once surgery has progressed (Figs. 18-6, 18-10, and 18-13).

The old adage, "A gadget or a machine is only as good as the man who uses it," certainly applies to a surgical instrument, only more so. Any type of measuring instrument that purports to guide the surgeon in determining the size of the nose and the angles of the nose can only be as good as the interpretation that the surgeon gives the measurements, the judgment to which these measurements are put, and the accuracy with which the surgery is performed. The usefulness of the rhinometer, and specifically the Straith profilometer, is limited by the surgeon's ability and judgment. It is a worthwhile additional instrument in the surgeon's armamentarium and specifically gives a quick way of judging the profile angle, the tip angle, and the degree to which the nose or any part of it may need raising, lowering, lengthening, or shortening.

CONCLUSION

The plastic surgeon's work is both an art and a science. He must study human anatomy, and art as well, to more nearly perfect his own art. To make his work more of an artistic science, he must take advantage of any planning, any study, and any instruments that may make his work more nearly perfect.

REFERENCES

1. Aufricht, G.: Combined plastic surgery of nose and chin, Am. J. Surg. **95:**231, 1958.
2. Conroy, W. C.: Simple nasal tip set back, Plast. Reconstr. Surg. **36:**48, 1965.
3. Gonzalez-Ulloa, M.: Planning the integral correction of the human profile, J. Internat. Coll. Surgeons **36:**364, 1961.
4. Joseph J.: Nasenplastik und Sonstige Gesichtsplastik, Leipzig, Germany, 1931, Curt Kabitzsch.
5. Lewis, J. R., Jr.: The surgery of scars, New York, 1963, McGraw-Hill Book Co.
6. Lewis, J. R., Jr.: An atlas of aesthetic plastic surgery, Boston, 1973, Little, Brown & Co.
7. Lewis, J. R., Jr.: The nasal profile, Panminerva Med. **2:**170, 1969.
8. Masters, F. W., and Lewis, J. R., Jr., editors: Symposium on aesthetic surgery of the nose, ears, and chin, vol. 6, St. Louis, 1973, The C. V. Mosby Co.
9. Millard, D. R.: Adjuncts in augmentation mentoplasty and corrective rhinoplasty, Plast. Reconstr. Surg. **36:**48, 1965.
10. Peck, G.: Corrective rhinoplasty: taaching session of American Society for Aesthetic Plastic Surgery, New Orleans, March, 1974.
11. Rees, T. D., and Wood-Smith, D.: Cosmetic facial surgery, Philadelphia, 1973, W. B. Saunders Co.
12. Safian, J.: Fact and fallacy in rhinoplasty surgery, Br. J. Surg. **11:**45, 1958.
13. Straith, C. L.: Personal communication, 1948.
14. Straith, C. L.: Reconstruction about the nasal tip, Am. J. Surg. **43:**223, 1939.
15. Straith, R. E.: Personal communication, 1963.

Chapter 19

Primary and secondary correction of the nasal tip

Franklin L. Ashley, M.D.

Many procedures have been advocated through the years for the correction of the deformed nasal tip, both primarily and secondarily. The multiplicity of these procedures would indicate that no one of them is the complete answer to the problem. In the following pages I have outlined my procedures for the primary correction of the deformed nasal tip and the secondary correction after surgery, including a procedure for augmenting the nasal tip and for removing the scar tissue in the region of the nasal tip and between the upper and lower lateral cartilages.

ROUTINE NASAL TIP PROCEDURE

This procedure of reduction rhinoplasty is accomplished after the nasal dorsum has been contoured but before the lateral nasal osteotomies and infracturing are performed.

The initial incisions are made in the intercartilaginous grooves and are extended onto the nasal septum at the junction of the membranous and cartilaginous septum. The septal incisions are continued inferiorly to the nasal spine, thus separating the membranous and cartilaginous septum. The dorsal bone, septal cartilage, and medial aspect of the upper lateral cartilages are appropriately contoured with scissors, osteotomes, and rasps. An 11 mm double hook is placed in the nasal ala near the dome, and pressure is exerted on the dome with the operator's middle finger to provide the proper exposure for the rim incision, which is made in the nasal vestibule at the free caudal border of the lower lateral cartilage (Fig. 19-1, *A* and *B*). This incision is also carried onto the membranous septum along the caudal border of the medial crus for a distance of 3 or 4 mm. While maintaining traction on the double hook and external finger pressure on the dome, the skin over-

lying the lower lateral cartilage is easily elevated from the cartilage by sharp and blunt dissection with the Ragnell scissors (Fig. 19-1, *C*). It is particularly important to the patient with thick skin and abundant fibrous tissue in the nasal tip to keep this dissection as close to the dermis as possible. This dissection continues well into the dome and frees the first few millimeters of the medial crus.

A retractor is then inserted in the intercartilaginous incision, and the tip of the retractor is pushed forward between the lower lateral cartilage and the skin and emerges from the rim incision (Fig. 19-1, *D*). This maneuver will evert the lower lateral cartilage into the nostril opening for maximal exposure. The fibroareolar tissue attached to the superior surface of the lower lateral cartilage is carefully removed from the cartilage with Stephens strabismus scissors (Fig. 19-1, *E*). Once this tissue has been removed, the entire lateral crus and dome of the lower lateral cartilage will be visible. An incision is then made in the lateral crus parallel to and 1 or 2 mm above the inferior rim of the cartilage (Fig. 19-1, *F*). The incision is continued into the dome and a few millimeters down on the medial crus. A small 2 mm double hook is placed in the midportion of the free inferior margin of the lower lateral cartilage for countertraction while the portion of the cartilage superior to the cartilage incision is separated from the underlying mucosa with Ragnell scissors (primarily a spreading rather than cutting action of the scissors) (Fig. 19-1, *G* to *I*). This results in resection of the superior four fifths to seven eighths of the lateral crus and dome of the lower lateral cartilage. An incision is then made in the mucosa of the dome from the upper margin of the cartilage to the intercartilaginous incision. This allows the nasal mucosa to conform readily to the new tip contour. The inferior

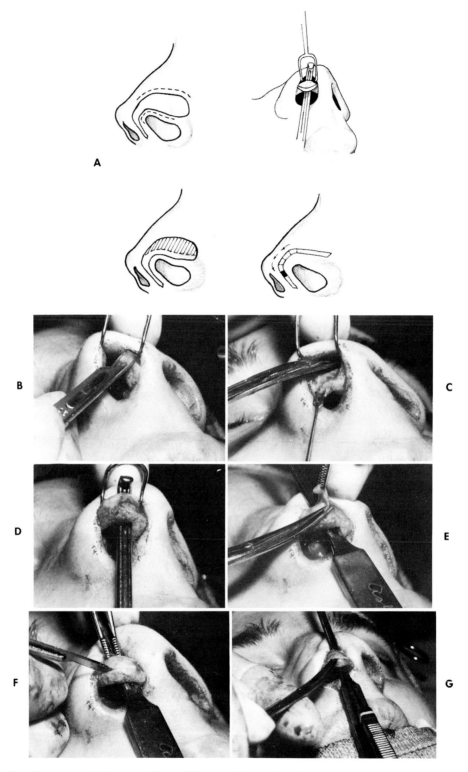

Fig. 19-1. A, Technique of tip revision and tip reduction. **B,** Rim incision. **C,** Freeing up bipedicle flap by blunt dissection. **D,** Everting and delivering bipedicle flap. **E,** Excision of subcutaneous soft tissue. **F,** Incising caudal margin, leaving 1 mm of cartilage. **G,** Freeing up dorsal segment of alar cartilage to be removed. **H,** Removing dorsal segment of alar cartilage. **I,** Incising mucosa but not removing it.

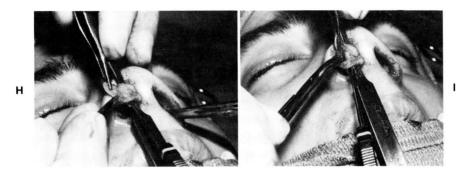

Fig. 19-1, cont'd. For legend see opposite page.

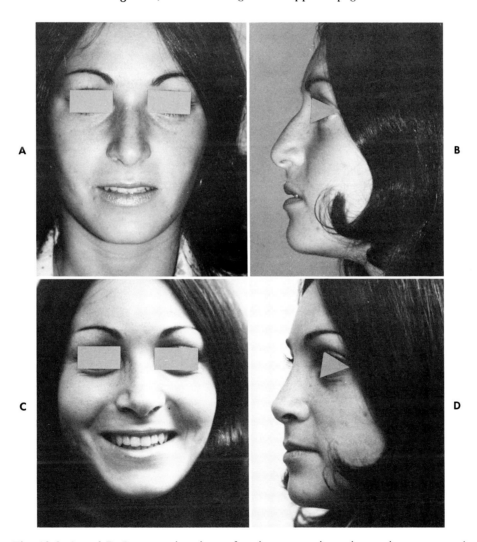

Fig. 19-2. A and **B,** Preoperative views of patient to receive primary tip reconstruction along with remainder of rhinoplasty. **C** and **D,** Postoperative views of same patient.

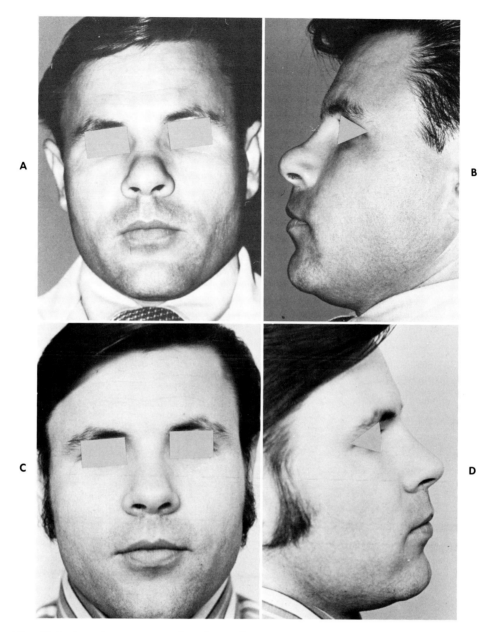

Fig. 19-3. A and **B,** Preoperative views of patient to receive tip reconstruction only. **C** and **D,** Postoperative views of same patient.

1 or 2 mm rim of the lower lateral cartilage remains intact and provides sufficient support to the ala to prevent postoperative collapse (Figs. 19-2 and 19-3).

If the nasal tip projects excessively, this may be corrected by resecting 1 to 4 mm of the medial crus just below the dome (Fig. 19-1, *A, lower right*). When this procedure is used, the dome must be recontoured by making three or four incisions part way through the remaining rim of cartilage in the area of the new dome. These incisions are spaced

1 or 2 mm apart and are perpendicular to the free inferior margin of the cartilage. The continuity of the medial crus is reestablished with a single suture of 5-0 catgut. It is unnecessary and unwise to remove any nasal lining in the area of cartilage resection in the medial crus.

If elevation of the nasal tip is desired, the appropriate amount of cartilage is excised from the free caudal margin of the nasal septum at the junction of the superior and caudal borders.

Lateral nasal osteotomies and infracturing are

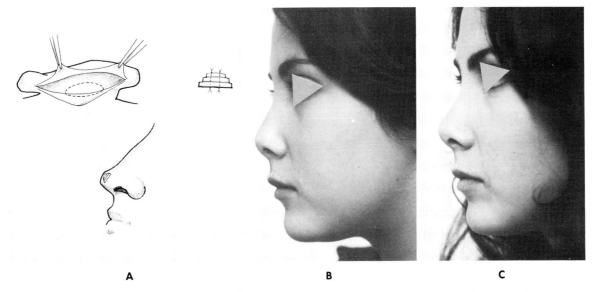

Fig. 19-4. A, Formation of autogenous cartilage grafts from ear and its placement in nasal tip by rim incision. **B,** Preoperative view of patient to receive cartilaginous augmentation to nasal tip. **C,** Postoperative view of same patient.

performed next. The rhinoplasty is completed by excising an elliptical wedge of membranous septum, approximating the membranous and cartilaginous septum with two 4-0 chromic mattress sutures, and closing the rim incisions with one or two 5-0 plain catgut sutures. A dorsal nasal splint of tape and aluminum is applied, and Polysporin ointment is placed in both nostrils. No nasal packs are used unless major septal resection to correct airway obstruction has been performed.

SECONDARY RHINOPLASTY
Correction of shortened tip

A 5 to 10 mm incision is made in the dome of the right nostril, and a subcutaneous pocket is dissected with a Ragnell scissors in the tip of the nose. A postauricular incision is made over the concha of the ear, and a generous ellipse of conchal cartilage is excised. This cartilage is cut into three or four pieces of decreasing size, and the segments are placed on top of each other to form a pyramid. Two sutures of 5-0 plain catgut are used to unite this pyramidal autogenous cartilage graft. The pyramid is placed in the preformed pocket with the base resting on the tip of the nasal septum. The nasal mucosa is closed with 5-0 plain catgut, and Polysporin ointment is placed in the nostril. We routinely administer 500 mg of erythromycin intravenously during the operative procedure and continue oral administration of 250 mg of erythromycin, qid, for 5 days postoperatively (Fig. 19-4).

Correction of the supratip hump

This procedure consists of a composite resection of scar, fibroareolar tissue, and a portion of the cephalad segment of the medial crus and dome of the lower lateral cartilages. Bilateral incisions are made in the medial portion of the intercartilaginous septum and are carried down onto the nasal septum at the junction of the cartilaginous and membranous septum, and a through-and-through V-shaped portion of the membranous septum is resected. The apex of the V is directed inferiorly toward the nasal spine. The base of the V usually includes a portion of the cephalad edge of the medial crus and dome of the lower lateral cartilage. The dissection proceeds upward into the supratip hump immediately beneath the skin, removing all scar and excessive fibrous tissue in this area. A small V-shaped wedge of nasal mucosa is also removed from the intercartilaginous groove. The apex of this V is directed laterally, and the base of the V is the area of the supratip hump. The entire mass of tissue is removed as a single specimen. The columella is sutured to the septum with two 4-0 chromic mattress sutures. Polysporin ointment is placed in both nares, and a dorsal tape splint is applied to the nose (Fig. 19-5).

Combined procedure

Fig. 19-6 represents a combination of the routine nasal tip procedure, secondary rhinoplasty, and autogenous cartilage graft to nasal tip.

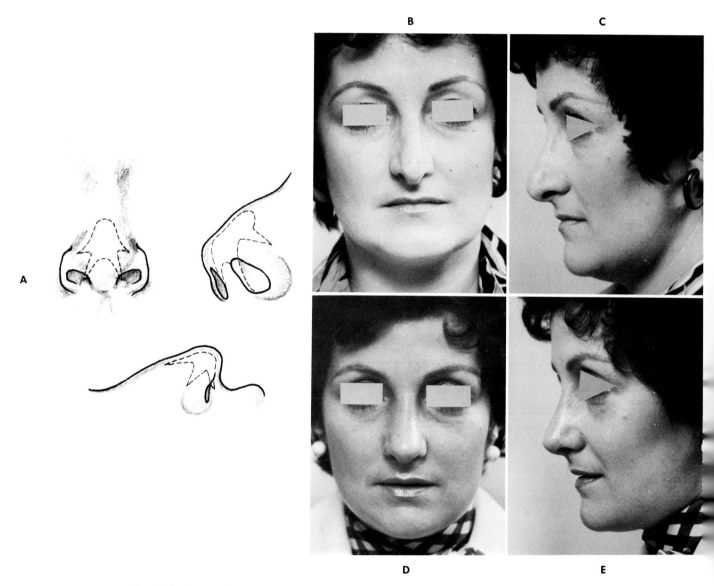

Fig. 19-5. A, Double-wing excision of scar, soft tissue, and dorsum of septum for secondary supratip hump correction. **B** and **C,** Preoperative views of patient to receive double-wing procedure. **D** and **E,** Postoperative views of same patient.

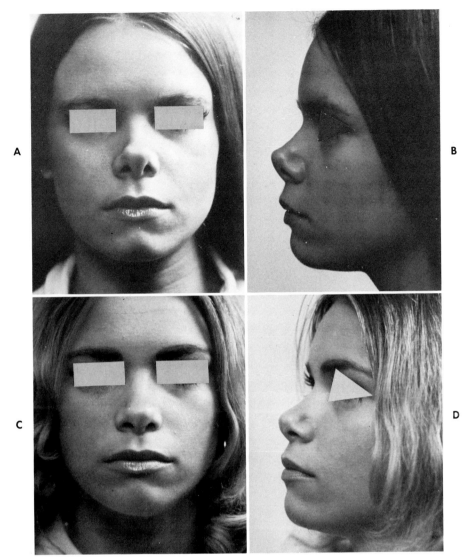

Fig. 19-6. A and **B,** Preoperative views of patient to receive combined procedure. **C** and **D,** Postoperative views of same patient.

SUMMARY

In the preceding pages I have outlined my procedures for the primary and secondary correction of the nasal tip, both before and after surgery, and for the correction of the congenitally deformed nasal tip. These procedures have been simplified, and I hope they will be of help to some of the younger surgeons in our specialty, but by no means do they offer the complete answer to these complex problems.

Discussion

Sheen: I enjoyed Dr. Ashley's pictures. There is one thing I would like to point out, and this is on the supratip area. Whenever you lack skeletal support, I don't care how much scar tissue you find, you're not going to correct the problem. The problem is that you're always saying to the patient, "You're forming scar tissue," when actually the contractility of the tissue is not such that it will drape over the skeleton. So I say, never attempt this in the supratip area, as it lacks skeletal support. I think we showed this morning that skeletal support was lacking and the supratip was there, yet the supratip area already had been thinned out. If you keep thinning out a supratip area, you can only add to the scarring. These supratip areas have been thinned out three times without the doctor realizing the fundamental point I'm trying to make, and that is you must have skeletal support for the tissues to drape properly. Thank you.

Millard: There are ways and ways of excising supratip scarring, and, of course, if you leave it in the right place and take it in the right place, as you saw in the case that Frank showed, you can improve the condition. But if you take it from the wrong place, you get what Jack is warning you about.

Peterson: Ralph, let me make one comment. I don't do this on all cases. I've been interested in the procedure described by Ashley and have been trying to compare it to see whether it really did have any advantages.

Millard: What do you think?

Peterson: I think it's a good operation for holding the tip of the nose up, but I don't think that's the whole answer. You saw Peck resolve the problem in a couple of these and they're just as good—intracartilaginous or by any other technique, whether it is Ralph's or Jack Anderson's, is probably as good or superior.

Millard: So what would you tell your young residents? What is their reaction? Most of my residents think the intracartilaginous incision is the easiest.

Peterson: I might say one other thing about Dr. Ashley. You know, we have experts in the world on China and Russia, but I'm one of the world's experts on Ashley because I was one of his residents. His first 800 rhinoplasties took him an hour and sometimes an hour and a half to do as a real superperfectionist. Now having done many thousands more, he has reduced it to 20 minutes, and that's okay.

Peck: Over the last 10 to 15 years, we have come to realize that we don't like to violate the nasal tip, that we like to leave the alar cartilage continuity. This is possible when using the transcartilaginous or intracartilaginous incision, whichever you prefer to call it. Dr. Ashley has just shown us a rimming incision, and with a rimming incision, you expose the cartilage so it can be seen better. However, at one point, Rex came to me and said that he had watched our procedure and had gone home and tried it. He mentioned that he had some problems with the rimming incision. Well, maybe Dr. Ashley doesn't have a problem, and maybe we can learn something that would make it easier. Let us remember that in the nose, where there is a slightly bulbous tip and where we don't need a tremendous reduction as in a Pinocchio tip or the real wide bulbous tip, I feel that we should not violate the tip. Maybe we can get some kind of answer about the advantages or disadvantages of a rimming incision versus the transcartilaginous incision.

Peterson: May I give a 30-second talk on this? I believe with all my heart that any time you can avoid a rimming incision, it is better. I think you should get less scar on the tip, and you preserve one part of the tip of the nose that is unviolated. And if you can do the rhinoplasty and reduce that tip without the rim incision, as well as an intracartilaginous or intercartilaginous, I think the patient will be better off.

Millard: I see absolutely no need for rim incision. I find it difficult besides it being very close to the edge and possibly a little bit dangerous; it is difficult to dissect your tissues if you cut in front of the cartilage. If you cut through the cartilage, you get to the perichondrium, and several sweeps and you're free. Now, if you've done a cartilage splitting, intra instead of intercartilaginous incision, you cut through the cartilage at the point at which you will probably reduce all above it. And with three sweeps, you've got it clear and all is easy. Then you take your two-pronged hook and turn this inside out, and with two sweeps you've got the anterior part exposed completely. You can trim it as you wish under direct vision. If you have to take away the medial crus, which is usually not necessary, you can get at it. It is not necessary in my opinion to cut it free as a dangling flap or strap and bring it out in your hand. You can see it just as well from this incision, and you've made one less scar.

Sheen: Can I say a word? I have used the rimming incision now for about twelve years, and I use Dr. Peck's incision. I feel that the intracartilaginous incision applies to perhaps 10% or 15% of those cases that have ideal tip configuration. Now, when you make an intracartilaginous incision, you are committed, and if you use the Peck technique where you shove a cotton swab under the cupula and you make that incision, you are committed, and if you make it thin enough, you've attenuated the dome. If it actually changes the basal perimeter, you've got unnatural length, in fact. Furthermore, if you make the intracartilaginous incision, you have no chance of changing the basal perimeter to a softly triangular one. Now, to say that doing a rim incision violates tissues is really not quite true because thousands of rhinoplasties are being done every year using this technique successfully. I could show you—in fact, when I present my case on finesse, every case I show you will be through a rim incision, and many of them will have tissue resected from the dome. So I would just like to have a plug for the rim incision.

Millard: Fine. I want to correct one point, Jack. I didn't mean trauma in the sense of cutting or making an incision. I make marginal incisions quite often. What I mean is when you've made an incision that close to the rim and freed the lining, your actual marginal rim is at the mercy

of that flap, and if you take out too much cartilage or lining and produce any tension, the discrepancy will cause a greater effect on that rim. If you've gotten back a bit and left your skin, subcutaneous tissue, and a little rim of cartilage intact, a little further up, that's your safety margin.

Lewis: I feel as Ralph does that an intracartilaginous or an intercartilaginous incision gives you an adequate exposure of the cartilage. You simply turn it down and work on the outside of the cartilage rather than the underside of the cartilage. I don't think you commit yourself any more; Ralph and I seem to do a number of noses and actually do a little trimming in front of that incision, and are not committed. There is another thing I wanted to mention. There are two reasons for the dimpling in Rex's surgical technique of the split cartilage. One, you take too much lining or else you take cartilage a little too far down so that you're getting scar tissue formation with contraction. If you leave the cartilage a little longer and preferably bevel it from the tip down towards the alar rather than straight across, and leave a little more mucosa—less lining out than cartilage, in other words—there should be no problem.

Conroy: I just wanted to say that the dimpling I saw preoperatively was dimpling over the sesamoid cartilage and not over the lateral crus at all. Even if you took the entire lateral crus out, it wouldn't effect the dimpling.

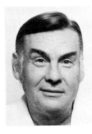

Dr. Ashley

Ashley: I think as I said at the beginning of my talk, we are all talking about pretty much the same thing. We're just approaching it a little differently. For instance, I've tried several hundred of the modified eversion techniques that others are using, but in my hands, it didn't give me enough exposure so that I could do the things that I wanted to when I worked on the cartilage. If I wanted to raise that tip out from the face and the columella diameter, I could do it much more accurately when I was looking right at it— the margin—rather than having it everted. If I wanted to depress it, I could do the same thing.

So it gave me a lot more leeway than using the everted technique that I used in several hundred cases. Since then, I've done several hundred more, maybe more than that, using the rim incision, and it isn't exactly at the rim. If you study anatomy of this lower lateral cartilage and the anatomy of the nose, its anterior margins are further than you think from the margin of the ala. I don't think it is difficult to dissect at all, as Ralph said. You just go in on one side of the midseptum toward the tip and the other side, and cut that with the scissors, it comes right out.

All you have to do is remove the fat. So as I say, in my hands and in the hands of some of my residents who use this technique and others, we've had very few complications. We suture the margins after we get everything in position so that we don't have any overlap or any failure in apposition. I think that the younger ones of you, especially when you're learning, might examine this approach carefully, because it certainly gives you a better view of what you intend to do if you want a little leeway.

Chapter 20

Tip rhinoplasty by composite alar resection

Rex A. Peterson, M.D.

Reduction of the alar cartilages to remodel the nasal tip by a simultaneous resection of desired portions of the alar cartilages and their contiguous mucosal lining may produce aesthetic results comparable to any other method of tip rhinoplasty.

This, or similar, operative maneuvers have been described by Webster[2] as a "lateral crural flap" (of alar cartilage) and by Serson-Neto[1] in a presentation at the American Society for Aesthetic Plastic Surgery in 1971. Both surgeons reported excellent tip contours, which stimulated me to use the operation in fifty-two cases.

In this series of patients the nasal tip reduction was the first step in the aesthetic rhinoplasty, excepting those who had a septoplasty or submucous resection, in which the septal surgery was completed first.

Reduction of the tip before the other osseocartilaginous portions of the nose allows the surgeon to adjust the profile of the septum, lateral cartilages, and nasal bones to whatever position is aesthetically pleasing in relation to the tip. If the tip is reduced at the end of the operation, one may encounter difficulty adapting the tip to the already reduced profile.

OPERATIVE TECHNIQUE: COMPOSITE ALAR RESECTION

1. The first maneuver is an incision in the membranous septum at the caudal edge of the quadrilateral cartilage, first on one side, then on the other to free the columella. These are individually extended laterally as intercartilaginous incisions to separate the alar from the lateral cartilages and the caudal end of the septum.

2. Next, a cartilage-splitting incision is made in the lateral crus of each side. These are extended medially to remove approximately half the width of each alar dome and continued inferiorly in the medial crura to remove 3 or 4 mm of these. Then the lateral crural flaps are incised transversely, *superior to the cartilage-splitting incision,* to join the intracartilaginous incision at a place that is about the midpoint of the lateral crus (Fig. 20-1). Then this island of the superior portion of the alar cartilage is removed with its mucosal lining *attached and intact.* Fine judgment is required to place the cartilage-splitting incisions and lateral crural flap dividing incisions at the best levels. Certainly adequate alar cartilage and nasal lining must be preserved. One would not want a deficiency of mucosa in the area of the alar domes.

3. Composite alar reduction of the nasal tip alters what may be called the dynamics of the interrelationship of the structures about the nasal tip. The tip will assume a higher, more upward-tilted position just by the maneuvers already described. One should *rarely* resect any portion of the caudal edge of the septum in this operation and almost *never* remove a triangle of the caudal angle of the septum to tilt the nose, or it will be too short with an excessive, objectionable upward tilt.

The septum usually should be reduced only along the profile line and its mucosa left high to attach to the lining at the alar domes (Figs. 20-2 and 20-3).

The caudal edges of the lateral cartilages should not be reduced (or excised) to avoid valvular pinching.

In my cases, the lateral cartilages and their mucosal attachments were divided from the septum by scissors cutting before lowering the profile by removing a portion of septum and osseocartilaginous junction with an osteotome.

However, I am now convinced that it is highly desirable to leave intact the mucosal junction of the lateral

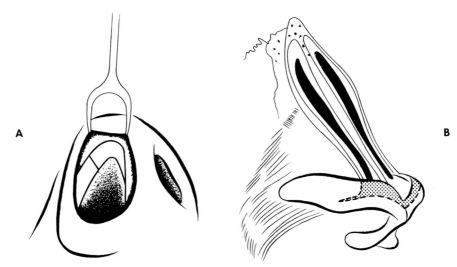

Fig. 20-1. A, Incision lines for composite alar resection showing *intercartilaginous* incision (lower curve), *cartilage-splitting* incision (upper curve), and vertical or lateral crural flap incision all joining to form *island* of alar mucosa and lining to be resected intact. **B,** Stippled area reveals that portion of alar cartilage and mucosa incised and to be removed. Also shown is profile of nose lowered by quadrilateral cartilage resection and osteotomy.

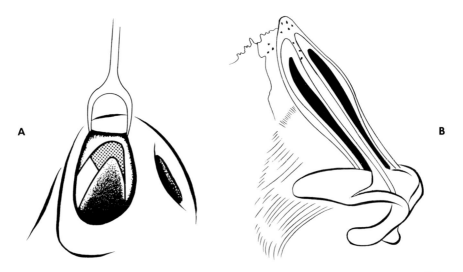

Fig. 20-2. A, Stippled area represents alar mucosa and cartilage to be removed. Sufficient alar rim and dome are preserved for support. Usually preserved rim is about 5 mm wide laterally (but may be more) and at least half width of alar dome. **B,** Composite alar resection completed, with lateral crural flap remaining.

cartilages with the septum to preserve normal valvular architecture and avoid supra-alar pinching that results from contracture of scar binding the laterals to the septum. Any reduction of the lateral cartilages along the profile line is best accomplished after dissecting the mucoperichondrium away from the cartilages and septum—before resection—no matter what methods are employed for reducing and remodeling the nasal tip and other nasal parts.

4. After reduction of the profile and lateral osteotomies to remodel the nasal bones, the composite flaps of the superior portions of the lateral crura are trimmed slightly to shape the cartilage tips. The mucosal edges of the alar domes are sutured to the mucosa at the caudal angle of the septum bilaterally (Fig. 20-4, *A*). These are the key sutures for anchoring the position of the tip (Fig. 20-4, *B*). The septum is then sutured, and other

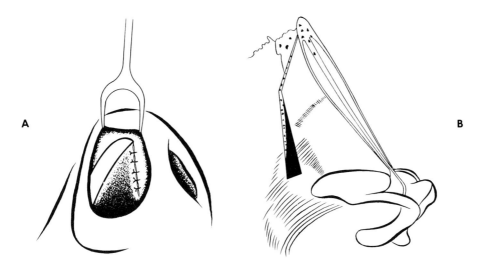

Fig. 20-3. A, Columella has been sutured to septum. Key suture, placed first, is stitch anchoring mucosa of caudal angle of septum to alar dome area. Lateral crura flap moves medially adjacent to septum. **B,** Lateral osteotomies have been completed. Lateral crural flaps are in medial positions. In taping nose for splinting, one must *not* permit these flaps to overlap septum.

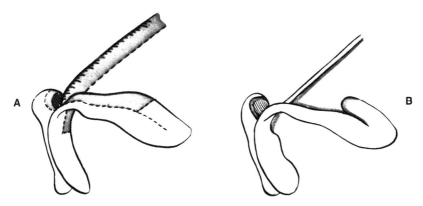

Fig. 20-4. Resection of alar cartilage and mucosa and lateral crural flap. *Most importantly,* none of caudal edge of quadrilateral cartilage or its mucosa has been removed. To do so would cause tip of nose to be too high.

sutures may be placed in osteotomy incisions if desired. The flaps of the superior portions of the alars drift medially, and supra-alar pinching does not occur unless the caudal edges of the lateral cartilages have been shortened, the mucosa of the laterals have been separated from the septum, or there was an overzealous composite alar resection.

The composite alar resection has an unusual lifting power, which can produce a fine, nicely tilted nose without complication if the dynamics of the procedure are understood.

PROBLEMS AND COMPLICATIONS

Four types of problems occurred in these fifty-two patients:

Tip drop. In three patients over 45 years of age, all of whom had long noses and inelastic skin, the tip dropped slightly so that the nasolabial angle was 90 degrees or less.

Supraalar dimples. Eight patients had mild dimpling or indentation in the supraalar areas, none of which could be considered disfiguring or detracting from the aesthetic result as judged by the patient. However, the surgeon was more critical.

Two patients had supra-alar pinching or indentation to a degree considered a poor result by the surgeon. These may have resulted from detachment of the lateral cartilages and mucosa from the septum combined with excision of some of the caudal margins of the lateral cartilages. These maneuvers and the composite excision of alar lining and cartilage may well have caused the contracture and lateral wall indentation.

Asymmetry of alar cartilages. One patient with pinching deformity described above had objectionable asymmetry of the alar domes; another had mild asymmetry.

Supratip convexity. Five patients had objectionable supratip convexity and subcutaneous scarring. Three of these had open-flap rhinoplasties, which contributes to this problem. Four of the five required minor secondary excision of scar between the skin and the quadrilateral cartilage.

DISCUSSION: SOME CAUSES OF SUPRA-ALAR PINCHING

Many people who never had a rhinoplasty have deep indentations above the alar cartilages, but when this occurs after rhinoplasty, it is a sure clue that the nose has been operated on. This stigma should be avoided because any postoperative nasal deformity tends to worsen with the passage of time. Years later, the alar domes become more pointed and the supra-alar indentations deeper.

Supra-alar indentation may be only a dimple, but it can be severe and deforming. In my opinion, it may most often result from overresection (or any resection) of the inferior (or caudal) edges of the

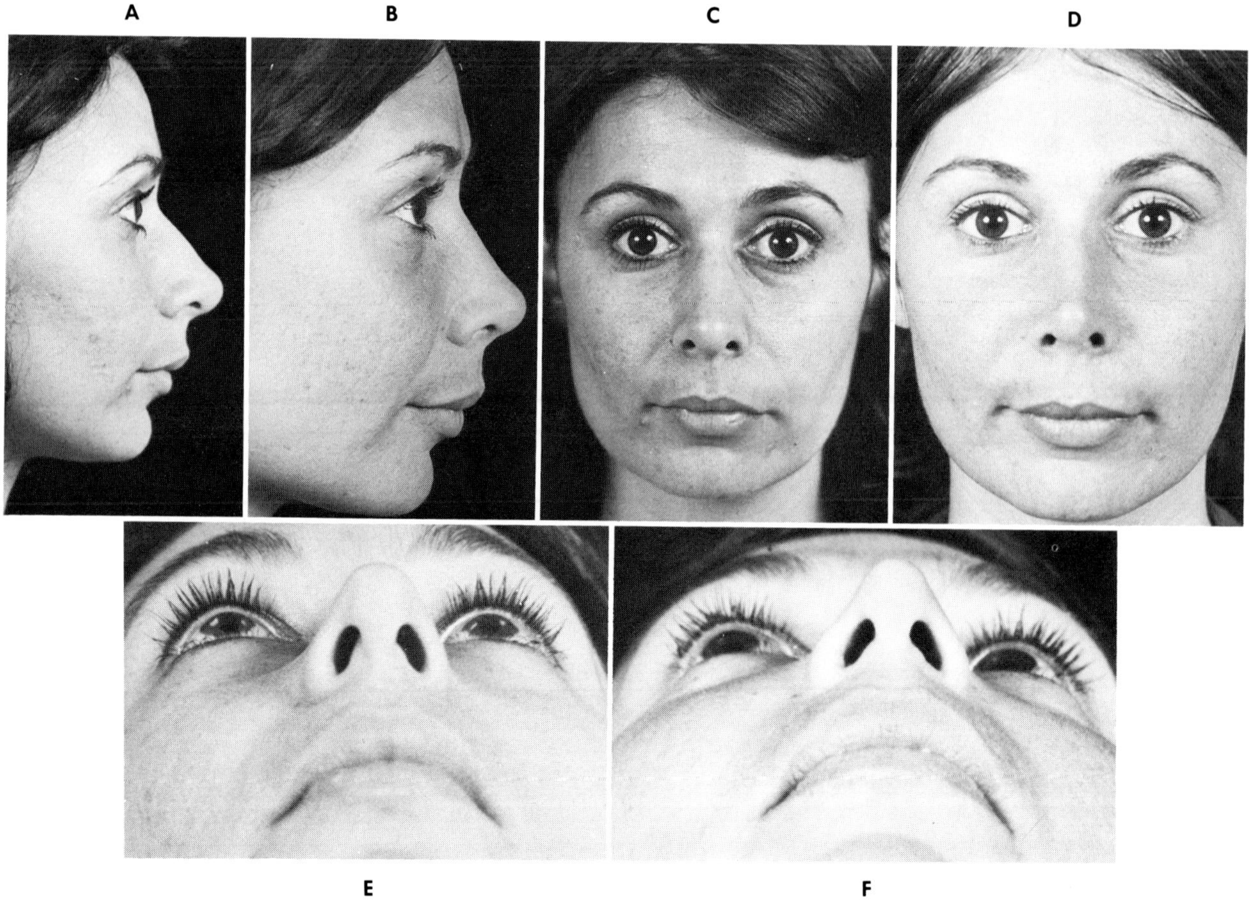

Fig. 20-5. P. A., 26 years old, with old nasal fracture with deviated septum and nasal obstruction, wide medial alar crura, and narrow lateral alar crura. Submucous resection, septoplasty, and rhinoplasty were performed; minimal portions of alar cartilages were removed by Serson technique. Patient did not want chin implant. Postoperative photographs were taken 3 months after surgery. **A,** Lateral preoperative view. **B,** Lateral postoperative view. **C,** Frontal preoperative view. **D,** Frontal postoperative view. **E,** Basal preoperative view. **F,** Basal postoperative view.

lateral cartilages and/or mucosa, which scar to the superior edges of partially resected lateral alar crura. Both together contract inward to the cut edge of the lowered quadrilateral cartilage. This may result in bilateral supra-alar pinching, valvular airway obstruction, and a contracting scar under the skin that thickens and raises the skin profile (although the quadrilateral cartilage is low enough).

This sequential contracture and the pinching deformity can be avoided principally by maintaining after operation a close-to-normal architecture at the junction of the caudal edge of the lateral cartilages and the quadrilateral cartilage. This can be aided by preserving undamaged the mucoperichondrial continuity at these areas and by avoiding any resection of the caudal edges of the lateral cartilages, by not resecting too much quadrilateral cartilage, and by avoiding taking out too much of any structure in the tip area.

Supra-alar pinching may thus occur from removing too much lateral cartilage, too much alar cartilage, too much quadrilateral cartilage, *too much mucosa* in any of these areas, or too much of *both* cartilage and mucosa.

How does this concept relate to the composite alar resection? Although mucosal lining may not be removed in some rhinoplasties by some surgeons, it does not necessarily occur that removing alar mucosa with alar cartilage, if the amount is judicious and the design for excision appropriate, will result in any deformity of the nasal tip. In fact, the amount of mucosa removed in the composite alar resection does not differ significantly from that excised in the single cartilage-splitting incision operation; however, the design or shape of the lining removed in the latter procedure may be more anatomically appropriate.

The composite alar cartilage resection for tip rhinoplasty may well give excellent contours of the

Text continued on p. 178.

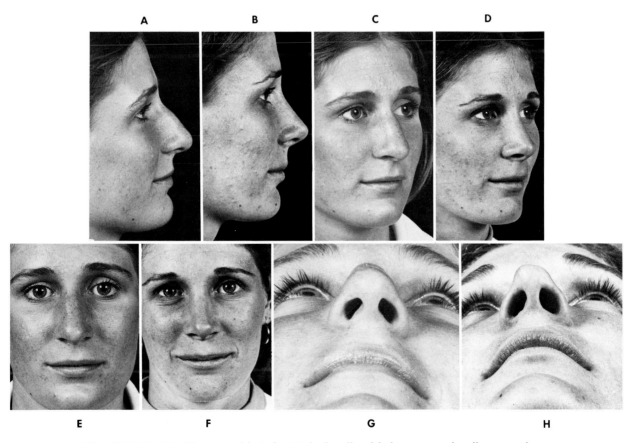

Fig. 20-6. M. K., 19 years old, 5 feet 1 inch tall, with large nose in all proportions. Rhinoplasty was performed. Postoperative photographs were taken 3 years after surgery. **A,** Lateral preoperative view. **B,** Lateral postoperative view. **C,** Oblique preoperative view. **D,** Oblique postoperative view. **E,** Frontal preoperative view. **F,** Frontal postoperative view. **G,** Basal preoperative view. **H,** Basal postoperative view.

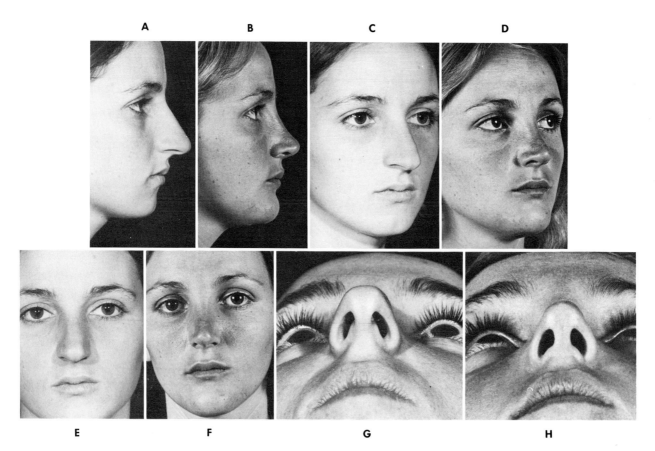

Fig. 20-7. K. D., 24 years old, with long thrusting nasal tip, alar domes separated, large alar cartilages, acute nasolabial angle, short upper lip, and small chin. Rhinoplasty was performed with alar wedges and chin augmentation. Postoperative photographs were taken 18 months after surgery. **A,** Lateral preoperative view. **B,** Lateral postoperative view. **C,** Oblique preoperative view. **D,** Oblique postoperative view. **E,** Frontal preoperative view. **F,** Frontal postoperative view. **G,** Basal preoperative view. **H,** Basal postoperative view.

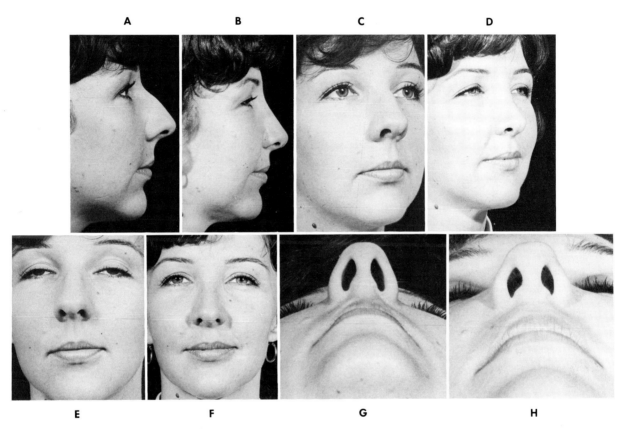

Fig. 20-8. D. L. H., 31 years old, 5 feet 9 inches tall, with nasal obstruction due to deviated septum and good nasolabial angle. Patient desired preservation of crease between alar cartilages. Simultaneous submucous resection, septoplasty, and rhinoplasty with alar wedges were performed. Postoperative photographs were taken 18 months after surgery. **A,** Lateral preoperative view. **B,** Lateral postoperative view. **C,** Oblique preoperative view. **D,** Oblique postoperative view. **E,** Frontal preoperative view. **F,** Frontal postoperative view. **G,** Basal preoperative view. **H,** Basal postoperative view.

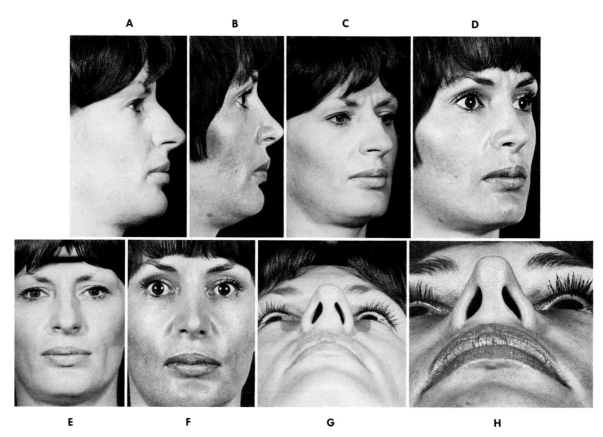

Fig. 20-9. C. W., 31 years old, had history of childhood nasal fracture and had nasal obstruction due to deviated septum and asymmetric alae and nares. Simultaneous submucous resection, septoplasty, and rhinoplasty with alar wedges were performed. Postoperative photographs were taken 18 months after surgery. **A,** Lateral preoperative view. **B,** Lateral postoperative view. **C,** Oblique preoperative view. **D,** Oblique postoperative view. **E,** Frontal preoperative view. **F,** Frontal postoperative view. **G,** Basal preoperative view. **H,** Basal postoperative view.

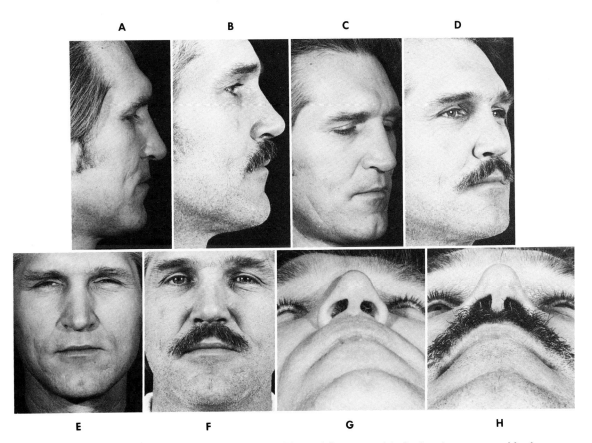

Fig. 20-10. R. D. L., 42 years old, had old nasal fracture with deviated septum residual after previous submucous resection, rhinoplasty, and removal of right frontal boss (over frontal sinus). Postoperative photographs were taken a year after surgery. **A,** Lateral preoperative view. **B,** Lateral postoperative view. **C,** Oblique preoperative view. **D,** Oblique postoperative view. **E,** Frontal preoperative view. **F,** Frontal postoperative view. **G,** Basal preoperative view. **H,** Basal postoperative view.

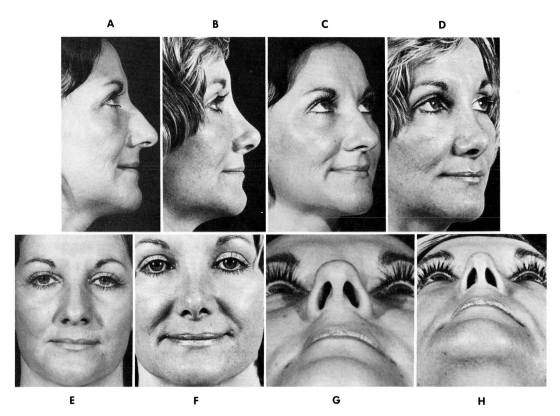

Fig. 20-11. G. M., 30 years old, with nose large in all proportions and deviated nasal septum with nasal airway obstruction. Submucous resection, septoplasty, and rhinoplasty were performed. Postoperative photographs were taken 8 months after surgery. **A,** Lateral preoperative view. **B,** Lateral postoperative view. **C,** Oblique preoperative view. **D,** Oblique postoperative view. **E,** Frontal preoperative view. **F,** Frontal postoperative view. **G,** Basal preoperative view. **H,** Basal postoperative view.

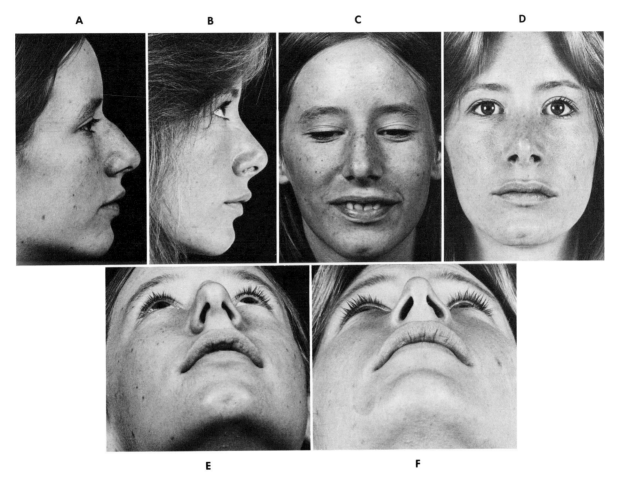

Fig. 20-12. K. C., 15 years old, with deviated nasal septum and nasal obstruction. Submucous resection, septoplasty, and rhinoplasty were performed. Postoperative photographs were taken 4 years after surgery. **A,** Lateral preoperative view. **B,** Lateral postoperative view. **C,** Frontal preoperative view. **D,** Frontal postoperative view. **E,** Basal preoperative view. **F,** Basal postoperative view.

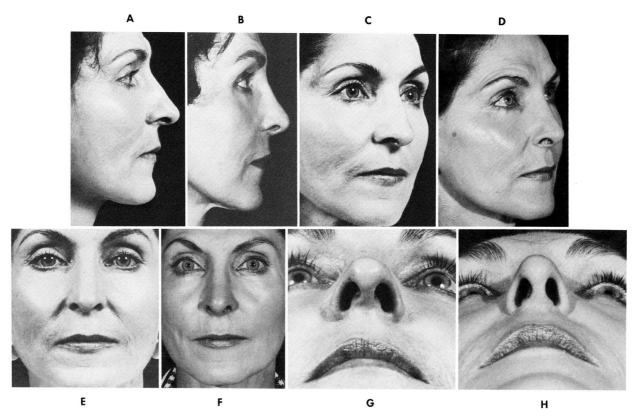

A
B
C
D

E
F
G
H

Fig. 20-13. J. K., 50 years old, with long projecting tip. Rhinoplasty was performed. Postoperative photographs were taken 6 months after surgery. **A,** Lateral preoperative view. **B,** Lateral postoperative view. **C,** Oblique preoperative view. **D,** Oblique postoperative view. **E,** Frontal preoperative view. **F,** Frontal postoperative view. **G,** Basal preoperative view. **H,** Basal postoperative view.

nasal tip and prevent drop of the tip postoperatively. It is most important, if one uses this method, to avoid removing a triangle of quadrilateral cartilage and mucosa at its caudal angle, or there will be insufficient mucosa for repair without deforming the nasal tip. Rarely is any portion of the caudal end of the septum excised, and then only if there is an unusually long convexity of the columella.

Figs. 20-5 to 20-13 illustrate a spectrum of good results that may be expected from this method.

CHANGE IN TECHNIQUE

Since the symposium at which this subject was presented, I have changed my nasal tip plasty technique, but not because of any dissatisfaction with the alar composite resection.

I prefer now a single alar cartilage-splitting incision for removal of the desired portions of the alar cartilage (as in Millard's method) and a submucoperichondrial dissection of the upper lateral cartilage and that portion of the profile edge of

the quadrilateral cartilage to be removed (as in Jack Anderson's method) to keep the mucosa in continuity. I do not resect the caudal edges of the lateral cartilages and seldom make a medial osteotomy between the nasal bones and the vertical plate of the ethmoid (as in Sheen's method). Lateral osteotomies alone *do* narrow the nose, as Sheen says, and I could not agree more with his level of osteotomy, since I have for years kept my osteotomies low at the pyriform apertures and aimed for the medial ends of the brows, which gives great facility in accomplishing clean osteotomy fractures.

There were many other ideas at the symposium that I have found to have excellent merit in rhinoplastic surgery.

REFERENCES

1. Serson-Neto, D.: Presentation, American Society of Aesthetic Plastic Surgery, Boston, 1971.
2. Webster, R. C.: Study course on rhinoplasty, American Society of Aesthetic Plastic Surgery, Newport Beach, Calif., 1973.

Discussion

Participant: Am I to believe that in the fifty-two cases from Dr. Peterson there was no airway problem?

Peterson: There is no airway problem, no stenosis, and I should have had and don't have some intranasal pictures of that lining afterward. There is absolutely no stenosis.

Millard: Dr. Converse?

Converse: I haven't said anything much during the discussion, but I do want to say that I think one of the things we must think of is that if a surgeon uses a certain type of technique and uses that technique all the time, he gets very good at it. Many surgeons, who in essence are rhinoplasticians, have techniques they prefer. We try to be selective in the different types of tip operations. I think this is something you must bear in mind. You use a certain technique, and you get good at it. There is one thing that I would like to point out which in my way of thinking is absolutely essential. One of the basic rules of rhinoplasty is not to remove any lining of the vestibule, which risks the creation of raw areas, open to infection, eventually causing scar tissue and other complications. Now, in the large noses, occasionally you can, but very rarely.

Chapter 21

The septum in rhinoplasty
form and function

Mark Gorney, M.D.

Form follows function.
> Frank Lloyd Wright

In contrast to Frank Lloyd Wright's classic architectural dictum, quite the opposite applies in rhinoseptoplasty: function is almost wholly dependent on form.

No one's septum is really straight. Hereditary, birth, and repetitive trauma all combine to give most of us some degree of septal irregularity[13] (Fig. 21-1). As long as the nasal vault is adequate, it does not bother us. However, it is self-evident that any narrowing or lowering of that vault without simultaneous correction will lead to some limitation of air flow. The externally deviated nose cries for both aesthetic as well as functional correction. What we are concerned with here is the essentially straight or slightly deviated nose inside of which there is a potential for both functional and aesthetic disaster. You cannot straighten a crooked nose without correcting the septum; you can create a crooked nose if you do not correct the septum.

A structurally sound and straight septum is the foundation of a satisfactory rhinoplasty result. As obvious as this may seem, there is still a substantial degree of disagreement among plastic surgeons on appropriate corrective techniques. There is also some misunderstanding of nasal physiology, particularly around the valve area, and sometimes there is a cavalier disregard for the integrity of the nasal airway. I suspect a much higher degree of obstructive complications than those officially reported in the literature. In other words, it's nice to make them beautiful, but can they breathe?

The ear, nose, and throat literature is replete

with references going back to the turn of the century. The key articles* have been reviewed.

In the plastic surgery literature, Converse's masterful and detailed coverage of the subject stands out.[2,15] Peer,[18] Steffensen,[21] Dingman,[3] and Horton[14] have all written knowledgeably and well on this subject. There are volumes written on the functional aspects of nasal surgery. Neither this material nor the internal anatomy or physiology of the nose will be belabored here. Rather I will limit my attention to one facet of a broad field: a simplified overview of the structural aspects of septoplasty as it relates to cosmetic rhinoplasty.

INFORMED CONSENT

In my "Informed Consent" session with the patient who has a potential nasal obstruction, I draw the following metaphor:

Your nose is like an **A**-frame cottage. The front half of the cottage is made of canvas and the back is made of wood. Down the middle from front to back there is a main bearing wall that supports the spine of the roof. If a giant tree were to fall on the house, it would cave in the roof and probably bend the main bearing wall to a much greater degree on the soft front than on the hard back. The bearing wall will buckle to variable degrees, thereby obstructing the rooms on either side. Imagine further that this wall at its bottom is set into a trough several inches high and also running from the front to the back of the house. Both sides of the central bearing wall and the sides of the trough are covered with thick red velvet wallpaper. On the slanting

---

*References 1, 5, 6, 11, 12, 16, 17, 20.

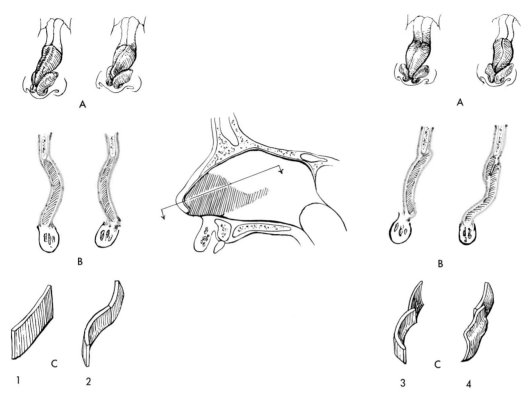

Fig. 21-1. Deviation may or may not produce external deformity. Mechanism of injury is significant. Lateral lower nasal trauma may result in deformity in column *1,* upper lateral nasal trauma in column *2,* blow from above in column *3,* and one from below in column *4* (note fracture/telescoping). Cross section in center shows level of sagittal section indicated in all figures *B.*

side walls of the house there are some broad shelves that protrude into the room. If the wall is bulging into the space on either side, it would be difficult to pass from one end to the other. If the wall is crooked enough that the shelves on each side touch it, there is no passage at all. If the wall is only partly crooked and I wish to make the house narrower by moving the side walls in, I will achieve the same effect (no passage) unless I straighten out the main bearing wall first. To do this I must raise up the wallpaper, get under it, and remove the crooked portion of the dividing wall. However, I cannot remove all of it, because then the roof might collapse. I must leave at least an L-shaped support at the front and under the roof. If this portion is also crooked, I must then straighten it out. The wallpaper on both sides then goes back together, back to back, then there will be better passage on either side.

Although this may seem an oversimplified version, it has served me well over the past 15 years, even in cases where results have been less than optimal. Patients have always proved to be understanding when a minor secondary correction is required.

NASAL PHYSIOLOGY

For the purposes of this discussion I will focus on several limited but important facets of internal nasal physiology[4,19] of significance to the plastic surgeon.

1. The way in which air currents traverse the nasal conduits, their direction, their shape, and speed of the stream are determined as much by nasal configuration as by the natural anatomic constriction found approximately 2 cm inside the nostrils. This area, commonly referred to as the valve, is the confluence of the caudal edge of the upper lateral cartilages and the septum (under the overlap of the upper border of the alar cartilages). This constriction acts like the nozzle of a hose. The length and capacity of the hose mean nothing; the stream it throws and its direction are characterized by the shape of the nozzle.

2. On normal inspiration in the intact nose, the air is directed upward and backward, arching up

between the septum and turbinates to the face of the sphenoid, down through the choana and into the pharynx. Relatively little passes along the floor. The choana has essentially no effect on the stream.

3. Over the turbinates air becomes humidified to approximately 90% relative humidity before reaching the larynx.

4. On expiration air passes through the lower choana and is thrown into eddies by the baffle effect of the posterior aspect of the turbinates and the nozzle effect of the nostrils.

5. As the air currents are moved over the ciliated surfaces particulate matter is deposited, probably by electrostatic principles. The mucosal glands deposit a lubricating blanket, which is moved by the cilia and carries off debris. Tear flow assists.

6. The physiology of the nasal cilia has been detailed by Proetz.[19] Cilia line the inner surface of the nose except for the olfactory areas. Going back to the metaphor, one can visualize a house through the center of which run two corridors covered with thick velvet pile wallpaper. The dust entering the house is passed along the wall, ceiling and floor, down the corridor, through the back door, and into the ashcan; it makes a complete trip in 20 minutes. Thus self-cleaning wallpaper works 24 hours a day unless something happens. Cilia are tough and have only one natural enemy: drying. This incapacitates their ability to function and move mucus.

7. The principal iatrogenic enemy of cilia is scar tissue, which makes hurdles over which cilia cannot move the mucosal blanket. Annular scars not only bar the flow but further narrow the nozzle, thus creating not only a mechanical but also a physiologic barrier.

8. The valves must be of sufficient size to allow free flow of respiration, and both should be nearly alike. If disproportionate amounts of air are allowed to enter one side only, it will tend to dry and undergo metaplasia. This so-called rhinitis

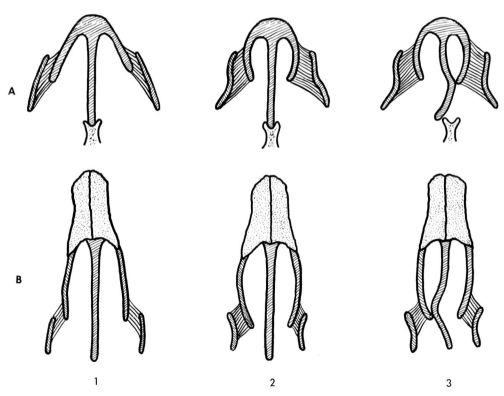

Fig. 21-2. Anatomic/physiologic relationships in valve area. Upper edge of the alar cartilage slightly overlaps lower edge of upper laterals. There is tenuous fibrous attachment between them. **A,** Cross sections. **B,** Sagittal sections. Column *1,* quiet inspiration, midsagittal septum; column *2,* forceful inspiration, midsagittal septum; column *3,* forceful inspiration, deviated septum. There need be no external deviation visible. When nose is narrowed, problem becomes more disturbing.

sicca may be reported by the patient as a feeling of nasal obstruction. Underventilation will lead to constant mucus accumulation.

9. The important relationship of the upper edge of the alar cartilage and the caudal edge of the upper laterals is illustrated in Fig. 21-2. The legend explains the anatomic-physiologic correlation as well as the valve or nozzle concept. Any uncorrected or iatrogenic septal deviation at this point automatically aggravates obstruction on inspiration and virtually assures dissatisfaction.

ARCHITECTURAL SIGNIFICANCE OF THE SEPTUM

Converse[2] and others have thoroughly detailed the role of the septum in nasal architecture. I would like to reemphasize a few vital points.

1. It is generally agreed that if one drops an imaginary line from the nasion to the nasal spine, anything posterior to that line can be resected from floor to ceiling without fear of collapse. Anything anterior to it must resected with discretion and forethought lest insufficient support and subsequent functional (and aesthetic) distortion occur. Even if there seems to be an adequate dorsal cartilaginous support remaining, beware of the effect of contracture of the mucosal leaves and the plane of scar between them. If there have been perforations, this will be even more significant.

2. If one considers the upper laterals as the wings sprouting from the upper edge of the septum (an embryologically correct concept), then if the upper edge of the septum is deviated, it must be freed from the wings that tether it. If one fails to do this, their guy-wire effect will eventually redeviate the dorsum. This separation should be

done at a submucoperichondrial level. If one keeps the mucoperichondrial flap attached to the underside of the upper laterals, except where they join the septum, then the mucoperichondrial flaps will not sag. In this way one can avoid cutting away the upper laterals, mucosa and all. In my opinion, this maneuver always creates scar and synechiae, which later may restrict inspiratory air flow (Fig. 21-3).

3. High septal deflection, often undetected, can frustrate a perfect rhinoplasty. The hump, which is in the normal midsagittal plane, may be covering a crooked septum just under it. (It is easy to miss these in cursory preoperative examinations.) Operative edema may deceive the surgeon. When infracture has been finished, one has then brought together the nasal bones and upper laterals against an undiscovered deviation of the new upper border of the septum. Two weeks later, when the edema recedes, the beautiful result at the end of the operation may look distinctly off center.

4. The sequence of the septal correction at surgery is important. Fig. 21-4 shows a typical subluxation and override of the septovomerine junction at the anterior inferior corner of the quadrilateral cartilage. What happens here can have a profound effect on the new profile line. If one frees up the dislocated lower edge of the cartilage within it, this will tend to lift the lower end of the nose. On the other hand, if one has to cut off the extremely deviated lower edge of the septum, chisel the vomer groove out to replace the septum in the center, or both, one may end up lowering the end of the nose, whose support depends on the remaining cartilaginous strut. Thus the surgeon

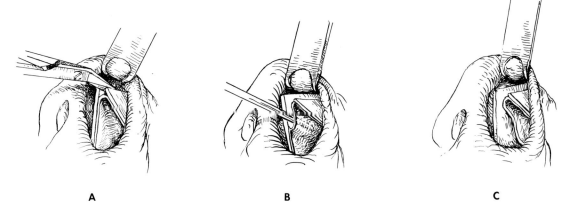

| A | B | C |

Fig. 21-3. A, Cutting upper laterals away at subperichondrial level. **B,** Separating mucoperichondrial flap. **C,** Flap will not sag if left attached to underside of upper lateral. (Modified from Converse, J. M.: Arch. Otolaryngol. **52:**671, 1950.)

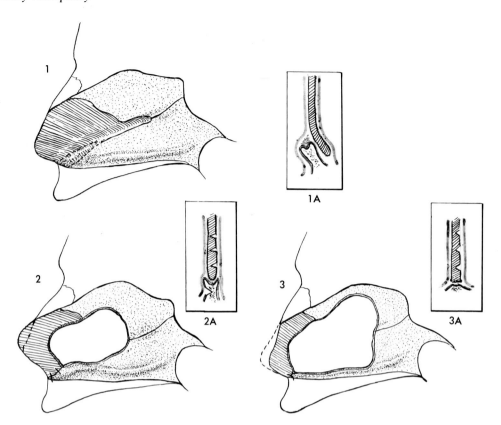

Fig. 21-4. *1* and *1A,* Typical subluxation with override at anterior inferior junction of septal cartilage and vomer groove. Note that cartilage and vomer are each separately enveloped in perichondrium and periosteum respectively. *2* and *2A,* Assuming correction of both vomerine and lower cartilaginous deflection, if current anatomic relationship can be restored, tip of nose will be lifted. *3* and *3A,* Resection of lower cartilaginous edge or vomer groove to restore alignment may result in tip droop.

must know what he is going to do ahead of time. It is poor planning to make a beautiful profile and then fix the septum only to find it lowered in the tip area. I try to do my correction first, leaving more than adequate dorsal buttress so that corrections along the profile line or shortening the nose can still be done at the end of the rhinoplasty without weakening the remaining support. If in doubt, the hump resection and dorsal correction must be done first and then the septoplasty, so that enough cartilage is left behind to guarantee integrity of the profile line. I also find that doing the septum first, particularly if it is badly bent, is much easier from the standpoint of visibility, neatness, and safety.

5. The hump may be a relative or absolute one. A large Arabic or a romanesque hump can be characterized as an absolute one. If the profile line suddenly dips below the end of the nasal bones, this is a relative hump, which is almost invariably caused by septal abnormality. If the septum has

been distorted severely enough to be noticeable externally, oftentimes almost total removal of the septum will barely affect the profile line significantly. This is the nose in which it is wise to consider using the resected septum to bridge the sag between the self-supporting tip and the end of the nasal bones.

6. In severe internal deviations, the remaining L-shaped strut may remain deviated. If the surgeon fails to straighten it out, he is guaranteed a deviated nose. Until recent years, most authors advised various maneuvers to score, cut, crosshatch, or remove strips vertically from the convex side of the deformity with the idea of allowing the remaining septum to swing back into the midline (Fig. 21-5, *2B* and *2C*). There are also a number of maneuvers described to keep it there, too. In my experience this has been, at the best, chancy. At least as many have redeviated as have stayed improved. Gibson[10] and, more recently, Fry[7,8,9] have effectively demonstrated the existence

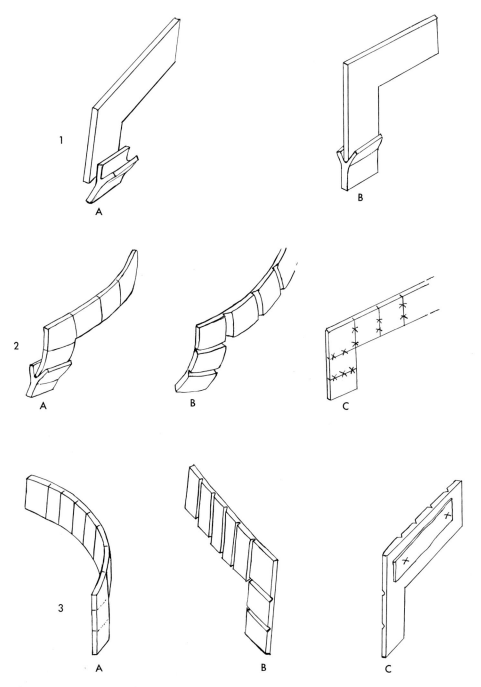

Fig. 21-5. *1A,* Schematic representation of typical dislocation of remaining L strip from vomer groove; *1B,* ideal restoration. *2A,* Commonly seen situation at end of procedure or months later; *2B* and *2C,* Popular correction by scoring, crosshatching, strip removal, hinging, or other means, always on convex side and often recurring. *3A* and *3B,* Scoring on concave side results in deviation toward intact side. *3C,* If in doubt, reinforce with small cartilage batten on intact side.

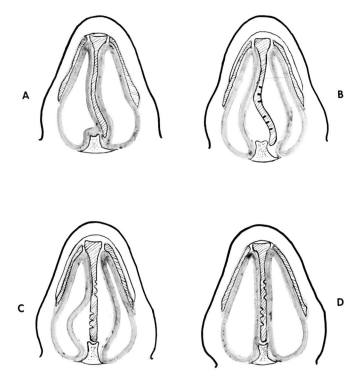

Fig. 21-6. A, Typical biconvex deviation with subluxation. **B,** Mucoperichondrial flap elevated on left side. Note release of upper lateral cartilage guy wires. Right side is left partially attached for blood supply. **C,** Release of interlocking stresses by scoring on each concave surface and restoration on vomer groove. Trimming may be necessary to allow septal cartilage to swing back.

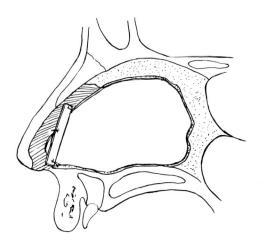

Fig. 21-7. If in doubt, splint remaining L strut with surplus septal cartilage or ethmoid plate batten. Apply against convex side where curve is most noticeable.

of interlocking stresses within cartilage. Most significantly, Fry has dramatically illustrated the tendency of cartilage to curl to the opposite side from which it is scored. For the past few years I have always scored on the concave side (Fig. 21-5, *3A* and *3B*). If the deviation is a complex one, I score both sides but always on the concave portion (Fig. 21-6, *C*), and I have been gratified by the obvious improvement in long-term follow-ups (Figs. 21-14 to 21-16).

7. Recently, in particularly badly deviated septums I have taken to reinforcing my scoring by placing a small batten of surplus septal cartilage or vomerine bone on the unscored side to act as a reinforcement. I have been gratified with the results so far. This maneuver is illustrated in Fig. 21-5, *3C,* and Fig. 21-7.

TECHNICAL SUGGESTIONS

I agree with Converse[2] that no one operation can correct a deformity so infinite in its variables. Horton[14] and others have pointed out that the classic submucous resection, as such, is hardly ever the complete answer. What must be done is an opera-

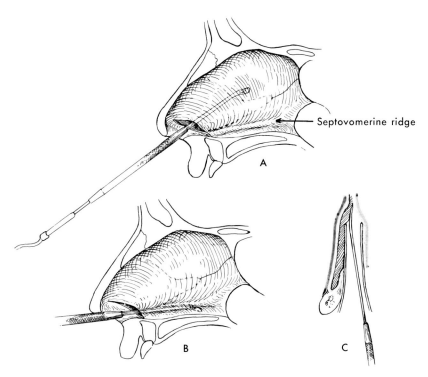

Septovomerine ridge

Fig. 21-8. A, Incision along protrusive caudal margin of cartilaginous septum (note typical septovomerine shelf). Subperichondrial elevation (look for blue-gray reflex) to roof of nose, as far posteriorly as possible, but inferiorly only down to septovomerine ridge. Do not attempt to dissect over it. **B,** Subperiosteal incision and elevation or new tunnel up to septovomerine ridge. The two spaces are then gradually joined from back to front. **C,** Sagittal section showing speculum blades retracting while suction elevator does its work under perichondrium and periosteum.

tion that will (1) restore function, (2) correct deviation, and (3) prevent saddling, columella retraction, and tip droop. The principle of the operation is to divide every attachment of the cartilaginous septum except for a mucosal flap on one side (to maintain the blood supply) and to release the interlocking stresses in the twisted cartilage. The goal should be maximum mobility with the least removal of tissue possible. My approach to the problem is an amalgam of many standard techniques with a few personal modifications. These are shown in the illustrations and legends.

A few caveats may be in order (Figs. 21-8 to 21-13):

1. The secret to avoiding perforations is to undermine at the right level: subperichondrially. In the distal 1 or 2 cm of cartilaginous septum, the mucosa is intimately attached to the cartilage. After incising along the protrusive leading edge, a pair of Converse scissors or a sharp elevator is useful in finding the correct plane. It is easy to start down the wrong one, and this virtually guarantees perforations and tears, particularly along

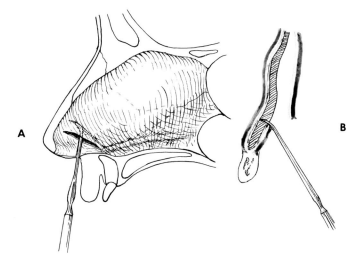

Fig. 21-9. A, Freer knife passes under flap and makes vertical cut through cartilage only up to what will be lower margin of dorsal buttress. **B,** Sagittal section. Knife does not penetrate opposite perichondrium.

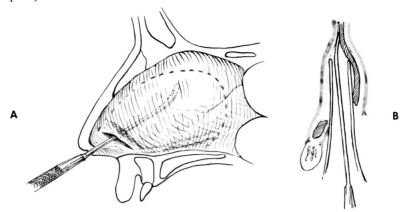

Fig. 21-10. A, Suction elevator now lifts off mucoperichondrium and periosteum from opposite side from nasal floor to limits of cartilaginous resection. Mucosa remains attached to cartilage that is to be left as support, but on only one side. **B,** Cross section.

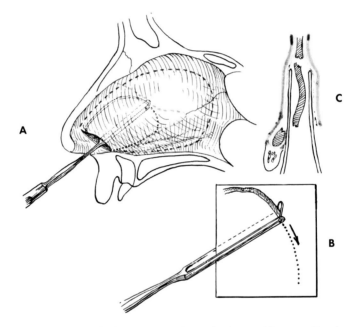

Fig. 21-11. A, If swivel knife is to be used, begin by making small scissors cut (not shown) at upper anterior limits of resection. Swivel knife then moves backward to rostrum of ethmoid and then down. **B,** Swivel knife cuts back and down. **C,** Cross section. If septal material is to be used in tip or nasal dorsum, it is better to use stout scissors instead of swivel knife.

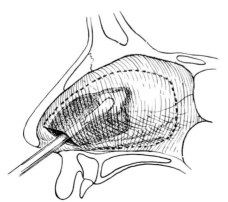

Fig. 21-12. Blakely forceps removes deviated bony septum.

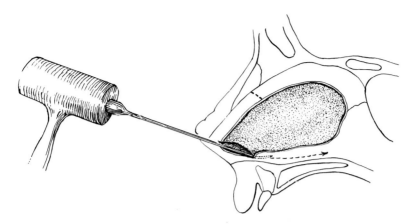

Fig. 21-13. If vomer groove is deflected, an attempt should be made to score along one side and crack it into midline (Fig. 21-4). If this is not possible, it must be chiseled out to allow cartilaginous septum to swing into midline.

the spurs, crests, and ridges where the mucosa is as thin as wet tissue paper. There is a characteristic gray-bluish reflex visible on entering the right plane ("If it ain't blue, it ain't true"). There is also a clean smooth feel on the instrument, which will glide along easily. When the instrument passes from the cartilage to the vertical plate of the ethmoid, there is a characteristic change in the feel of the scraping. It is best to proceed in semicircular upward motions rather than pushing straight and back. Do not try to go past the angle of deviation or around ridges. This will also produce perforations. (Small perforations are of no consequence unless they are back to back on both mucosal leaves; this will produce a permanent perforation.)

2. Along the inferior anterior aspect of the cartilaginous septum, where it fits in the vomerine ridge, it is difficult to pass down from the subperichondrial space of the cartilage to the subperiosteal space of the vomer. Fig. 21-4, *A,* shows why. The quadrilateral septal cartilage is invested completely by perichondrium, even along its lower edge, which may or may not sit in the vomer groove. The vomer ridge, in turn, has periosteum tightly adherent over it. Therefore after undermining from the roof of the nose to the septovomerine ridge, one should not try to continue inferiorly but back off and begin a new tunnel under the periosteum of the vomer. It is much easier to join these two spaces without tearing once they have been independently developed. It is easier if one proceeds from posterior (ethmoid-vomer) to anterior (cartilage-vomer) (Fig. 21-8).

3. If you use a swivel knife, do not proceed along the vomer first and then up, anteriorly, and out. You may come up too high and not leave

enough dorsal buttress for support. It is much safer to make the vertical cut up to a preselected point in the cartilaginous septum about 1 or 2 cm back from the leading edge. Do not perforate to the opposite perichondrium. Under direct vision, after undermining the subperichondrial space on the opposite side, one can push aside the septal leaves by opening up a speculum with the cartilage between the blades (Fig. 21-11). The dorsal incision line in the cartilage can be started with a pair of angled scissors. Then insert the swivel knife into this cut and proceed posteriorly along a preselected line parallel and about 2 cm below the dorsal profile. When the rostrum of the vertical plate of the ethmoid is reached, the swivel knife then swings down to the vomer and then back out along the vomer ridge and out.

4. Doing this operation is like making a watch in a drainpipe. The most useful instruments I have found to ease this sometimes difficult procedure are a no. RH850 combination suction-elevator made by V. Mueller and a no. N3000 Blakeley alligator forceps made by Storz. The former eliminates the need to keep changing instruments at critical moments. The latter is much easier to use because its fulcrum is at the tip of the instrument and only the business end opens, making it easier to work in restricted posterior spaces. Both will save a lot of time.

5. Often a deflected vomer can be greensticked into the midline by placing a 1 mm chisel on the nasal floor and scoring along one side of the base of the deviated vomer ridge. A little pressure by opening a long thin speculum along the floor of the nose will often do the trick.

6. If the vertical element of the remaining L-

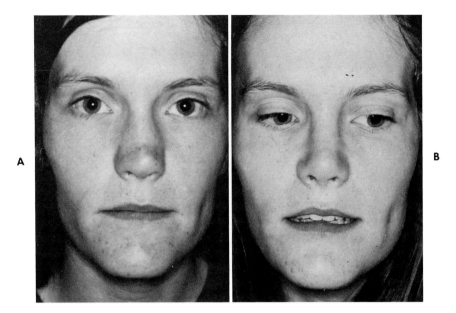

Fig. 21-14. Typical complex deviation with external manifestations **A,** Preoperative view. **B,** Postoperative view after long-term follow-up.

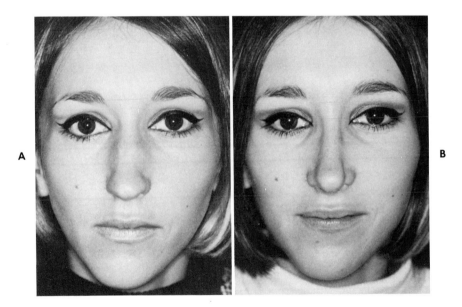

Fig. 21-15, Typical complex deviation with external manifestations. **A,** Preoperative view. **B,** Postoperative view after long-term follow-up.

shaped cartilage support is still crooked, do not depend on columellar pockets or transfixation devices to straighten it. It will not only not work, but it will also carry the tip of the nose with it when it redeviates. Score it on its concave side, and, if need be, stiffen it on the intact (convex) side with a thin cartilage batten (Figs. 21-5, *C,* and 21-7).

7. At the end of the procedure, pack what was the convex side first. (If the nose deviates to the right, pack the left side first.) Do not use the cram-jam technique. Pack carefully from the floor up using just enough material to put the mucosal leaves back to back. Put in one nasal length at a time and tamp it down by opening your speculum. Bear in mind that an overall splint will bring things further together and too much packing may tend

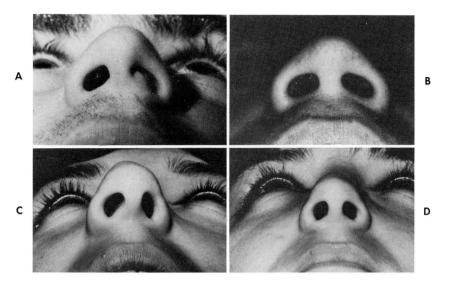

Fig. 21-16. Deviations of tip with severe obstruction. **A** and **C,** Preoperative views. **B** and **D,** Postoperative views after long-term follow-up.

to separate the nasal bones. I have been using Neosporin-soaked half-inch Adaptic. The pack stays in 3 or 4 days. If there is bad deviation and obstruction, I may pull the pack from the old obstructed side a day later than the other.

8. Totally intact, accurately closed mucoperichondrial leaves, if inadequately packed, may be dangerous. Septal hematomas are not uncommon, and if not evacuated properly can give a thick, obstructive septum. If in doubt, there is no harm in making a couple of stab wounds with a no. 5 blade at separate sites on either side at the base of the mucoperichondrial flaps for drainage.

9. The turbinates are often part of the problem. Time and space do not permit a detailed account of this aspect. However, it may be appropriate to deal with troublesome turbinates at the time of surgery by several simple maneuvers. They can be outfractured by forceful pressure with a long speculum, cauterized along their edge, or trimmed away. Beware of overly enthusiastic treatment for fear of rhinitis sicca as a consequence. Postoperatively they also respond nicely to intranasal corticoids injected directly into the submucosa.

REFERENCES

1. Becker, O. J.: Problems of septum in rhinoplastic surgery, Arch. Otolaryngol. **53:**622, 1951.
2. Converse, J. M.: Corrective surgery of nasal deviations, Arch. Otolaryngol. **52:**671, 1950.
3. Dingman, R.: Correction of nasal deformities due to defects of the septum, Plast. Reconstr. Surg. **18:**291, 1956.
4. Fomon, S., Sayad, W. Y., Schattner, A., and Neivert, H.: Physiological principles in rhinoplasty, Arch. Otolaryngol. **53:**256, 1951.
5. Fomon, S., et al.: New approach to ventral deflections of nasal septum, Arch. Otolaryngol. **54:**356, 1951.
6. Fomon, S., Gilbert, J. G., Silver, A. G., and Syracuse, V. R.: Plastic repair of obstructing nasal septum, Arch. Otolaryngol. **47:**7, 1948.
7. Fry, H. J. H.: Interlocked stresses in human nasal septal cartilage, Br. J. Plast. Surg. **19:**276, 1966.
8. Fry, H. J. H.: Nasal skeletal trauma and the interlocked stresses of the nasal septal cartilages, Br. J. Plast. Surg. **20:**146, 1967.
9. Fry, H. J. H.: The importance of the septal cartilage in nasal trauma, Br. J. Plast. Surg. **20:**392, 1967.
10. Gibson, T., and David, W. B.: The distortion of autogenous cartilage grafts: its cause and prevention, Br. J. Plast. Surg. **10:**257, 1958.
11. Goldman, I. B.: New techniques in surgery of deviated nasal septum, Arch. Otolaryngol. **64:**183, 1956.
12. Goldman, I. B.: Rhinoplastic sequelae causing nasal obstruction, Arch. Otolaryngol. **83:**151, 1966.
13. Gray, L.: The deviated nasal septum, J. Laryngol. Otolaryngol. **79:**567, 1965.
14. Horton, C. E.: Combined septoplasty and rhinoplasty. In Masters, F. W., and Lewis, J. R., Jr., editors: Symposium on aesthetic surgery of the nose, ears, and chin, St. Louis, 1973, The C. V. Mosby Co.
15. Kazanjian, V. H., and Converse, J. M.: Surgical treatment of facial injuries, Baltimore, 1974, The Williams & Wilkins Co.
16. Killian, G.: Die submucöse Fensterresektion der Nasenscheidewand, Arch. Laryngol. Rhinol. (Berlin) **16:**362, 1904; The submucous window resection of the nasal septum, Ann. Otol. Rhinol. Laryngol. **14:**363, 1905.

17. Metzenbaum, M.: Replacement of lower end of dislocated septal cartilage versus submucous resection of dislocated end of septal cartilage, Otolaryngol. **9:**282, 1929.

18. Peer, L. A.: Operation to repair lateral displacement of lower border of septal cartilage, Arch. Otolaryngol. **25:**475, 1937.

19. Proetz, A. W.: Physiology of nose from the standpoint of plastic surgeon, Arch. Otolaryngol. **39:**514, 1944.

20. Seltzer, A. P.: Nasal septum; plastic repair of deviated septum associated with deflected tip, Arch. Otolaryngol. **40:**433, 1944.

21. Steffensen, W. H.: Reconstruction of the nasal septum, Plast. Reconstr. Surg. **2:**66, 1947.

Chapter 22

Septoplasty with pin fixation

William C. Conroy, M.D.

Although respiratory physiologists agree that the main inspiratory nasal airway is chiefly past the upper half of the septum by way of the olfactory fissure or the middle meatus, the average submucous resection emphasizes removal of cartilaginous bony septum in the lower half with increased size of available airway as the chief goal. If the size of the airway alone were the prime end, we would all be mouth breathers. Rather, the goal should be a laminar airflow without eddies along a straight septum passing high to the olfactory sense organs and back to the pharynx without excessive drying or irritation of the sidewalls. For the plastic surgeon this should be accomplished with a minimum of time and conservation of all available support and circulation to allow him to make all the other necessary alterations in the shape of the external nose.

PHYSIOLOGY

Inspiration results in an oval column of air directed medially upward hugging the septum with a laminar flow. Regardless of whether the stream of air that passes medial to the anterior tip of the middle turbinate traverses the olfactory fissure or the middle meatus, the major flow is through the upper half of the nose, and distortions here such as septal angulation and impaction of the upper lateral cartilage against the septum are more important than septal ridges and spurs lying along the crest of the vomer, and even these are apt to be streamlined to the current. Frank dislocation of the septum from the vomer groove into the nasal gutter, however, causes significant obstruction. Inspired air directed against the sidewalls by a deviated septum causes excessive drying, crusting, interference with ciliary action, and blockage of sinus ostia. Constriction of the stream of air causes deposits and drying beyond the narrowed area, and Bernoulli's phenomenon results

in decreased pressure at the constriction with consequent further narrowing due to edema. The effects of allergy, infection, posture, and cyclical autonomic influences on the turbinates are well recognized but are beyond this discussion. A properly directed laminar airflow without eddies is the important consideration, since overpatency can be accompanied by stuffiness due to overdrying and air eddies. Some make much of baffles and valves. In our experience the internal valve is either unimportant or indestructible, since the intercartilaginous incision and detachment of the upper lateral cartilage from the septum insult this structure on two sides with no apparent breathing difficulty resulting in our cases.

ANATOMY

The most common nasal fracture with displaced nasal bones and fractured ethmoid plate frequently has a straight septum presenting no problems in correction. When the nasal bones are not displaced but present at most a distal tip fracture, deformities of the quadrilateral plate fall into fairly predictable patterns. Our experience agrees with Sawney that only a small percentage of septa are of the C or S variety. Injuring forces from below cause fractures at the first buttress at the lower border of the lateral cartilage prolongation or at the second buttress at the lower end of the nasal bones, and septal fractures here are accompanied by dislocation of that portion of the lateral cartilage extending beneath the nasal bones. Blows from in front cause dislocation of the septum from the vomer groove or horizontal fractures higher up. Combinations may occur, and the nasal spine and tip cartilages may be injured. The posterior superior border of the septum is convex anteriorly in a strong $1/4$-inch-wide end-to-end relationship with the ethmoid plate, which readily accepts a pin. The inferior border of the septum is in a loose tongue-and-groove relationship with the vomer and easily displaced.

METHOD

Making sure to allow at least 5 mm of intact septum to remain along the dorsum, we cut the cartilage along the furrow on the concave side of the deflection, using the opposite index finger to cut against to prevent damage to the opposite mucoperichondrium. In a similar manner on the convex side, the cartilage is incised along the vomer crest, again sparing the opposite mucoperichondrium; anteriorly, we sever the connections of the septum to the nasal spine.

Now the septum is thoroughly bent on itself, opposite to the bend of the original deflection, until it remains overcorrected without fixation. The distorted relationships between the septum and the upper lateral cartilages are corrected by cutting the latter loose from the septum.

When all distorting forces are released, a stab wound incision is made in the membranous septum on the concave side at the nasal spine, and the inferior border of the septum is exposed. A 2¹/₄-inch Vitallium needle impales the straightened septum as, grasped in a heavy needle holder, it is passed subperichondrially superiorly in the exact midline as judged by the central incisors and the midpoint between the eyebrows (Fig. 22-1).

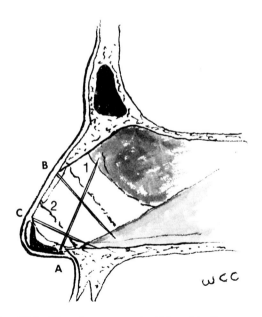

Fig. 22-1. Pin placement. *A*, Ethmoid; *B*, vomer; *C*, short vomer. *1*, Proximal septal fracture; *2*, distal septal fracture.

The ethmoid plate should be engaged when about 1 cm of the needle still protrudes from the naris. If it does not, the needle should be redirected. The distal end of the ethmoid plate widens to ¹/₄ inch at its articulation with the cartilage. With a twisting motion the needle is started into the bone and then tapped with a mallet for a few millimeters into place. Slight overcorrection is desirable. The end of the needle is nipped off, allowing about 2 mm or more to recede into the soft tissues.

As with otoplasty techniques, any overriding of the cartilage must be controlled by restoring alignment with 4-0 catgut or Dexon sutures.

Should inspection now show a residual tendency of the inferior border to drift toward its previously dislocated position, a small nick is made in the dorsum, the convex mucoperichondrium is expanded with saline or anesthetic solution, and a second needle is passed from the dorsum subperichondrially on the convex side. While holding the septum in the corrected position with a spread nasal speculum on the convex side, the second needle is embedded into the vomer and bitten off, leaving just sufficient protrusion for later identification.

When a rhinoplasty is being done, the septum is corrected last. This is a skeletal fixation; it must engage cartilage and bone, and it must be subperichondrial.

Submucous resection of any residual obstructing cartilage is accomplished through the orignal incisions. Anteroposterior and lateral x-ray films of the nose are taken before the patient is discharged from the hospital.

Pin removal is accomplished easily by palpating the end of the ethmoid pin where it protrudes into the membranous septum, injecting a small amount of anesthetic solution, making a stab wound, and grasping the needle in a hemostat. The vomer pin is removed by injecting the septum and skin over the pin, incising the mucoperichondrium and feeling the blade strike metal, grasping the needle with a hemostat, and backing it out until it protrudes under the skin. A small stab wound is made, and the needle is grasped and removed. (The x-ray films taken after the original procedure should be at hand.)

The informed consent should state that the pin must be removed within 6 months. There have been reports of Vitallium needles migrating into the brain cavity if this precaution is neglected.

RESULTS

Extrusion of the pin is not a problem. Since 1968, seventy-one pins have been placed in sixty-one patients, and five have been extruded. They have been remarkably asymptomatic without pain or discharge except as noted here. Eight patients have pins in place 3 years or more against advice and promising to return if trouble develops. Most of these pins are carbide steel, since the point of the stainless did not penetrate bone well, and carbide steel will disintegrate. Problems of corrosion and occasional fracture of carbide steel pins have caused us to return to stainless steel. Since we were unable to obtain stainless steel carbide–tipped needles, we are now using fine Kirschner wire pins prepared for us by Howmedica, Inc.

The septal deformity in thirty-one cases consisted of deviation at the distal end of the nasal bones, and seven of these cases had associated dislocation of the inferior border from the vomer groove. Results in these cases were uniformly excellent with straight noses and free breathing consistently achieved in observations over 2 years. Associated dislocations at times required conservative cartilage excision and dorsal pinning into the vomer. The needles were usually removed in 4 to 6 months.

Distal deflections in ten cases remained excellent until the pin was removed, and then some return of buckling of the free-lying septum was observed in three cases. Two patients under observation for about a year have maintained a straight septum with indwelling pins passed from the dorsum into the vomer. The short pins are visualized under the intact mucoperichondrium, are asymptomatic, and are solidly embedded on palpation. Associated deformity of alar cartilages must be corrected. Pins placed in the vomer may produce transient discomfort in incisor teeth, and, anteriorly, incisor roots should be avoided.

Dislocations of the inferior border from the vomer groove, even when severe, were effectively returned to good anatomic position by pinning the vomer from the dorsum. The less frequent higher horizontal fracture was better treated by excision.

Use of the pin in acute fractures in four cases returned equivocal results due to reluctance to complete the septal fracture by open reduction, thus allowing forces described by Fry to operate. The only infection was in this group.

Multiple and complex septal deformities in four cases did not lend themselves to pinning. Although a straight septum was initially obtained, multiple distorting forces inevitably created deformity with time and extrusion rate was high, but these pins were introduced into the vomer from the spine incision, and dorsal pinning was not used. Our approach here is to accept a shorter goal, removing obstruction by excision, hoping to get a sufficiently long straight piece of septum to place on the dorsum.

Four unilateral cleft lip nose repairs were attempted, with two extrusions and three poor re-

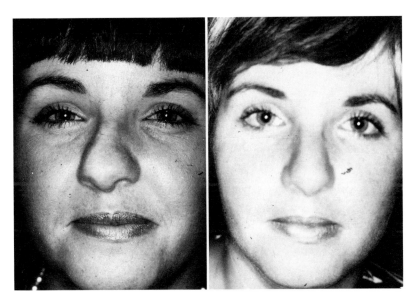

Fig. 22-2. Proximal septal fracture; pin in ethmoid.

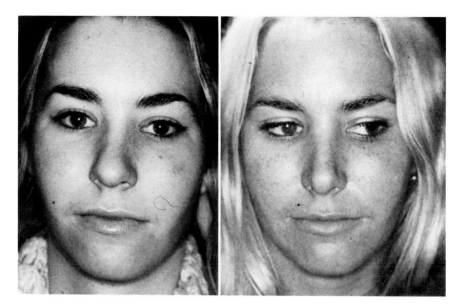

Fig. 22-3. Proximal septal fracture; pin in ethmoid.

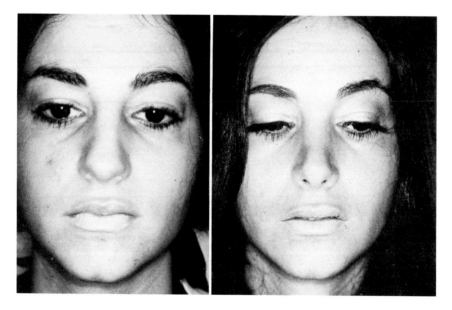

Fig. 22-4. Proximal septal fracture; pin in ethmoid.

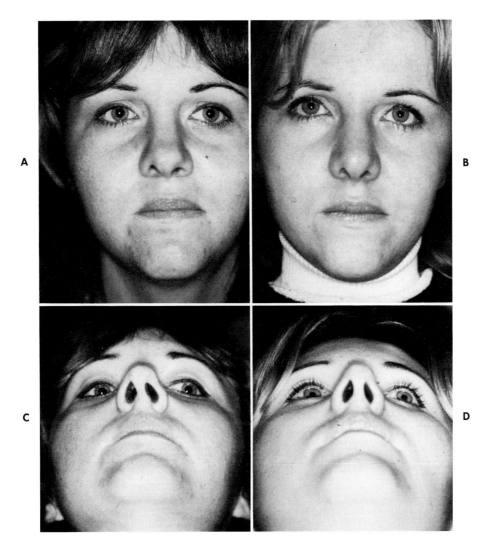

Fig. 22-5. A and **C,** Distal septal fracture; short pin in vomer. **B** and **D,** Tip cartilages realigned.

sults due to primarily the lack of a midline vomer to pin against. Failure to preserve 0.5 cm of dorsal septum in an early case was accompanied by loss of tip support.

DISCUSSION

One has but to read the enthusiastic and confident presentation on the permanent correction of septal deformities by means of cartilage scissors and a few weeks of packing and septal straightening over 80 years ago by Asch and similar positivism for distal septal deflections by Metzenbaum 50 years ago to beware of extravagant claims for the management of septal deformities. It is enough to state that a method of fixing the septum asymptomatically in a straightened position for long periods of time and perhaps permanently is suggested.

SUMMARY

The management of septal deviations by release of distorting forces, conservative cartilage excision, and fixation of the septum with a steel pin is presented.

REFERENCES

1. Adams, W.: On the treatment of broken nose by forcible straightening and mechanical retentive apparatus, Br. Med. J., p. 421, Oct., 1875.
2. Adamson, J. E., Horton, C. E., Crawford, H. H., and Taddeo, R. J.: Acute submucous resection, Plast. Reconstr. Surg. **42:**152, 1968.
3. Asch, M. J.: A new operation for deviation of the

nasal septum with a report of cases, Trans. Am. Laryngol. Assoc. **12:**76, 1891.

4. Bernstein, D.: The twisted nose and the submental film, Eye Ear Nose Throat Mon. **45:**92, Oct., 1966.

5. Brown, J. B., and McDowell, F.: Plastic surgery of the nose, St. Louis, 1951, The C. V. Mosby Co.

6. Clark, G. M., and Wallace, C. S.: Analysis of nasal support, Arch. Otolaryngol. **92:**118, Aug., 1970.

7. Converse, J. M.: Reconstructive plastic surgery, vol. 1, Philadelphia, 1964, W. B. Saunders Co., p. 691.

8. Drehner, B.: Pathophysiological relationship between the upper and lower airways, Ann. Otol. Rhinol. Laryngol. **79:**499, 1970.

9. Dupont, C.: Autogenous vomer bone graft for permanent correction of the cartilaginous septal deviation, Plast. Reconst. Surg. **38:**243, 1966.

10. Fomon, S., Goldman, I. B., Neivert, H., Schattner, A., Bell, J. W., and Berger, E. L.: New approach to ventral deflections of nasal septum, Arch. Otolaryngol. **54:**356, 1951.

11. Fry, H. J. H.: Nasal skeletal trauma and the interlocked stresses of the nasal septal cartilages, Br. J. Plast. Surg. **20:**146, 1967.

12. Fry, H. J. H.: The distorted residual cartilage strut after submucous resection of the nasal septum, Br. J. Plast. Surg. **21:**170, 1968.

13. Goldman, I. B.: Rhinoplastic sequelae causing nasal obstruction, Arch. Otolaryngol. **83:**93, 1965.

14. Goldman, I. B.: New technique in surgery of the deviated nasal septum, Arch. Otolaryngol. **64:**183, 1956.

15. Gray, L.: Deviated nasal septum. III. Its influence on the physiology and disease of the nose and ear, J. Laryngol. Otol. **81:**953, 1967.

16. Griffin, C. J.: The architecture of the congenitally dislocated nasal septum, Aust. Dent. J. **10:**20, Feb., 1965.

17. Ingals, E. F.: Deflection of septum narium, Trans. Am. Laryngol. Assoc. **4:**61, 1882.

18. Klaff, D. D.: Surgical correction of septal deformities in newborn infants and children, South. Med. J. **58:**1276, 1965.

19. Koch, W., and Kaplan, D.: A simple method for measuring nasal resistance, Acta Allergol. **21:**351, 1966.

20. Konno, A.: Surgical physiology of the nose. In Rees, T. D., and Wood-Smith, D: Cosmetic facial surgery, Philadelphia, 1973, W. B. Saunders Co.

21. Metzenbaum, M.: Dislocation of the lower end of the nasal septal cartilage, Arch. Otolaryngol. **24:**78, July, 1936.

22. O'Brien, M. A.: Current concepts of nasal surgery, J. Laryngol. Otol. **82:**987, 1968.

23. Ogura, J. H., Dammkoehler, R., Nelson, J. R., Togawa, K., and Kawasaki, M.: Nasal obstruction and the mechanics of breathing: physiologic relationships and the effects of nasal surgery, Arch. Otolaryngol. **83:**135, 1966.

24. Papisier, S. C.: Correction of deviated nose, Arch. Otolaryngol. **92:**60, 1970.

25. Patterson, C. N.: Physiologic septoplasty and rhinoplasty, N.C. Med. J. **27:**74, Feb., 1966.

26. Peer, L. A.: A method to correct saddle nose associated with retracted columella, Plast. Reconstr. Surg. **38:**477, 1966.

27. Pollock, W. J.: Rhinoplasty following repeated nasal fractures, J. La. State Med. Soc. **121:**46, Feb., 1969.

28. Proetz, A. W.: Respiratory air currents and their clinical aspects, J. Laryngol. Otol. **67:**1, Jan., 1953.

29. Reich, J.: Post-traumatic deformity of the nasal skeleton, Med. J. Aust. **1:**821, 1966.

30. Reidy, J. P.: The nasal septum, Hunterian Lecture, 1968.

31. Roydhouse, N.: A new look at the crooked nasal septum or septoplasty in children, N.Z. Med. J. **65:**686, 1966.

32. Rubin, F. F.: Permanent change in shape of cartilage by morselization, Arch. Otolaryngol. **89:**602, 1969.

33. Sawhney, K. L., and Sinha, A.: Diagnosis of deviated nasal septum, J. Otolaryngol. Soc. Aust. **1:**261, 1964.

34. Seltzer, A. P.: The use of magnets to maintain centralization of the nasal septum following submucous resection, J. Natl. Med. Assoc. **60:**210, 1968.

35. Smithdeal, C. D.: The significance of correction of the anterior septum in rhinoplasty, South. Med. J. **61:**931, 1968.

36. Stoksted, P.: The physiologic cycle of the nose under normal and pathologic condition, Acta Otolaryngol. **42:**175, 1952.

37. Unger, M.: Architecture of the nasal septum; how deviations are formed, Laryngoscope **75:**322, 1965.

38. Williams, R. I.: Hemitransfixion approach to problems of the nasal septum, Laryngoscope **77:**1116, 1967.

39. Wright, W. K.: Principles of nasal septum reconstruction, Trans. Am. Acad. Opthalmol. Otolaryngol. **73:**252, 1969.

Discussion

Millard: These have been two very interesting and informative papers on a subject on which sometimes plastic surgeons are not strong. How about some discussion?

Converse: Dr. Gorney says he forgot to mention probably the most important thing to facilitate your submucous resection. Balloon out the mucoperichondrium and periosteum with procaine (Novocain), using an 18- to 20-gauge needle with a short bevel. We call it the hydraulic resection. The whole thing just balloons up, and you can do your resection in less than a minute. Now there is a trend among the rhinologists to be more conservative when you do a submucous resection. Lately we have become much more conservative than we used to be, and there is a feeling that in a wide submucous resection, the flaps flapping in the breeze interfere with the nasal physiology. There is a mysterious aspect to the whole question of nasal breathing. The patients with severe nasal deviation, like some I will show later, when asked whether they have any trouble breathing, say no, they don't have any trouble breathing: "That's why I had my nose fixed." In true distinction is the patient with atrophic rhinitis. Here the turbinates shrink up, producing huge airways, and yet the patients say they can't breathe. There is a sensory aspect to nasal breathing that has never been elucidated. The patient must have the sensory feeling of air penetrating the nose, and if the patient doesn't have that sensation, he feels his nose is obstructed.

Millard: Thank you, John.

Friedman: I'd like to make a few comments. First of all, last year I recall in one of our problem clinics a patient was presented with the K-wire pin that had been placed in his midface at an undetermined time. The pin had somehow migrated posteriorly and was lying back against the brain near the sella turcica. Neurosurgical consultation and ENT consultation had been obtained, and nobody would touch it. So we don't know why it was there and the patient had no facial fractures, but it had to have been put there by some physician for some reason. So I would like to mention, before anybody puts K-wire in the face and plans to leave it forever, they might consider this possibility.

Millard: Bill, you don't know anything about that one, do you?

Conroy: Well, I'm very glad you mentioned that. I don't know about that one! As a matter of fact, when I use these pins, I study these things very carefully before I do it. You know the ethmoid plate comes out from the cribriform plate. One thing you must remember is that many times, x-ray men will take x-ray films without the sagittal plane being perpendicular to the plate, and you will get all kinds of reports from these x-ray men about a pin being in the ethmoid region or all over the head, depending upon where they project the perpendicular plate of ethmoid. I talk this over with my patients beforehand. If they seem to have any kind of apprehension about it, I tell them I'm going to use a pin and leave 2 mm projecting into the membranous septum where they can feel it. They tolerate it very well. One surgeon can put a pin in a patient and another surgeon, seeing the patient, may cause concern. The first thing you know, the patient will come back to you worried and say that they have heard the pin might go all over the place. Number 1, use a pin that will not cause any problem. Avoid the use of pins of carbide steel, which tend to disintegrate. Number 2, reassure the patient of the safety of this method and explain that pin cases have been hit in the head with baseballs without ill effect, and, in fact, no real problems have occurred with this pinning for me. It is important to remember that x-ray films, unless they are tomograms, do not always show the exact position of the pin.

Friedman: I have a couple of comments on Mark Gorney's excellent paper. First of all, on badly deviated and complicated septums, perhaps subluxated and thickened by scar tissue, it is very nice to score them on the concave surface to straighten them. But in some you can't do that, and you want to take out the entire or a significant portion of the septum, but you might otherwise jeopardize support of the nose. In these cases, you can take it out, morselize the entire thing, and slip it back between the leaves of perichondrium. Oftentimes we serve both purposes. Something that I recently learned from one of our ENT friends is that there are now triangular-shaped perforated Teflon plates, and they are available to slip in on each side of the nasal septum after your septoplasty. With a through-and-through horizontal mattress suture, you can keep everything lined up in the midline without the need of packing, avoid recreating an S-shaped curvature pattern, and prevent hematomas.

Millard: Thank you. Let me respond to the gentleman back there. You've been standing for so long.

Traub: How often would one see severe airway obstruction secondary to marked hypertrophy of the inferior turbinates in the postrhinoplasty SMR? Also, what do you do for this?

Millard: Which one of you experts is going to answer that? Mark?

Gorney: I didn't want to get into the turbinate thing because I know Jack Sheen is going to discuss it and because I think that's a whole separate subject. Turbinates play a part in your obstruction, and you've got to do something about the cartilage inside. Cauterizing in conjunction with corticoids are various maneuvers that you can do and I think are part and parcel of the operation. You should do something about it, and perhaps Dr. Converse will have some comments too. On Gary's comment, I am familiar with what you're saying, Gary, and this is all well and good if you have an intact septum. But if you end up with Belgian lace, then you can't put in a Teflon plate. While I'm on my feet, I would like to make one last comment on the issue of informed consent. Very often the patient will have severe obstruction on one side, and you relieve it and put the septum in the midline. Then the patient will come back and tell you that he can breathe real well on that side but he can't breathe on the other. The problem is that all of a sudden they're getting much more air on the obstructed side so that by comparison, the other side seems obstructed. Dr. Converse, who's sitting beside me, also remarked that oftentimes you get patients who interpret it as obstructed symptoms. I think if they have a badly complicated septum, you might warn the patient ahead of this problem and the relative improvement to be expected.

Kayfid: Richard Straith described the use of a Kirschner wire to keep the septum straight and I employed this method on several occasions and one time wound up with a pin in the cranial vault, which was removed by a neurosurgical team. I mentioned this interesting follow-up with Dr. Straith, who said, oh yes, that happened to us also, but we never reported it!

Millard: Thank you for reporting it.

Traub: Can my first question be answered? How often does one find in postrhinoplasty and SMR marked hypertrophy of the inferior turbinates when they weren't there before?

Millard: Mark doesn't find that to be a problem. Does anybody else find that to be a problem? Bernie?

Kaye: I was delighted to see Mark show a very handy gadget and an inexpensive one, namely, the Hamburg suction dissector. This is a device by which you can keep your way clear and dissect at the same time, as it has a semisharp edge so it can't gouge or cut unless you directly push it. Not only is it handy for submucous resection, but you find it very handy when you're exploring the orbital floor and want to get things up. It is also very handy for cleft palate work, too, where you dissect and suction simultaneously. It works in all but the most severe flood of blood. In regard to the septum where you've resected the ridge on the protruding bulge and you want to get the rest of it un-undulated, I agree that morselization is a very nice device. You don't have to make a free graft out of it. All you need to do is morselize but keep it intact. Then, a very handy way of holding it together is a relatively old way, by making two little Teflon sheet battens; this was described years ago in literature. Then suture them loosely together around the septum, and you can leave it there for a week or 2 weeks, as long as it is loose; it won't necrose the septum, and it doesn't obstruct like packing does. I wish I could claim originality for that, but it has been used for a long time.

Millard: Thank you. Any more? This is a very important subject and should go on for quite a while.

Pool: Dr. Gorney mentioned using internal splints. What does he mean by that term?

Gorney: When I said internal splint, I'm referring to that little batten of cartilage that I sew alongside once I've scored the septal cartilage—a thin straight piece of vomer that acts as an internal splint.

Chapter 23

Secondary and tertiary correction of postrhinoplastic deformities

some dos and don'ts

Blair O. Rogers, M.D.

The number of unsatisfactory results from primary rhinoplasties seems, unfortunately, to increase markedly with each passing year. The medical literature, however, contains surprisingly few articles describing secondary corrective rhinoplasty.*

In some cases, the postoperative deformities are caused by those complications which are the bane of every surgeon's practice—infection, hemorrhage, and excessive scarring. Some of them are avoidable; others are not avoidable, no matter how careful and meticulous the surgeon is.[18,20] An example of a condition that neither the surgeon nor the patient can control is the inability of extremely thick, inelastic skin with large pores to shrink and conform like a glove to the new, smaller skeletal framework. In a few cases the patient does not follow postoperative instructions, becomes a nose fiddler, and literally tampers, swabs, pinches, and physically assaults the nose to cause inordinate scarring, furrowing, dimpling, or thickening.

Under the aforementioned conditions it is almost impossible to indict any particular procedure or surgeon as responsible for the deformity. However, it would be shirking the issue to disregard the exceptionally large number of postrhinoplastic deformities caused by a surgeon who either does not understand the basic, well-described principles of rhinoplasty or has anthropologic blind spots[19] that prevent him from recognizing the normal relationships between the nose and the rest of the face. Although some of these deformities can be traced to lack of surgical skill on the part of accredited plastic surgeons, the majority are usually the

result of surgery performed by so-called plastic surgeons with inadequate training or no specialty certification whatsoever. When such a so-called surgeon adds insult to injury by operating again and again in a too-short period of time to correct the deformity he has created, the result is likely to be the crucified or butchered nose, which presents any skillful reconstructive plastic surgeon with perhaps the most difficult problem in aesthetic surgery.[10,11,13-18]

Although none of us will ever be free from revision rhinoplasties, we should not have a secondary operation rate of more than 5%. These revisions are usually minor adjustments, such as additional narrowing of wide nostrils, shortening of a drooped tip, modeling of the alar cartilages, or correction of a residual parrot's beak deformity.

Klabunde and Falces[7] recently emphasized that few articles are concerned with an analysis of complications and unsatisfactory results in cosmetic rhinoplasties. Their study of 300 patients revealed that approximately 10% "may have needed one or more secondary procedures." This figure seems somewhat excessive.

The surgeon who performs secondary rhinoplasties will be challenged by almost every conceivable nasal deformity. Secondary procedures are almost always more difficult than the primary surgery. Millard,[10] in his usual colorful and instructive manner, described secondary operations:

These problems range from difficult to insurmountable and usually present limited potential (if the secondary deformity is our own, we have already done the very best we could: if it is another surgeon's result, then often he has discarded what we would leave and has retained

*References 1, 2, 4, 5, 8, 10-18.

what we must take). This is particularly true if the primary surgeon's main focus has been on the airway and his radical submucous resection has removed all cartilage, which can be a trump card in a secondary reconstruction.*

Because of the difficulty in performing secondary rhinoplasties, it would probably be wise for the novice plastic surgeon to refer any postrhinoplastic deformities as a result of surgery by himself or others to senior surgeons.

If one is tempted to perform secondary or tertiary correction of a postrhinoplastic deformity, no matter how seemingly simple or obviously severe it may be, I would advise all of us to strictly adhere to the following three aphorisms of Sir Harold Gillies and Ralph Millard[6]:

1. "When in doubt, don't!"
2. "Replace what is normal in normal position, and retain it there!"
3. Most importantly, "Never do today what can honorably be put off till tomorrow!".

These aphorisms will now be discussed one at a time.

"When in doubt, don't!" This maxim applies chiefly to neurotic patients who expect us to repair deformities they attribute to another surgeon "elsewhere." In my experience, some of these patients are directly responsible for their deformities, but they strongly deny tampering or interfering with their postoperative care and shamelessly will place the blame on their surgeon. If you, therefore, *doubt* their sincerity and their clinical history even in the slightest, reject them as patients, and *don't* operate. If operated on, they are rarely satisfied and all too often inclined to instigate malpractice suits not only against their first surgeon but against you as well.

From another viewpoint, if you also *doubt* preoperatively the outcome of some small secondary procedure, sometimes called the *surgery of nuances*—doubts because of the patient's overly sebaceous tip tissue, poor blood supply, or exaggerated intranasal incisional scarring or adhesions—*don't* perform the procedure! It might and often does lead to just another deformity, for which the patient then demands a tertiary or quaternary corrective procedure, and then both you and the patient become the victims of frequently repeated surgical exercises, each successive one as unsatisfactory as its predecessor, until the patient becomes what we in our clinic refer to as a nasal

*From Millard, D. R., Jr.: Plast. Reconstr. Surg. **44**:545, 1969.

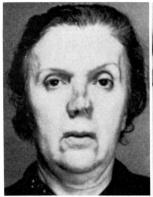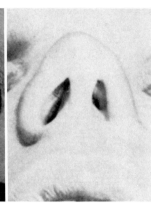

Fig. 23-1. Postoperative deformity of nose and airways after sixteen rhinoplastic operations performed in 20 years. Note partial stenosis of right airway and almost complete stenosis of left airway. (From Rogers, B. O.: The importance of "delay" in timing secondary and tertiary correction of post-rhinoplastic deformities. In Transactions of the Fourth International Congress of Plastic and Reconstructive Surgery [1967], Amsterdam, 1969, Excerpta Medica Foundation.)

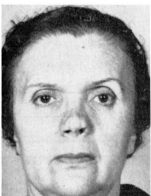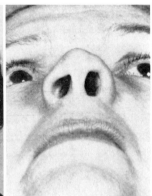

Fig. 23-2. Postoperative result obtained in patient in Fig. 23-1 after correction of left airway stenosis by retroauricular full-thickness skin grafting, which was subsequently followed by several liquid silicone injections to correct small irregular tip defects. (From Rogers, B. O.: The importance of "delay" in timing secondary and tertiary correction of post-rhinoplastic and Reconstructive Surgery [1967], Amsterdam, 1969, Excerpta Medica Foundation.)

cripple with a surgically mutilated nose (Fig. 23-1).

The woman in Fig. 23-1 had sixteen operations in 20 years before coming to our clinic for help. She also represents our adherence to the second aphorism: *"Replace what is normal in normal position, and retain it there!"* Excessive scar tissue in the left vestibule was widely excised. The remaining vestibular tissues then fell back into more normal anatomic positions. A retroauricular skin graft was

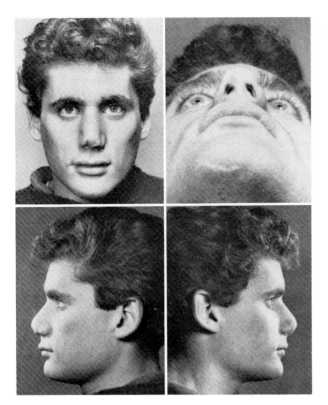

Fig. 23-3. Postoperative nasal disfigurement resulting from a single rhinoplasty performed by general surgical resident without adequate supervision. Note partial stenosis of both airways. (From Rogers, B. O.: The importance of "delay" in timing secondary and tertiary correction of post-rhinoplastic deformities. In Transactions of the Fourth International Congress of Plastic and Reconstructive Surgery [1967], Amsterdam, 1969, Excerpta Medica Foundation.)

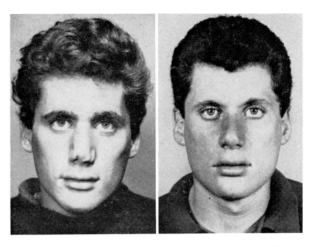

Fig. 23-4. *Left,* Preoperative photograph of postrhinoplastic deformity. *Right,* Photograph demonstrating improvement obtained by complete secondary nasoplasty with vestibular scar excision bilaterally, full-thickness skin grafting of both vestibular defects followed by several liquid silicone injections to improve tip contour defects. (From Rogers, B. O.: The importance of "delay" in timing secondary and tertiary correction of post-rhinoplastic deformities. In Transactions of the Fourth International Congress of Plastic and Reconstructive Surgery [1967], Amsterdam, 1969, Excerpta Medica Foundation.)

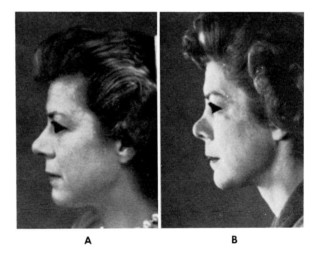

A   B

Fig. 23-5. A, Preoperative photograph of patient who consulted pseudo–plastic surgeon for correction of septal deviation and broad tip contours. **B,** Postrhinoplastic deformity after inadequate and unaesthetic surgery performed by pseudo–plastic surgeon. (From Rogers, B. O.: The importance of "delay" in timing secondary and tertiary correction of post-rhinoplastic deformities. In Transactions of the Fourth International Congress of Plastic and Reconstructive Surgery [1967], Amsterdam, 1969, Excerpta Medica Foundation.)

sewn into the denuded vestibule and *retained* in place by a dental compound mold (Fig. 23-2). This was subsequently replaced by a hollow acrylic mold, which the patient has worn daily for more than 2 years. Small irregular alar cartilage defects were partially disguised and better contoured by liquid silicone injections, because we assumed correctly that her sixteen previous operations had left her with little or no normal anatomic alar cartilage to remodel and reposition.

The young man in Fig. 23-3 had a nasal disfigurement that was the result of a single rhinoplasty performed by a general surgical resident without any supervision. The same sequence of surgery, including vestibular scar excision bilaterally, skin grafting of both vestibular defects, and subsequent liquid silicone injections, was utilized. His final satisfactory results (Fig. 23-4) were obtained with two conservative injections of 350 SCT soluble silicone.

The woman in Fig. 23-5 with a slightly gener-

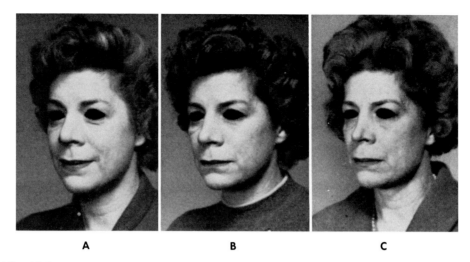

A   B   C

Fig. 23-6. A, Preoperative photograph of postrhinoplastic deformity with thickness of tip region and septal cartilaginous and alar cartilage irregularities. **B,** Early result after secondary correction of rhinoplastic deformity 1 year after secondary corrective procedure. **C,** Late result illustrating more marked contour improvement of tip region, which appeared postoperatively only after 2 years had elaspsed from secondary corrective procedure. (From Rogers, B. O.: The importance of "delay" in timing secondary and tertiary correction of post-rhinoplastic deformities. In Transactions of the Fourth International Congress of Plastic and Reconstructive Surgery [1967], Amsterdam, 1969, Excerpta Medica Foundation.)

ous nose preoperatively complained merely of a deviated septum to a pseudo–plastic surgeon famous for his drugstore paperbacks. He gave her the hideous postoperative deformity seen in Fig. 23-5, *B,* which made her look as if she was always sniffing something disagreeable. A secondary *complete* rhinoplasty was performed to restore her remaining nasal tissues to a more normal anatomic and aesthetically acceptable position, where they were retained in place by an external dental compound splint worn for 2 weeks postoperatively. She desired an extremely angular and narrow Anglo-Saxon nasal tip in keeping with her parental background. It did not appear postoperatively, however, until at least 2 years had elapsed, a time period illustrated between the preoperative photograph (Fig. 23-6, *A*) and the postoperative photograph (Fig. 23-6, *C*). Fig. 23-6, *B,* represents her appearance a year after the secondary corrective procedure, and, although some contour improvement can be seen, it was not of the degree requested by the patient or anticipated by the surgeon, and it only made its satisfactory appearance after the second postoperative year. Thus, instead of the customary 6 months to a year recommended by most surgeons as the time interval required before the final results of a rhinoplasty can be clearly detected and evaluated, this patient was typical of so many patients who have undergone secondary

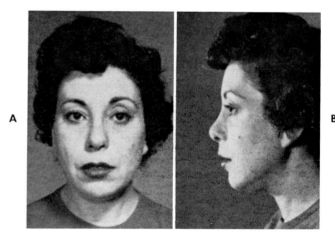

A   B

Fig. 23-7. Postrhinoplastic deformity of alar cartilages, tip contour, and profile disfigurement after primary rhinoplastic surgery performed by a pseudo–plastic surgeon. (From Rogers, B. O.: The importance of "delay" in timing secondary and tertiary correction of post-rhinoplastic deformities. In Transactions of the Fourth International Congress of Plastic and Reconstructive Surgery [1967], Amsterdam, 1969, Excerpta Medica Foundation.)

procedures whose final acceptable results may not be obtained in some cases until a minimum of at least 2 or 3 years has passed by.

The woman in Figs. 23-7 and 23-8 was similarly disfigured by another pseudo–plastic surgeon. The

A B C

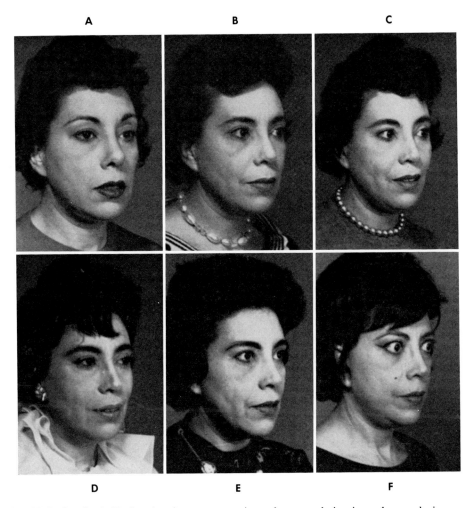

D E F

Fig. 23-8. Gradual diminution in postoperative edema and tip tissue hyperplasia over a 6-year time span after secondary and tertiary correction of postrhinoplastic deformity illustrated in Fig. 23-7. **A,** Postrhinoplastic deformity before secondary correction. **B,** Ten months after secondary surgery. **C,** Twenty months after secondary surgery. **D,** Two years after secondary surgery. **E,** Two and a half years after secondary surgery. **F,** Six years after secondary surgery. Change in patient's orbital region was due to sudden onset of hyperthyroidal exophthalmos, which was brought under control. (From Rogers, B. O.: The importance of "delay" in timing secondary and tertiary correction of post-rhinoplastic deformities. In Transactions of the Fourth International Congress of Plastic and Reconstructive Surgery [1967], Amsterdam, 1969, Excerpta Medica Foundation.)

postoperative photograph in Fig. 23-8, *F,* was taken 6 years later after one major secondary corrective procedure, which was followed by a minor tertiary procedure performed 3 years after the secondary. This delay between secondary and tertiary procedures is as important as the delay between primary and secondary rhinoplastic surgery and strictly adheres to the third aphorism, *"Never do today what can honorably be put off till tomorrow!"*

During this 6-year time span her nose underwent a slow, gradual diminution in postoperative edema and tip tissue hyperplasia, and, as in the case in Fig. 23-6, the benefits of secondary surgery

were not distinctly evident either to the patient or to her surgeon in the top row of photographs in Fig. 23-8. During the first 20 months after surgery, the patient was overly anxious and slightly disappointed.

A distinct improvement with narrowing of the edematous, hyperplastic tip tissues and the calloused osteotomy sites finally became apparent 2 years after secondary surgery (Fig. 23-8, *D*), more distinctly apparent 2½ years after surgery (Fig. 23-8, *E*), and definitely obvious 6 years after secondary surgery (Fig. 23-8, *F*). The change in the patient's orbital region in Fig. 23-8, *F,* was due to the sudden onset of hyperthyroidal exophthalmos, which was brought under control. She was also a difficult psychologic problem to handle during these prolonged periods of *delay* between the secondary and tertiary procedures, but eventually she was convinced, when she was shown these serial photographs and those of other similar patients, of the important value of delay, especially as soon as her photographs began to demonstrate an obvious but slow improvement in her appearance from year to year. Here again, the customary advice of waiting for 6 months to a year before performing a secondary or another corrective procedure had to be disregarded, because in this case, as in many other similar cases, a much longer period of time had to elapse before assessing the initial results of the primary and, even more importantly, of the secondary corrective procedure.

I now advise all patients seeking secondary correction of rhinoplastic deformities that such a correction will not be undertaken until a year or more has passed by after the primary surgery. Furthermore, they are also advised that, if it becomes necessary, a tertiary procedure will not be performed until another 1 or 1½ years or more have elapsed after the secondary operation. Of course, some patients will see the beneficial results of these operations sooner, and if they do, their subsequent procedure can be scheduled somewhat earlier.

When these principles and aphorisms of Gillies and Millard are ignored by a surgeon who surrenders to the emotional pressures of agitated patients or to his own ego-shattering disappointment with the results of his primary surgery, one can easily understand how and why severe postrhinoplastic deformities result, when the side effects of the primary operation such as edema, vestibular scarring, and tip hyperplasia, have hardly had time to subside before the surgeon superimposes on these side effects those side effects resulting from secondary, tertiary, and often quaternary surgery performed unfortunately only a mere interval of 2, 4, or 6 months after each preceding so-called corrective touching-up procedure. Is it any wonder, then, that patients with marked scarring and intranasal adhesions, dimpling, depressions, irregular and jagged alar cartilage marginal areas, and repeated inadequate lateral osteotomies are seen with increasing frequency today all over the world?

Figs. 23-11 to 23-15 will perhaps raise a somewhat controversial subject. As seen in the historical review (Chapter 1), the whole tendency in the development of corrective surgery of the nose was the avoidance of external incisions at any cost if possible. Fig. 23-9 shows the external incisions of Dieffenbach to reduce the overall size of a large nose, and Joseph (Fig. 23-10) in his very first case in 1898 used external incisions to accomplish the same reduction. There are, however, those rare cases which are a severe challenge to correct after secondary and sometimes tertiary procedures have failed to overcome the thick unsightly profile and tip contours (Fig. 23-11, *A* and *C*).

These deformities exist especially in patients with excessively thick, sebaceous, or oily tip skin with or without scarring secondary to acute or chronic acne, and these patients usually have a predictably poorer result after primary rhinoplasty than patients with thin, dry skin. Such patients should be advised beforehand or preoperatively of the possibility of poor results. Supratip hyperplasia of the connective tissue and the skin appendages usually results in a rounded, unpleasant tip contour after primary surgery. If a standard secondary nasoplasty gives little or no improvement to this polly tip deformity because the thick skin refuses to contract or settle down to the new skeletal framework, the only operative solution seems to be the external excision of some of this thick skin, as originally recommended by Brown and McDowell.[1] External incisions, therefore, although generally frowned on by most plastic surgeons, can be used successfully on occasion. The patients in Figs. 23-11 to 23-15 will demonstrate this type of surgery.

The patient in Fig. 23-11, *A* and *C*, had a thick, scarred, telangiectatic hyperplastic polly tip unimproved by myself in a routine secondary operation, which included scooping the cartilaginous dorsal profile according to the recommendations of Aufricht. His postoperative improvement can be seen in Figs. 23-11, *B* and *D*, after external excision in the nasal midline of a long vertical ellipse of the thick, scarred skin, and in Fig. 23-11, *D*, one can notice the minimal midline scar, which was further improved in a later operation by dermabrasion.

The young girl in Fig. 23-12 with a severely scarred bilateral harelip, which needs further repair, and a markedly disfigured nose with sebaceous thick scarred skin unresponsive to other surgery, also responded well to a midline external excision of the deformed tissue with a suturing together under direct exposure in the midline region of the newly created domes of the reshaped alar cartilages. In Fig. 23-12, *A* to *C*, one can follow the satisfactory progress of the gradual diminution

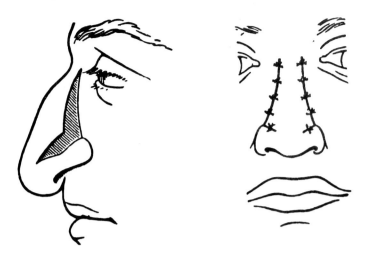

Fig. 23-9. Dieffenbach's external incisions used to reduce overall size of nose. (From Davis, J. S.: Plastic surgery: its principles and practice, Philadelphia, 1919, P. Blakiston's Son & Co.)

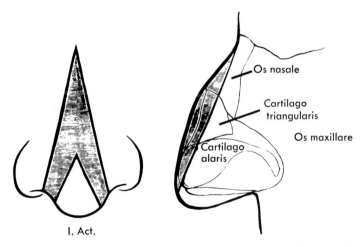

Fig. 23-10. Joseph's external incisions to reduce overall size of nose. (From Joseph, J.: Ueber die operative Verkleinerung einer Nase [Rhinomiosis], Berl. Klin. Wochenschr. **40**:882, 1898.)

in the visible appearance of the midline scar, which can be further improved at a later date by dermabrasion.

The young man in Figs. 23-13, 23-14, and 23-15, whose bilateral harelip was excellently repaired elsewhere, showed preoperatively a huge disfigured asymmetric nasal tip (Fig. 23-13, *A*) with thick skin, as well as septal and alar cartilages unimproved by many previous secondary, tertiary, and quaternary nasoplasties. His immediate postoperative result with a satisfactory contour improvement was obtained by the external longitudinal excision of a lateral-to-the-midline elliptical wedge of scarred, thick skin and cartilage together

with the repositioning under direct exposure of the underlying septal and alar cartilages, as can be seen in Figs. 23-13, *B*, 23-14, *B*, and 23-15, *B* to *D*. The remaining domes of the alar cartilages were remodeled and sutured together in the midline under direct vision. Fig. 23-15, *C* and *D*, demonstrates the intradermal nylon suturing reinforced by only a few 6-0 black silk sutures supported during the entire immediate postoperative course by external Dermicel taping applied directly over the entire incision site. In Figs. 23-13, *B*, 23-14, *B*, and 23-15, *B* to *D*, the Dermicel tape has been removed, the photographs having been taken on the tenth postoperative day.

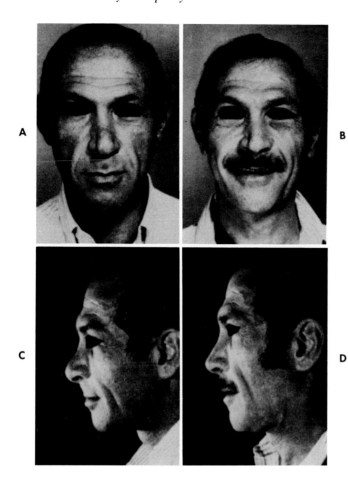

Fig. 23-11. A, Preoperative photograph. Thick, scarred, telangiectatic, hyperplastic poly tip was unimproved by routine secondary correction, which included scooping cartilaginous dorsal profile. B, Postoperative photograph. Note minimal midline scar, which was further improved by dermabrasion. C, Preoperative photograph. D, Postoperative photograph. Satisfactory contour improvement after external excision of midline, long, vertical ellipse of scarred thick skin. (From Rogers, B. O.: Rhinoplasty. In Goldwyn, R. M., editor: The unfavorable result in plastic surgery: avoidance and treatment, Boston, 1972, Little, Brown & Co.)

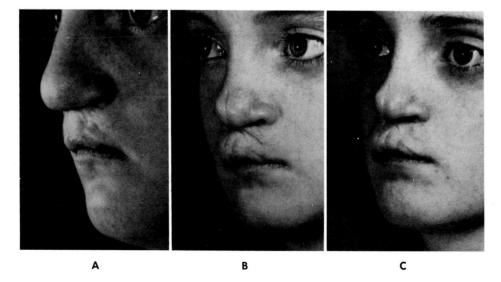

Fig. 23-12. A, Thick, scarred nose and nasal tip in patient with bilateral cleft lip deformity. B, Postoperative close-up view of nasal tip a year after midline external excision of nasal tip tissue. C, Postoperative close-up view of nasal tip 2 years after midline external excision.

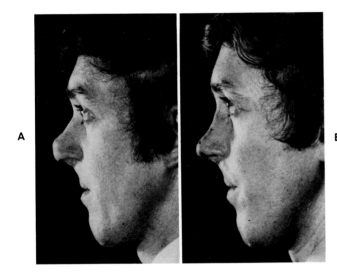

Fig. 23-13. A, Preoperative left profile view of scarred, distorted nose and nasal tip in patient with repaired bilateral cleft lip deformity. **B,** Postoperative photograph of immediate improvement in profile contour noted 10 days after external excision (just lateral to midline) of distorted and scarred nasal cartilage and skin.

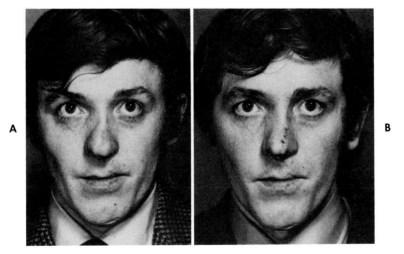

Fig. 23-14. A, Preoperative full-face view of nasal deformity in patient with repaired bilateral cleft lip. **B,** Postoperative photograph of immediate improvement in full-face appearance of nose 10 days after external excision of distorted and scarred nasal cartilage and skin. A few 6-0 black silk sutures can be seen along incisional line of closure.

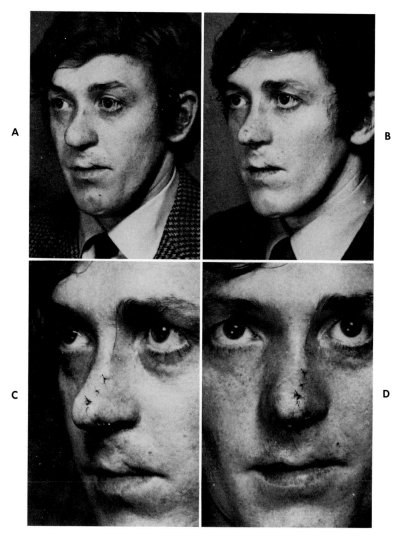

Fig. 23-15. A, Preoperative photograph. Huge disfigured asymmetric nasal tip, with skin and septal and alar cartilages unimproved by previous secondary and tertiary naso- plasties. **B,** Postoperative photograph. Satisfactory contour improvement obtained after external excision of midline wedge of scarred, thick skin together with underlying septal and alar cartilages. Remaining domes of alar cartilages were remodeled and sutured together in midline under direct vision. **C,** Postoperative three-quarters left close-up view demonstrating intradermal nylon suturing reinforced by only a few 6-0 black silk sutures supported by external Dermicel taping of entire incision site. Tape has been removed in this photograph taken on tenth postoperative day. **D,** Postoperative full-face photograph revealing same features of suturing technique explained in **C.**

SUMMARY

In summary, therefore, let us all remember again and again the aphorisms of Gillies and Millard when treating any patient with a postrhinoplastic deformity and in handling the patient's emotional pressures and pleas for a secondary correction. I would plead with all surgeons to follow the advice seen at railroad crossings in the United States countryside, with a slight paraphrasing of those railroad crossing signs as follows: STOP! LOOK! LISTEN! WAIT! and DELAY!

REFERENCES

1. Brown, J. B., and McDowell, F.: Plastic surgery of the nose, ed. 3, Springfield, Ill. 1965, Charles C Thomas, Publisher.
2. Denecke, H. J., and Meyer, R.: Plastic surgery of head and neck. I. Corrective and reconstructive rhinoplasty, New York, 1967, Springer-Verlag New York, Inc., p. 451.
3. Dieffenbach, J. F.: Die operative Chirurgie, Leipzig, Germany, 1845, F. A. Brockhaus.
4. Dingman, R. E., and Claus, W.: Use of composite ear grafts in correction of the short nose, Plast. Reconstr. Surg. **43:**117, 1969.
5. Fomon, S., and Bell, J.: Rhinoplasty—new concepts: evaluation and application, Springfield, Ill., 1970, Charles C Thomas, Publisher.
6. Gillies, H. D., and Millard, D. R., Jr.: The principles and art of plastic surgery, Boston, 1957, Little, Brown & Co.
7. Klabunde, E. H., and Falces, E.: Incidence of complications in cosmetic rhinoplasties, Plast. Reconstr. Surg. **34:**192, 1964.
8. McGregor, M. W., and Vistnes, L. M.: Unsatisfactory cosmetic rhinoplasty. In Masters, F. W., and Lewis, J. R., Jr., editors: Symposium on aesthetic surgery of the nose, ears, and chin, vol. 6, St. Louis, 1973, The C. V. Mosby Co., p. 50.
9. Millard, D. R., Jr.: The triad of columella deformities, Plast. Reconstr. Surg. **31:**370, 1963.
10. Millard, D. R., Jr.: Secondary corrective rhinoplasty, Plast. Reconstr. Surg. **44:**545, 1969.
11. Millard, D. R., Jr.: Problem cases in rhinoplasty. In Masters, F. W., and Lewis, J. R., Jr., editors: Symposium on aesthetic surgery of the nose, ears, and chin, vol. 6, St. Louis, 1973, The C. V. Mosby Co., p. 45.
12. O'Connor, G. B., and McGregor, M. W.: Secondary rhinoplasties: their cause and prevention, Plast. Reconstr. Surg. **15:**404, 1955.
13. Pollet, J., and Baudelot, S.: Sequelles de la chirurgie esthetique de la base du nez, Ann. Chir. Plast. **12:**185, 1967.
14. Rees, T. D., Krupp, S., and Wood-Smith, D.: Secondary rhinoplasty, Plast. Reconstr. Surg. **46:**332, 1970.
15. Rees, T. D.: Secondary rhinoplasty. In Masters, F. W., and Lewis, J. R., Jr., editors: Symposium on aesthetic surgery of the nose, ears, and chin, vol. 6, St. Louis, 1973, The C. V. Mosby Co., p. 58.
16. Rogers, B. O.: The importance of "delay" in timing secondary and tertiary correction of post-rhinoplastic deformities. In Transactions of the Fourth International Congress of Plastic and Reconstructive Surgery (1967), Amsterdam, 1969, Excerpta Medica Foundation, p. 1065.
17. Rogers, B. O.: Secondary and tertiary correction of postrhinoplastic deformities: the importance of "delay" in their timing. In Robbett, W. F., editor: Proceedings of the Centennial Symposium, Manhattan Eye, Ear and Throat Hospital, vol. 2, Otolaryngology, St. Louis, 1969, The C. V. Mosby Co., p. 237.
18. Rogers, B. O.: Rhinoplasty. In Goldwyn, R. M., editor: The unfavorable result in plastic surgery: avoidance and treatment, Boston, 1972, Little, Brown & Co., p. 283.
19. Rogers, B. O.: The role of physical anthropology in plastic surgery today, Clin. Plast. Surg. **1:**439, 1974.
20. Safian, J.: Uncontrollable factors in rhinoplasty, Plast. Reconstr. Surg. **12:**24, 1953.

Discussion

Millard: You asked how long to wait before secondary surgery? A year? Don't you think it might have gotten better eventually? Dr. Berkeley?

Berkeley: I don't know whether we were helped or hurt by the marginal incisions at the tip of the nose. But I hope that we got some men to do some thinking about external incisions. We are quite pleased with them.

Ungaro: I couldn't agree more wholeheartedly with Blair that a properly performed outfracture-infracture will increase the height of the nasal bones. I think the misunderstanding might be, and we've all seen it, is that frequently the infracture is performed too high, and if you look very carefully at the nasal bones as they more closely approach the apex of the septum, they become really relatively thinner. If the true infracture is performed in the maxilla, you get no ridging. You have quite a bit of distance medially to move those bones and still maintain bony contact. I've seen it repeatedly. The pictures that Blair showed there, we routinely use in our corrective device.

Kipp: I would like to bring up the point to the young men that isn't emphasized enough. I think you could do the same nose on an 18 year old and do it on a 45 year old, and you'd better not be as radical on the 45 year old. They have become fixed in their minds and are not willing to change their thinking. Just like some people won't employ someone over 40 because they won't change their way of thinking. If you do the same nose on a 45 year old that you would do on an 18 year old, the 18 year old may say for days that they are very upset about it and then in the next few days, they don't want it changed. The 45 year old will keep at you and she'll practically want the hump back. You've got to be awfully careful about trying to do a radical change on an older person.

Courtiss: I think we saw a very interesting principle in Ralph's demonstration this morning. When he wasn't 100% pleased with the way that dorsal cartilage graft sat in there, he still accepted it. An altruism that I believe important, particularly in secondaries, is that perfection can be the enemy of success. You may not get it 100% perfect, but sometimes it is the better part of valor not to go all the way.

[Applause]

Millard: Nonsense; I thought it might not be quite right, but Dr. Aufricht assured me it was!

[Much laughter]

Participant: Only one other pragmatic reason that Blair Rogers didn't mention on delaying secondaries up to 2 years is (1) they might get used to it, and (2) they might move away.

[Much laughter]

Millard: See if somebody else will operate on it in a year! Now, Dr. Reed Dingman, who some of us acknowledge as "Top Dog."

Chapter 24

Surgical correction of deformities secondary to rhinoplasty

Reed O. Dingman, M.D., F.A.C.S.

As a surgeon develops experience in his practice, he should have fewer of his own secondary deformities to correct, and by virtue of his reputation, he should have referral of patients with secondary deformities done by less experienced surgeons. Some surgeons refuse to see patients with complications who have had operations by other surgeons.

As one of the senior men in my community, I have an obligation to see patients with deformities incident to rhinoplastic procedures elsewhere. If the patient has been operated on by a competent surgeon capable of correcting the deformity, he is urged to return for further care. Most patients will return to the original surgeon, but some refuse to do so. There are instances in which it is probable that the original surgeon will further complicate the problem. To protect the patient from additional injury, usually I accept him for revision, providing the attitude is favorable and the deformity is correctable.

In accepting these patients, one assumes a great responsibility, and each case offers potential for legal action. In accepting the patient for care, it must be understood definitely by the patient and his family in the presence of witnesses that I will not become involved in problems between the patient and the original surgeon. The difficulty of doing secondary operations in the presence of scar and loss of tissue is explained. Nothing in the way of improvement is promised. If the patient has a correctable deformity and is willing to proceed on this basis, I accept him for treatment.

Most iatrogenic rhinoplasty deformities can be assessed to poor treatment planning or to ineptness of the surgeon in execution of the operation. Some deformities such as infection, hema-

toma, hypertrophic scar formation, and failure of integument to adjust to the revised supporting structures are beyond control of the surgeon. An occasional unfavorable result may be due to early postoperative trauma.

The surgeon must enter the operating room with a careful plan of procedure in mind. Photographs of the original preoperative condition may be helpful and, if possible, one should obtain operative records and discuss the patient with the original surgeon. A set of 1×1 black-and-white photographs should be made. Radiographs may be indicated, and a clinical and psychologic evaluation of the problem is imperative.

Some late deformities are due to inadequate removal or adjustment of supporting structures, and others are due to overenthusiastic removal of lining, cartilage, or bone. Some are due to lack of correction or inadequate management of septal deformities. In some, too much tissue has been removed in one area and insufficient tissue in another. Although most deformities are obvious and the cause is not difficult to determine, the patient's reaction to the deformity is necessary to ascertain his expectations from a revision operation. The treatment plan is formulated on assessment of many factors.

In case of underoperation, as may be present in the bulbous nasal tip, the operation consists of reexposure of the alar cartilages and adjustment or removal of cartilage as indicated. Some require replacement of cartilage for support. Septal deformities may require correction by bone or cartilage removal and osteotomy. In case of excess tissue removed, correction by moving in adjacent tissues or by replacing cartilage, lining, or bone from a distance may be necessary. Release of scar or Z-plasty of the vestibular lining may correct contractures of the nasal tip; in some cases skin grafts or composite grafts may be necessary. If the tip is bulbous due to thick skin and dense subcutaneous scar, then external skin excision, nasal base wedges, thinning of the alae or columella, or dorsal excision of tissue may be indicated. In some cases revision of osteotomy or bone grafts may correct the deformity.

Silastic implants to the tip or dorsum may give

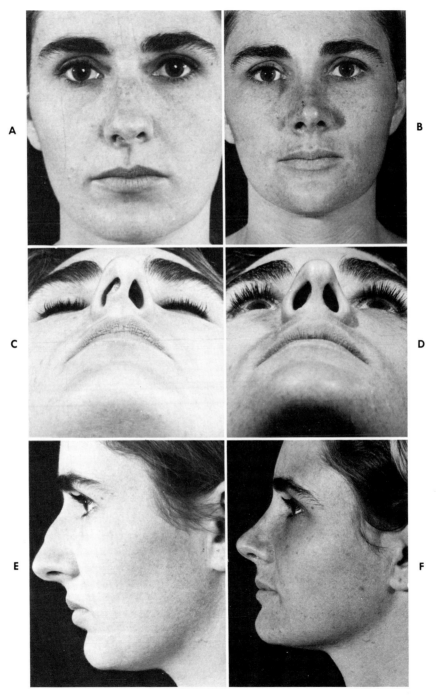

Fig. 24-1. A, Anterior preoperative view. **B,** Anterior postoperative view. **C,** Basal preoperative view. **D,** Basal postoperative view. **E,** Lateral preoperative view. **F,** Lateral postoperative view.

satisfactory results. My preference is autogenous tissue for reconstruction whenever possible. The following cases illustrate some of the common problems encountered secondary to rhinoplastic operations.

Case 1. S. S. had had a rhinoplasty and submucous resection previous to evaluation. She presented with partial removal of the bony dorsal hump, inadequate lowering of the bony and cartilaginous dorsum, prominence of the nasal tip, unequal elevation of the nasal alae, deviation of the columella and caudal septum with airway obstruction, and receding chin (Fig. 24-1). The operation was a total revision of rhinoplasty, consisting of intracartilaginous incisions and removal of the upper half of the lateral crus of greater alar cartilages, removal of the dorsal hump, septal reconstruction through transfixion incision, revision osteotomy, and preserved irradiated cartilage implant to the mandible through an intraoral approach.

Case 2. P. M. had had a rhinoplasty 2 years previously. She was unhappy about the bulbous tip, the wide bony base, depressed nasal bridge, and continual nasal drip from the tip of the nose (Fig. 24-2). Examination indicated inadequate management of alar cartilages, low bony dorsum, wide nasal base, retracted columella due to excessive excision of caudal cartilaginous septum, and webbing in the anterior nasal vestibule. The operation was a revision rhinoplasty, consisting of exposure and adjustment of alar cartilages, iliac bone graft to the nasal dorsum, and advancement of the nasal tip supported by a strut graft of septal cartilage between the medial crura through a midcolumellar incision. Postoperative photographs were taken 8 months after secondary corrective rhinoplasty.

Case 3. M. R. had had a rhinoplasty and submucous resection 5 years previously and revision 4 years later. The deformity consisted of deviation of the tip of the nose and supporting structures

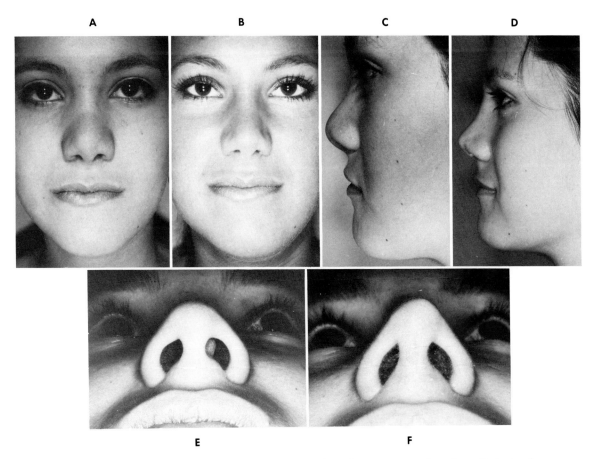

Fig. 24-2. A, Anterior preoperative view. **B,** Anterior postoperative view. **C,** Lateral preoperative view. **D,** Lateral postoperative view. **E,** Basal preoperative view. **F,** Basal postoperative view.

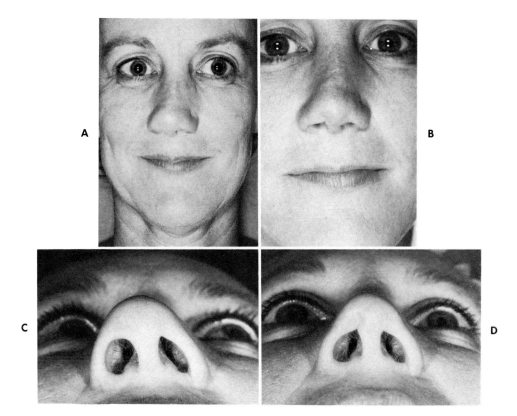

Fig. 24-3. A, Anterior preoperative view. **B,** Anterior postoperative view. **C,** Basal preoperative view. **D,** Basal postoperative view.

to the right with subcutaneous scar, bulbousness of the nasal tip, and deviation of nasal septum with overall elongation (Fig. 24-3). The operation consisted of revision of tip cartilages, lowering of the nasal dorsum, septal reconstruction with caudal edge shortening, and revision of osteotomy.

Case 4. B. W. had had four rhinoplastic operations. The first was a reduction, 3 weeks later a revision, and 10 months later a Silastic implant. The Silastic implant was removed because of erosion and exposure a year later. The patient was first seen a year after the last procedure. The deformity consisted of supratip prominence, depression of the bony dorsum, inadequate lowering of the cartilaginous dorsum, distortion of the nasal tip due to unequal excision of cartilage at the junction of medial and lateral crura, and septal deviation (Fig. 24-4). The operation consisted of revision of alar cartilages and lowering of the cartilaginous dorsum and iliac bone graft to nasal dorsum. Postoperative photographs were taken after 2½ years.

Case 5. N. S. had had a rhinoplasty 6 years before and revision a year later. Deformity consists

of pinched nasal tip, supratip prominence, collapsed alae, and an unbalanced tip (Fig. 24-5). The operation consisted of lowering of the dorsal edge of the quadrilateral cartilage and advancement of triangular cartilages upward and forward, exposure and adjustment of cartilage at the junction of the medial and lateral crus, Z-plasty release of scar contracture of the nasal vestibule, septal reconstruction, medial and lateral osteotomy with outfracture, and repositioning of nasal bone structures to widen the base.

Case 6. Rhinoplasty for reduction of J. D.'s large nose was done in a naval hospital; 3 weeks later a Silastic implant was inserted into the dorsum to correct an iatrogenic saddle defect. Six weeks later abscess of the nose was followed by continual purulent drainage for 3 months. The nose was draining when first seen (Fig. 24-6). In the operation, the Silastic implant was removed, and 6 months later the residual deformity was corrected by an iliac bone graft through a midcolumellar incision. Postoperative photographs were taken 2 years after the iliac bone graft.

Case 7. Two operations were done on G. I. to

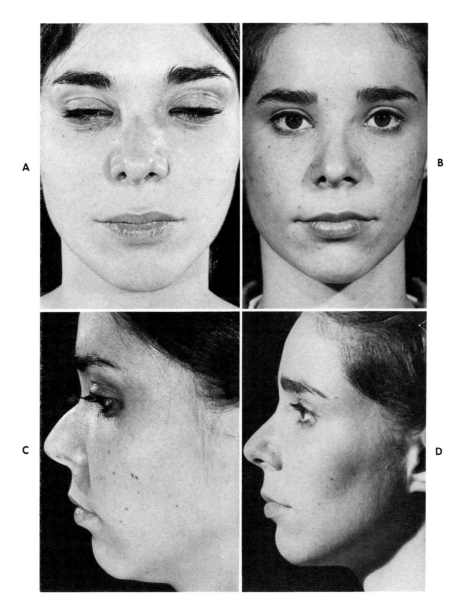

Fig. 24-4. A, Anterior preoperative view. **B,** Anterior postoperative view. **C,** Lateral preoperative view. **D,** Lateral postoperative view.

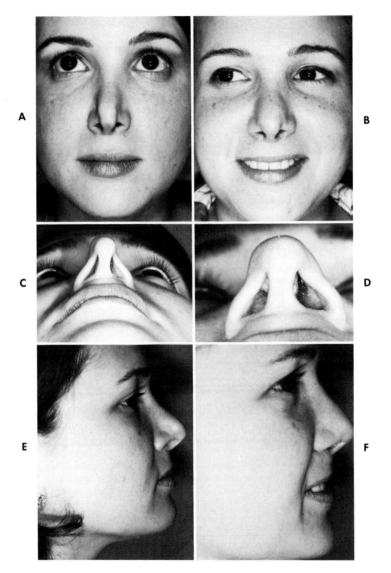

Fig. 24-5. A, Anterior preoperative view. **B,** Anterior postoperative view. **C,** Basal preoperative view. **D,** Basal postoperative view. **E,** Lateral preoperative view. **F,** Lateral postoperative view.

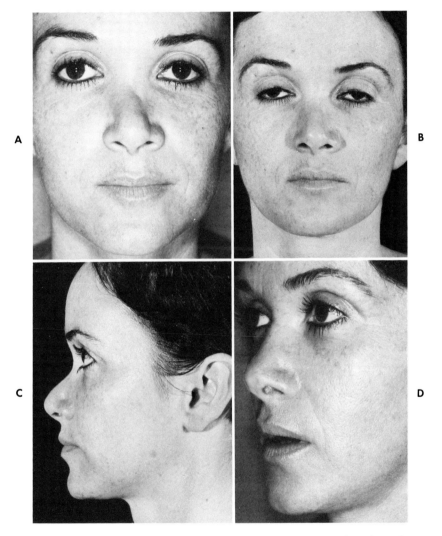

Fig. 24-6. A, Anterior preoperative view. **B,** Anterior postoperative view. **C,** Lateral preoperative view. **D,** Lateral postoperative view.

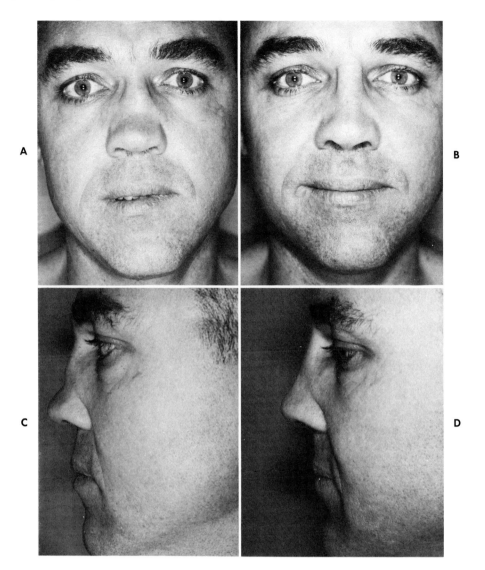

Fig. 24-7. A, Anterior preoperative view. **B,** Anterior postoperative view. **C,** Lateral preoperative view. **D,** Lateral postoperative view.

correct nasal deformity and nasal obstruction 18 years previously. There was no nasal tip support and total loss of septal cartilage. He complained of airway obstruction, postnasal drip, continual sore throat, and a poor cosmetic result (Fig. 24-7). Correction was done by an L-shaped iliac bone graft with dorsal and columellar strut. The columellar strut had lateral flanges to fill in the region of the nasal spine to correct acute nasolabial angle. Postoperative photographs were taken after 3 months.

Discussion

Musgrave: I want to warn about that midline excision of the thick skin. Willie White, whom I'm sure most of you know, recently was sued by a black lady who had an external excision done by Willie. The statute of limitations had run out, but her attorney brought it up as breach of contract. Willie won the case, but be very, very careful and make sure if you're going to do excision of heavy dorsal skin that the patients are thoroughly aware that this is going to leave a scar. She has a beautiful result, but she said she went in without a scar and when she left, Dr. White made this scar!

Dingman: It is true that with the thick sebaceous skin, you may get an objectionable scar. I have had occasion to revise them. You can dermabrade and get improvement of the scar, but waiting for a long period of time usually improves the scar. It is not an objectionable scar in most cases and is preferable to the original condition.

McGibbon: I'd like to suggest for consideration an alternative donor site for the autogenous bone graft. The ulna is easily exposed and gives the patient less discomfort than the hip or rib. With a small incision, an adequate bone graft can be obtained.

Musgrave: Do you do that with a Hall drill?

McGibbon: Yes, a Hall drill.

Musgrave: Anybody else here try that? You did and you did? Good!

Gorney: I've never used that, Ross, but I can recall the days when we used to take the tibia, which would be more or less similar type of bone, and it is very difficult to work with, difficult to contour, and for that reason, I like to use the iliac bone because it is nice to work with and I think the percentage of take will be much greater.

Cameron: Dr. Dingman mentioned the rhinorrhea and postnasal drip. I wonder if he saw any improvement after the secondary procedure? If so, what does he attribute it to?

Musgrave: Did you all hear the question? Some-

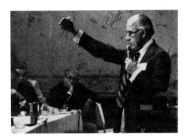

Dr. Musgrave

times the people in the back don't hear the questions well. Okay? To what did he attribute the improvement in dripping?

Dingman: We have had improvement in two cases where there was scar inside the nasal vestibule. As the mucus runs down to that area, it spills into the tip instead of running back into the floor of the nose. A Z-plasty in that area may be helpful, or, if there is not enough skin for a Z-plasty, a free graft from the postauricular area is indicated. I want to say a word about that and about the septum, which is not a uniformly thick structure. You will note bulges in the septum and areas below the bulges in which the septum is thin. These are roughly opposite the turbinates. These are ridges, so to speak. They are not sharp ridges but nice, rolled ridges in which there is increased thickness of the cartilaginous and bony septum above and posteriorly. They make troughs down which the mucus passes. If you get too radical with the excision of cartilage and bone from the nasal septum, you end up with an absolutely flaccid curtain of tissue that has no ridges in it, and mucus may run anteriorly, producing a sniffy patient. When we do septum work, we should retain all the septum that we possibly can and keep in mind the physiology of the nose and those pathways along which mucus passes from the upper anterior portion of the nose down to the posterior portion. We secrete over 1 liter a day of mucus, and if the physiology of the structures

221

is disturbed, instead of running backward into the nasal cavity where it is swallowed, it runs forward into the nasal vestibule, and we have a sniffing patient with a drippy-tipped nose!

Musgrave: Dr. Aufricht?

Aufricht: Regarding the necessity of secondary correction, I would like to recall my experience at my age of 40 or 50, when I was very busy during the summertime operating three rhinoplasties a day, 6 days a week. Most of my secondary corrections came from that period. If you do three cases a day, 6 days a week, you get up early and try to hurry through the operations. Therefore, it is my advice from this experience not to hurry plastic surgery. Do it slowly. I hope this will not be taken as a personal remark, but yesterday, during a very expert operation by George Peck, you noticed how carefully he went back and back to take a little bit more and a little bit more cartilage from the septal dorsum, and once he found a big chunk of tissue, and I'm sure he didn't expect it was still there. As Millard remarked, "You sneaked something out there on us, George." So if he hadn't taken his time and gone back and back,

a few months later, the patient would have felt something amiss. So please don't hurry plastic operations.

Musgrave: Thank you, Dr. Aufricht. Bill?

Conroy: I certinly consider iliac bone grafts to be the best bone to use. How frequently do you encounter absorption?

Dingman: I can't tell you how frequently we encounter absorption, but not very often. I can recall some. But how to gauge the amount of absorption you're going to have, I don't know. I usually overcorrect them a little bit, expecting them to absorb some, but I saw a patient in my office 2 days ago that I did 18 years ago with a bone graft, and I couldn't detect any absorption. I suppose it varies with different people. If you have good contact between the bone graft and the nasal bone (I usually flatten out the surface to get good contact), then there will not be much resorption. Even with a cantilever running down into the nasal tip, you will find that the bone will not resorb, even though the entire graft is not in contact with the bone. I think it's rather important to have bone at the distal end.

Chapter 25

The deviated nose

John Marquis Converse, M.D.

The deviated or twisted nose is most often of traumatic origin. In the unblemished nose, the nasal dorsum lies in the midsagittal plane of the face (Fig. 25-1, *A*). In partial deviations, only a portion of the nose is involved. When the nasal dorsum is curved to one side (Fig. 25-1, *B*), when two portions of the dorsum are twisted in opposite directions, as in an S-shaped deformity (Fig. 25-1, *C*), or when the entire nose veers to one side, the condition is referred to as a generalized or total deviation (Fig. 25-1, *D*). Whereas in most deviated noses the tip remains in the midline, in the last type (Fig. 25-1, *D*), the tip of the nose is also deviated.

There is also a vast number of congenital devia-tions of the nose caused by congenital clefts and other anomalies associated with craniofacial ano-malies; these will not be discussed.

CLASSIFICATION OF DEVIATIONS BY TIME OF ACQUISITION

Because of infinite variations, each deviated nose must be studied individually to determine the surgical measures required for correction. Nasal deviations may be classified into three broad cate-gories.

Congenital (prenatal) deviations

Some nasal deviations are caused by intrau-terine injury and do not correct themselves sponta-

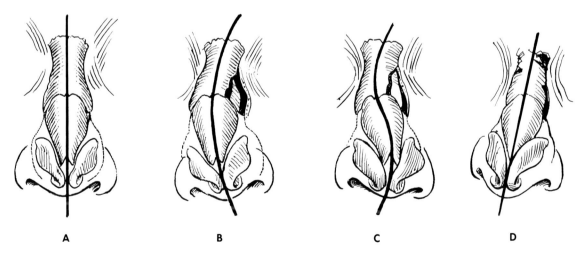

A   B   C   D

Fig. 25-1. Straight nose and three principal types of nasal deviations. **A,** In straight nose dorsum is aligned with midsagittal plane of face, which passes through nasion, above, and subnasale, below. **B,** C-shaped deviation. **C,** S-shaped deviation. **D,** General-ized deviation to one side. Whereas in other types of deviation, tip of nose is often in midline, in generalized deviation tip is often also deviated. (Modified from Converse, J. M.: Deformities of the nose. In Kazanjian, V. H., and Converse, J. M.: Surgical treat-ment of facial injuries, ed. 3, Baltimore, 1974, The Williams & Wilkins Co.)

neously. A genetic component is suggested when the parents or grandparents also show a similar deformity; a familial trend has been noted, especially in cases of dislocation of the caudal portion of the septal cartilage.

Deviations acquired in childhood

Deviation of the nose occurs not infrequently in the newborn during the trauma of delivery. Kirschner[6] has observed severe compression of the nose in every normal delivery. In posterior presentation, a greater amount of injury results from more extensive rotation of the head. Some degree of deviation of the nasal pyramid to the right and of the septal cartilage, which is dislocated from the vomer groove, to the left, has been observed. Most of these deviations tend to return to the midline spontaneously at the end of 3 months.

Another aspect that is generally overlooked is the injury occurring in the infant or young child as a result of a fall out of the crib or during the period when the child is undergoing the struggle to learn to walk. Studies have been made of the frequency of accidents in early childhood by Kravits and associates.[7] The battered-baby syndrome is another problem; I have fortunately seen few such cases, but, undoubtedly, the injuries suffered by the battered child are another cause of nasal deviation.

Injuries suffered in early childhood cause deviation by fracture, hypertrophic callus, or dislocation of the bones at a time when sutures are not yet closed. Deviation may also result from the disproportionate growth caused by the trauma,

and the deviation becomes more accentuated as the nose grows and becomes progressively more conspicuous in the adolescent. Developmental changes in the child result in greater anatomic disturbances than those which occur in the adult; this type of nasal deviation is often referred to as a developmental nasal deviation.

Deviations acquired in adult life

These deformities are produced by injury in adolescence or in adult life after or near the completion of nasal growth. The tip of the nose usually is in the midline, despite severe deflection of the dorsum.

CLASSIFICATION OF DEVIATIONS BY PART OF NOSE AFFECTED

It is convenient to divide the nose into upper (cephalic) and lower (caudal) portions; thus partial deviations may be designated according to the affected bony or cartilaginous portions. Such a division is arbitrary because both bony and cartilaginous portions of the nose are deviated in most cases and require straightening to obtain a satisfactory result.

Deviations of the bony portion of the nose

These usually show a one-sided dorsal hump, often thinly ridged and prolonged downward by a cartilaginous portion that is formed by the septal and lateral cartilages and is particularly prominent in the developmental type of nasal deviation. The deformities are varied and include such conditions

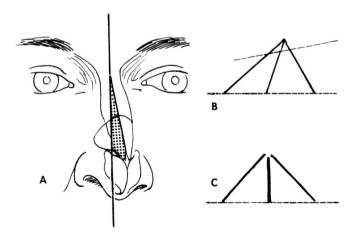

Fig. 25-2. Disproportion between lateral walls of nose in nasal deviation. **A,** Shaded area represents amount of bone and lateral cartilage excision required to equalize lateral walls. **B,** Resection of hump in beveled manner equalizes lateral walls. **C,** After correction of disproportion between lateral walls, dorsum of nose is realigned with midsagittal plane of face. Note also disproportion between lateral cartilages.

as simple deviations of the bony ridge, deviation with a dorsal hump due to hypertrophic callus or overriding fragments, widening, flattening, saddle deformity, or a combination of these deformities. The essential anatomic feature in such conditions is the disproportionate width of the lateral walls of the nose, the side of the deviation being narrower (Fig. 25-2). Deflection of the septum is a common occurrence because of the close association of the nasal bones with the lateral and septal cartilages.

Deviations of the cartilaginous portion of the nose

In addition to intranasal inspection, digital palpation of the dorsum of the deviated nose from the nasal bones to the tip provides information concerning the shape and position of the dorsal border of the septal cartilage; finger pressure just above the tip of the nose discloses the position of the septal angle (the anterosuperior [anterocaudal] angle of the septal cartilage). The dorsal portion of the septal cartilage may be C-shaped, or it may show an S-shaped curvature or a generalized deviation to one side. The position and shape of the septal angle and the caudal portion of the septum can be determined by placing the tip of the thumb in one vestibule and the tip of the forefinger in the other. When the nasal tip is gently elevated, the cephalic borders of the alar cartilages can also be seen protruding beneath the skin. The size, shape, and position of the alar cartilages can thus be determined.

The position and shape of the septum is con-firmed by intranasal examination. Hypertrophy of the middle turbinate (and of the inferior turbinate) on the side opposite the deviation is noted in patients with severe deviation of the septum; the hypertrophy is a compensatory phenomenon to fill the void caused by the deviated septum. Spurs are also a frequent finding near the vomer–septal cartilage junction.

Because of long-standing deflection, the lateral cartilages may be asymmetric, the cartilage on the side opposite the deviation being wider in developmental deviations (Fig. 25-2). The nasal tip feels soft to the touch and can be depressed by digital pressure when the septal angle is situated lateral to its midline position. A depression is noted just above the tip of the nose. The septal angle may protrude beneath one alar cartilage (Fig. 25-3), splaying out the alar cartilages and broadening the tip (Fig. 25-19), which is usually also asymmetric in shape. The caudal septal border, protruding in the narial opening, causes widening and distortion of the columella; the medial crus is separated from its counterpart, its lower portion forming a protrusion. In another less frequently encountered condition, the tip, the septum, and the entire nasal pyramid are deflected to one side (Fig. 25-12).

When the septum has been crushed or fractured, it loses its supportive function. In such cases the tip of the nose may be pressed backward against the face without encountering the septal angle; the septum no longer supports the tip of the nose (Fig. 25-4).

Variations also occur in the angulation or curvature of the septal cartilage in the sagittal and

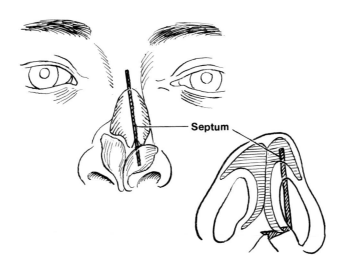

Fig. 25-3. Severe lateral deviation of septum and disproportionate size and shape of lateral and alar cartilages resulting from deviation of developmental type. Septal angle no longer being in midline elevates dome of left alar cartilage.

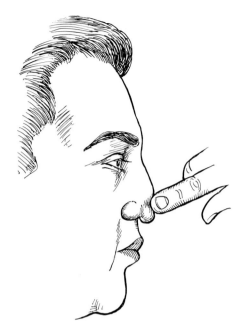

Fig. 25-4. Septum has lost its supportive function. Palpation demonstrates that tip of nose is depressed by digital pressure.

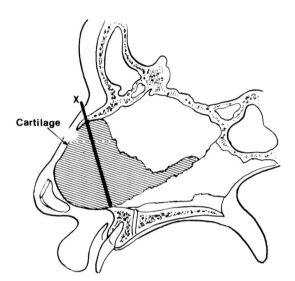

Fig. 25-5. Component parts of septal framework. Posterior to line *X*, septum is rigid.

vertical planes. The anterocaudal portion of the cartilage may be dislocated to one side of the vomer and the cephalic portion of the cartilage deviated toward the opposite side. The angulation may be such that the caudal portion of the septal cartilage lies transversely across one vestibule, with the free border of the cartilage protruding into the opposite vestibule, thus obstructing the airway.

More severe angulations occur along a line extending from the tip of the nasal bones or posteriorly at the junction with the perpendicular plate of the ethmoid. The posterior part of the septum is often seen to be fairly straight in severe deflection of the caudal portion of the septum. The reverse condition also occurs; a septum with severe posterior deflection may be relatively straight in its anterior portion.

Deviations of the septum may be complicated by a considerable increase in the thickness of the septum and by vomer-cartilage spurs in traumatic conditions. Thickening is caused by overlapping fractured cartilaginous fragments, with lamination of the cartilage, and by fibrous tissue thickening after hematoma of the septum. The curvature or angulation of the septal cartilage, its dislocation from the vomer groove, or a change in shape as a result of fracture may result in a decrease of the anteroposterior or vertical dimensions of the septum. The contraction after the healing of lac-

erated or destroyed mucous membrane can also cause a change in the position of the remaining portions of the septal cartilage after submucous resection. Characteristic deformities such as retraction of the columella and depression or flatness of the cartilaginous dorsum cephalad to the alar cartilages accompany these changes.

SEPTUM OF THE DEVIATED NOSE

The correction of septal deflection is the key to the straightening of the deviated nose. Deviations that occur in the cartilaginous portion of the nose can be explained by a brief review of some anatomic characteristics of the nasal septum. The component parts of the septal framework are illustrated in Fig. 25-5. The septal cartilage has two areas of fixation. The first is on the undersurface of the nasal bones, where it has an intimate relationship with the lateral cartilages and a shallow bony groove; septal cartilage, lateral cartilages and nasal bones are closely held together by the blending of the perichondrium and periosteum. The second area is the vomer groove; this area of fixation extends backward by means of a posterior extension of the septal cartilage into the perpendicular plate of the ethmoid (the ethmoid plate).

The caudal portion of the septal cartilage is mobile. This shock-absorbing anatomic feature protects the cartilaginous nose from trauma. The flexibility of the caudal portion of the septal cartilage is explained by the laxity of the attachments to the lateral cartilages, premaxillary wings, and anterior nasal spine.

The ethmoid plate plays a relatively unimportant role in supporting the osseous nasal vault. The area where the septal cartilage joins the perpendicular plate bone is usually thick, a resistant pillar that supports the portion of the vault formed by the lower part of the nasal bones and the lateral cartilages. This portion of the septal cartilage, the central pillar supporting the dorsal vault, must be preserved, if possible, to prevent the collapse of the dorsum. It is the pillar of support after the other nasal structures have been loosened from the adjacent attachments by the osteotomies in corrective rhinoplasty.

The cartilaginous septum plays a varying role in different types of noses. In the long, thin, straight nose the border of the septal cartilage may be distinctly felt along the entire dorsum to the junction of the septal angle and alar cartilages; the septal angle is immediately subcutaneous in the area between the lateral and alar cartilages. The septal angle prevents further depression if one attempts to depress the nasal tip. When the septum has been fractured, or when the septal support is lost by excessive submucous resection of the septal framework, the septal angle does not support the nasal tip. Septal angle support may also be absent in other ethnic or racial groups (Asiatic, black).

The alar cartilages are dislocated from the poorly developed septal angle, and this dislocation is a characteristic of this type of nose. The black nose is more rarely subjected to deviation, its anatomy being such that the nose is more protected against trauma.

As stated earlier in the text, the septum is required as a fixed structure, a central pillar, for the stabilization of the mobilized nasal structures after corrective nasal plastic surgery. After the nasal dorsal hump is resected, the profile line modified, the nose shortened, and the lateral walls mobilized, only the septum remains as a stable structure.

Collapse of the septal skeletal framework may occur after an extensive submucous resection in conjunction with a corrective rhinoplasty if the caudal portion of the septal cartilage is removed. After the osteotomy of the lateral walls of the nose, the remaining portion of the septum remains as a cantilever at the mercy of a fracture of the perpendicular plate of the ethmoid and may collapse into the nasal cavity. When this unfortunate complication occurs, it is necessary to suspend the remaining dorsal portion of the septum and suture it to the lateral cartilages (Fig. 25-6).

The situation is different when the continuity of the dorsal vault of the nose is undisturbed. In certain types of deviated noses, after a malunited fracture of the nasal bones, for example, when the continuity between the lateral cartilages over the dorsum of the nose is undisturbed, septal cartilage

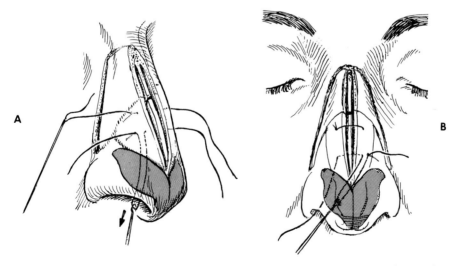

Fig. 25-6. A, Technique of fixation after fracture of septum and collapse of nose. Septal cartilage is sutured to lateral cartilages by transfixion sutures placed through skin. After exposing sutures intranasally, each suture is drawn out by means of hook as shown in drawing. **B,** Sutures are tied intranasally. An alternative technique is to obtain fixation to lateral cartilages by means of externally placed mattress sutures tied over bolsters (small dental rolls or pieces of gauze).

may be removed more extensively, without danger of a depression developing during the postoperative period. The present trend is to be more sparing in resecting cartilage.

Submucous resection and other techniques to straighten the septum

The classic submucous resection of the nasal septum is usually a partial resection that includes a portion of the septal framework consisting of septal cartilage, vomer, and perpendicular plate of the ethmoid. My technique is described in a recently published textbook.[2] The most important single operative step is to inject local anesthetic solution through a needle with a large bore and a short beveled point between the mucoperichondrium and the cartilage, thus separating the structures and facilitating the operation. Extensive resection of the septal framework is unnecessary as a therapeutic measure; the operation should be done only in cases in which there are specific indications, and, in many cases, more limited resection will give more satisfactory clinical results. A particular objection to the wide resection of the framework is the resulting flaccid septum (the "flapping flaps"). The replacement of resected septal cartilage fragments between the mucoperichondrial flaps has been advocated to avoid this complication, but it is hazardous, since complications such as twisting of the transplanted cartilage may interfere with the airway.

There are also techniques for straightening the septal framework that do not require extensive resection of the septal cartilage and bone.

In straightening a deviated nose, the surgeon has a dual objective: straightening the nasal pyramid and relieving obstructions of the nasal airways. This dual objective must be achieved by a corrective rhinoplasty without endangering the stability of the nasal structures. A submucous resection of the septum done before a corrective rhinoplasty is particularly undesirable since the preliminary sacrifice of the septal framework may leave inadequate support during the subsequent corrective operation of the external nose, and the necessary secondary septal surgery is more difficult because of the residual scar tissue.

An approach to the treatment of the deviated nose and septum is to perform the septal surgery necessary to realign the septum and straighten the nose. Various conservative techniques are available and are described later in the text. If nasal obstruction is not completely relieved, a secondary conservative submucous resection a few months later will complete the treatment. This compromise approach will avoid loss of cartilaginous vault support in most cases.

It is not always necessary to do a complete transfixion incision in operating on a deviated nose. If the nose does not require shortening and if the dorsal profile does not require modification, that is, when the nose requires only straightening, the transfixion incision may be interrupted slightly beyond the septal angle. In such cases, the approach to the septum is through a hemitransfixion incision. The tip of the nose and the columella are retracted with a double-pronged retractor to tense the membranous septum. An incision is then made along the caudal margin of the septal cartilage to the floor of the nose. Another horizontal incision through the mucoperiosteum along the base of the vomer ensures drainage. Nasal packing is occasionally necessary but usually not necessary. It is important to avoid incising the posterior vestibular fold, which delimits the floor of the vestibule from the nasal fossa proper. Failure to take this precaution may result in scar contracture, the formation of a web, which may interfere with the inflow of air currents into the nose.

When a complete transfixion procedure is performed along the caudal border of the septal cartilage, the septal framework may be approached through the transfixion incision.

If the caudal portion of the septum is straight, an L-shaped incision is made, leaving the caudal septum undisturbed and incising the mucoperichondrium posterior to the posterior vestibular fold.

Conservative septal procedures

After the mucoperichondrium is raised on one side, a wide exposure of the septal framework is obtained by retraction of the mucoperichondrial flap. A conservative submucous resection of the nasal framework is done, removing only the most obstructive portion. The important technical point in the deviated nose is to straighten the septum while preserving the dorsal and caudal portions of the septum. The perpendicular plate of the ethmoid may be straightened by fracturing it with Bruening forceps. The vomer may be detached from the floor of the nose by means of an osteotome and replaced into the midline.

As stated earlier, the inferior turbinates and particularly the middle turbinates may be hypertrophied, filling the void in the nasal cavity produced by the deviated septum. They may require outfracture, trimming, or electrocoagulation to

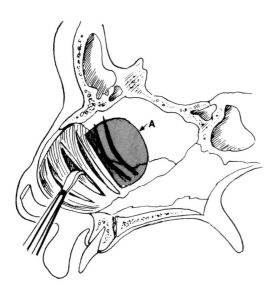

Fig. 25-7. Septal cartilage has been exposed by subperichondrial elevation on one side. Straightening is obtained by multiple incisions with minimal removal of cartilage. Mucoperichondrium on contralateral side is undisturbed. This technique ensures straightening of septal cartilage without endangering support of nasal dorsum. *A,* Area where deviated ethmoid plate is straightened by fracturing it.

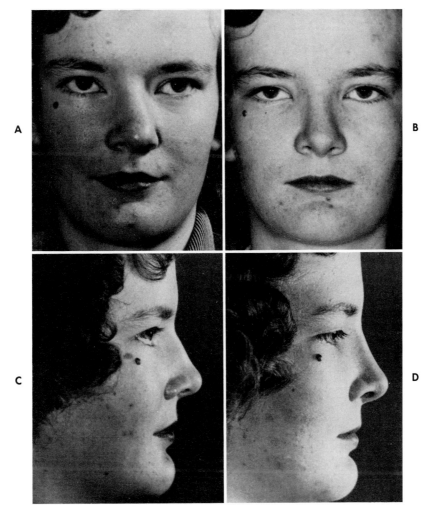

Fig. 25-8. Developmental nasal deviation with C-shaped deformity of dorsum (Fig. 25-1, **B**). **A,** Nasal deviation as result of trauma in infancy. Note protrusion of septal angle beneath left alar cartilage. Despite disparity in shape of alar cartilages, tip is in midline. **B,** Photograph taken after corrective rhinoplasty and straightening of septum according to type of technique shown in Fig. 25-7. **C,** Preoperative view. **D,** Postoperative view. Adequate projection of columella was obtained by inserting septal cartilage transplant into columella according to technique shown in Fig. 25-14.

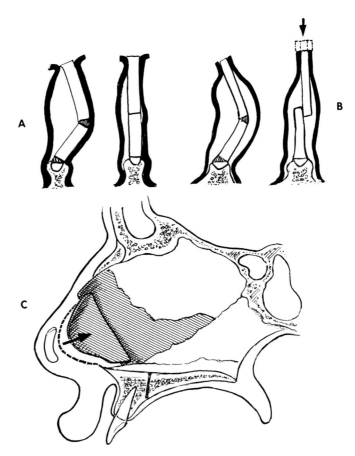

Fig. 25-9. Principle of mucoperichondrial splint. **A,** In angulated deformity of septum, wedge is removed at angulation; septal cartilage is thus straightened. **B,** Mucoperichondrium left attached on one side prevents overlapping of fragments shown in drawing. **C,** Same principle applies in preventing anteroposterior overlapping after incision through septal cartilage. Intact mucoperichondrium on one side prevents overlap and shortening of septal cartilage.

complete the restoration of the airway after the septum has been straightened.

Principle of the mucoperichondrial splint

If the caudal portion of the septum is in the midline, straightening of the remaining dorsal and caudal portions of the septal cartilage may be done by means of incisions extending through the cartilage but not through the mucoperichondrium on the contralateral side (Figs. 25-7 and 25-8).

When the septal framework is angulated or curved, selective incisions through the cartilage and strip excisions may straighten it (Fig. 25-7). The incisions may extend to the dorsal border of the septal cartilage if the lateral cartilages have not been separated from the septum. In most rhinoplastic operations, at this stage, the cartilages have already been separated from the septum, and such incisions should be avoided to avoid disrupting the continuity of the dorsal border of the septum.

The mucoperichondrium is elevated on one side of the remaining septal cartilage to obtain exposure. The mucoperichondrial elevation is limited on the contralateral side of the septum, sufficient only to permit excision of an angulated portion of the septum. When possible, the mucoperichondrium is left completely undisturbed; this ensures the continued nourishment of the septal cartilage, but, more importantly, the undisturbed mucoperichondrium acts as a splint, preventing overlapping of cartilage fragments after incision (Fig. 25-9). Such overlapping would result in a change in the vertical or horizontal dimensions of the septal cartilage and in a change in the contour of the nasal profile.

When both sides of the septal cartilage must be exposed, mattress sutures of chromic catgut may be employed to avoid overlapping of cartilage fragments.

The septal framework is exposed by raising the

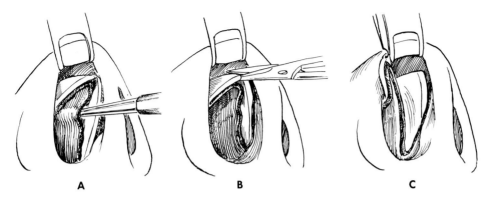

Fig. 25-10. Complete exposure of septal cartilage. **A,** Mucoperichondrium is being raised from septal cartilage. **B,** Lateral cartilage is detached from dorsal border of septum without incising through mucoperichondrium. **C,** Exposure is obtained.

mucoperichondrium and the mucoperiosteum on the side *opposite* the direction of the deviation; if the nose is deviated to the right, the septal framework is exposed on the left, and vice versa. The entire framework may be exposed and the lateral cartilage detached, since it usually must be trimmed to allow the return of the structures to the midline (Fig. 25-10).

The swinging door operation permits straightening the septal framework with a minimal resection of the septum (Fig. 25-11). This type of operation should be reserved for septal deflections in which the caudal half (or more) of the septal cartilage or the entire nasal pyramid is angulated to one side (Fig. 25-12). The septal deflection is also characterized by a dislocation of the septal cartilage to one side of the vomer (Fig. 25-13, *A*). The septal cartilage is retracted, an incision is made into the vomer groove, and fibrous tissue that fills the vomer groove is resected. The cartilage is separated from its vomer attachments and replaced into the groove (Fig. 25-13, *B* to *D*).

The flap of septal cartilage with mucoperichondrium attached, which has been freed by incisions separating the lateral cartilages from the septum and the septal cartilage from the vomer, has been swung into the midline like a door swinging on its hinges (Fig. 25-11).

If the vomer is also deviated, it must be detached from the floor of the nose by means of an osteotome and replaced in the midline (Fig. 25-13, *C* and *D*). If the septal cartilage shows a curvature in the frontal plane, a wedge excision may be required to replace the septal angle into the midline (Fig. 25-13, *C* and *D*). As previously mentioned, the attached mucoperichondrium on one side prevents overlapping of cartilage fragments and the danger of a loss of the vertical dimension of the

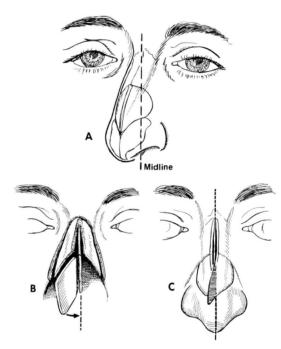

Fig. 25-11. Swinging-door operation. **A,** Entire nose is deflected to one side. **B,** Strip of septal cartilage has been resected at point of angulation, and caudal portion of the cartilage is swung into midline; fixation is established into vomer groove (Fig. 25-13). Mucoperichondrium on right side of septal cartilage remains attached. **C,** Restoration of symmetry between two lateral cartilages after replacement of structures in midline; portion of dorsal border of overlapping lateral cartilage must be excised.

septum. The structures should remain in the midline after the corrective surgery without any tendency to fall back into their previously deviated position. It is essential to provide fixation of the septal cartilage; a hole is drilled through the nasal spine or the premaxillary wings (or both) by means

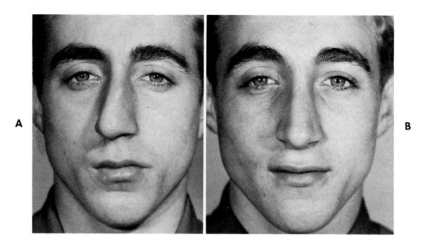

Fig. 25-12. A, Developmental deviation of nose. **B,** Result obtained by swinging-door operation technique.

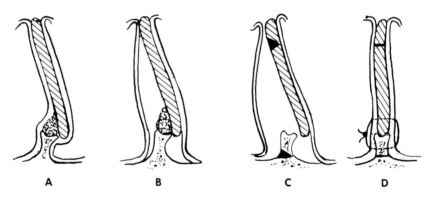

Fig. 25-13. Correction of dislocated caudal portion of septal cartilage. **A,** Frontal section showing dislocated caudal portion of septal cartilage. Vomer groove has filled with fibrous tissue. **B,** Mucoperichondrium and mucoperiosteum on side *opposite* deviation are raised. **C,** Fibrous tissue filling vomer groove has been resected. Septal cartilage is free. Wedge is resected to permit straightening septal cartilage. Mucoperichondrium over deviated side of septal cartilage is not raised. In unusual cases vomer must also be either fractured into midline or straightened by wedge excision. **D,** Cartilage has been straightened. An important point is to maintain position of lower portion of straightened septal cartilage by means of suture that is passed through drill hole made either in vomer or in nasal spine or anterior edge of pyriform aperture for permanent fixation.

of a small round drill point activated by an air turbine. The caudal portion is maintained in fixation with a nonabsorbable or stainless steel wire (Fig. 25-13, *D*).

Reshaping the deformed columella may require section or resection of a portion of the lower end of one or both medial crura.

The vomer and the anterior nasal spine may be in the midline, the cartilage being dislocated from the vomer groove, or the vomer may participate in the deviation (Fig. 25-13, *A*).

It is possible to preserve the entire septal cartilage, straightening it and replacing it in the midline. After the usual exposure of the nasal framework

and the transfixion incision, which frees the septal cartilage along its dorsal and caudal borders, the lateral cartilage attachments to the septum are severed. The mucoperichondrium and mucoperiosteum are then raised from one side of the septum only (Fig. 25-13, *B*). One should choose the side opposite the deviation; thus if the septum is deviated toward the right side, the mucoperichondrium on the left side of the septum should be elevated; if the reverse situation exists and the deviation is toward the left side, the mucoperichondrium on the right side of the septum should be raised. The purpose of this technique is to benefit from the contraction of the raised flap during the period of postoperative healing; the contraction of the healing flap assists in maintaining the septum in its corrected central position.

After the septal mucoperichondrial and mucoperiosteal flaps have been raised on one side, the mucous membrane over the septal cartilage remains intact on the contralateral side. The mucoperiosteum is raised from the vomer, however, and the mucoperiosteal elevation is extended to include the floor of the nose.

The point of angulation of the septal cartilage in the sagittal plane is cut through or resected to straighten the cartilage. The incisions are made through cartilage and do not extend through the mucoperichondrium on the opposite side (Fig. 25-11).

Morselization by means of an instrument with asperities on one or both branches of the instrument, which grasps the septal cartilage, cutting through the cartilage at multiple points and thus weakening it, has not proved efficient. It may have some merit in septal cartilage deviations of lesser degree, and, combined with fracture and straightening of the perpendicular plate of the ethmoid and the vomer, it permits straightening without resection of cartilage, thus avoiding the flabby septal flaps that result from extensive resection of the framework. The technique has not proved to be as effective as incisions through the cartilage combined with judicious excision of obstructive portions of the septal framework.

Internal splint

When a number of incisions through the septal cartilage have been required, mattress sutures may assist in the fixation of the fragments, in addition to the mucoperichondrial splint.

Nasal gauze packing assists in supporting the straightened septum. The packing may be inconvenient, however, when a rhinoplasty is done concomitantly because, to be effective, a considerable amount of gauze packing is required. Sheets of plastic materials such as Teflon, polyethylene, or other materials that are nonreactive to the tissues may be cut to size and placed on each side of the septum and joined by a *loosely* tied mattress suture. This type of internal splinting was described by Johnson[5] and was used by him successfully. The splints are left in position for 7 to 14 days.

DISLOCATED CAUDAL END OF SEPTAL CARTILAGE: ANTERIOR COLUMELLAR APPROACH

Dislocation of the caudal end of the septal cartilage from its position in the vomer groove causes it to protrude to one side of the columella. The protrusion itself is objectionable from an aesthetic standpoint, obstructs the airway in some cases, and nearly always distorts the columella.

The swinging door procedure can be employed to replace the cartilage in the midline without resecting the cartilage (Fig. 25-11).

The caudal portion of the septal cartilage may be so distorted in some cases that any plan to straighten the septal framework by conservative surgery must be abandoned. The caudal portion of the septal cartilage is then resected; resection of the vomer spurs is often also required to ensure an adequate nasal airway. Retraction of the columella is prevented by the embedding of a strip of septal cartilage into the columella through *an incision along the caudal border of the medial crus* (Fig. 25-14, *A* to *D*). The skin covering the lateral surface of the columella is raised by the injection of local anesthetic solution. A pocket is prepared beneath the skin of the caudal surface of the columella. The cartilage transplant is then placed caudad to the medial crura, immediately beneath the skin extending downward over the nasal spine (Fig. 25-14, *E* to *G*).

TOTAL RESECTION AND TRANSPLANTATION OF SEPTAL CARTILAGE OVER THE DORSUM OF THE NOSE

There are two types of nasal and septal deviations in which a conservative type of septal straightening cannot be achieved.

The first is the deviated nose in which the septal cartilage is severely twisted in the frontal plane as well as in the sagittal plane; the dorsal border of the septal cartilage shows an accentuated S-shaped curvature in both the sagittal and frontal planes (Fig. 25-15). In this type, the cartilage must be resected because it cannot be straightened. From the excised cartilage it is always possible to recover strips of straight cartilage that are used as transplants into the columella (Fig. 25-14) and over the nasal dorsum (Fig. 25-16).

A second type in which the septum must be completely resected is in the flat and deviated nose often seen after repeated trauma. In this type of deformity, the septum has lost its supportive function. Septal resection is necessary because the septum is so thick that it obstructs the airway (the boxer's septum). Complete resection of the septum does not result in any change in the shape of the nose because the septum has already lost its role as a supporting structure. This type of nose may require reconstruction by means of cartilage (sep-

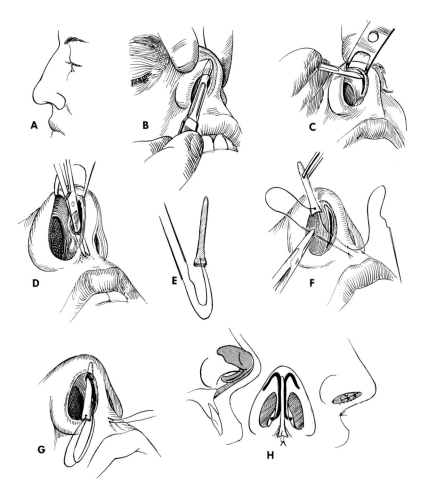

Fig. 25-14. Columellar strut placed through anterior incision. **A,** Retracted columella. **B,** Technique of making incision along caudal border of medial crus. Nasal tip is pinched. Scalpel is placed in recess of vestibule along caudal border of dome and sweeps down along caudal border of medial crus. **C,** Incision is being completed. **D,** Scissors establish pocket between two medial crura. Undermining is extended downward caudal to nasal spine. **E,** Septal strut with guide suture. **F,** Guide suture is being placed and brought out through skin below nasal spine. **G,** Septal cartilage graft is being introduced into columella. **H,** Position of septal cartilage graft in columella. Graft is placed anterior to nasal spine and is maintained in position by transcutaneous suture, which is removed after a few days. *Left insert,* Sagittal view of cartilage graft in position. *Right insert,* Incision along caudal border of medial crus is sutured. Note projection of columella.

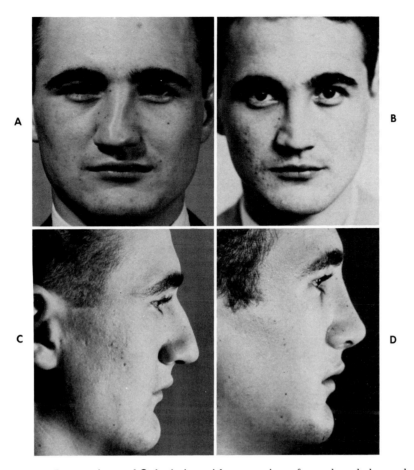

Fig. 25-15. A, Traumatic nasal S-deviation with protrusion of septal angle beneath right alar cartilage, causing distortion of tip. **B,** Result obtained by realignment of structures. Septal cartilage was resected completely, and strips of cartilage were transplanted over dorsum as illustrated in Fig. 25-16. **C,** Retraction of columella. **D,** Photograph taken after corrective surgery and columellar septal transplant, as illustrated in Fig. 25-14.

tal costal or bone) grafts to restore the contour of the dorsum when the nose has been flattened against the face (the boxer's nose).

Technique

The dorsal hump is resected. It is usually a small pseudohump resulting from the loss of contour of the cartilaginous dorsum of the nose. The continuity of the mucous membrane lining the lateral cartilages and the septum should be preserved (Fig. 25-10). Thus one avoids the collapse of the septal mucoperichondrial flaps, which may occur when the entire septal framework is exposed and the lateral cartilages and the mucous membrane are cut through and separated from the septum. Excision of tissue from one lateral cartilage to equalize both, a procedure often necessary in the deviated nose, may be accomplished without cutting through the mucous membrane.

In some cases it is possible to maintain the continuity of the cartilaginous vault by preserving a strip consisting of septal cartilage a few millimeters thick between the lateral cartilages. Thus a bed is prepared for the septal cartilage transplant.

It is possible to secure a sufficiently long straight piece of cartilage (or cartilage plus ethmoid plate as advocated by Sheen) for a suitable transplant even in the most deviated septal cartilage. The resected cartilage is placed in a moist saline sponge until all the other procedures of the nasal plastic operation have been completed; the cartilage transplantation is the final procedure. A single piece of cartilage or a number of superimposed pieces may be required. They should be meticulously carved, often a tedious procedure.

The cartilage graft is introduced through one of the incisions previously made to correct the tip and is placed over the lateral cartilages. The dorsal

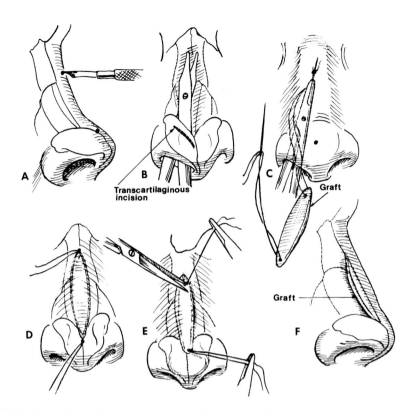

Fig. 25-16. Technique of transplantation of septal cartilage to dorsum of nose. **A,** Two ink dots on skin indicate upper and lower limits of transplant. **B,** Scissors undermining area over dorsum to be occupied by transplant. **C,** Transplant is held by guide sutures; upper guide sutures are introduced in position by means of straight needle, which pierces skin through upper ink dot. **D,** Traction exerted on upper guide sutures has introduced transplant into predetermined position along dorsum of nose. Guide sutures are tied. **E,** Guide sutures are removed. **F,** Graft is in position.

septal cartilage transplant may be placed with precision by the technique illustrated in Fig. 25-16, a technique I described in 1950.[1]

Two ink dots are made over the dorsum at points between which the cartilage is to be placed. The dots indicate the upper and lower limits of the transplantation site (Fig. 25-16, *A*), which is undermined with scissors (Fig. 25-16, *B*). Sutures of 5-0 plain catgut are threaded through the eye of a straight cutting needle, which is placed through each extremity of the cartilage transplant (Fig. 25-16, *C*). The needle carrying the cephalic traction sutures is placed into the subcutaneous pocket and out through the skin (Fig. 25-16, *C*); the needle with the caudal traction sutures is also placed into the pocket and through the skin. The sutures may be tied over a small piece of gauze over the dorsum of the nose (Fig. 25-16, *D*), or they may be cut and removed after the operation has been completed and before adhesive paper tape is placed over the dorsum to stabilize the transplant (Fig. 25-16, *E*).

The advantage of plain catgut is twofold: the buried sutures may be left to dissolve spontaneously, and the nasal splint need not be removed. Another procedure can also be employed. Instead of exerting force on the suture, which may displace the transplant, slight tension is placed on the sutures while the flat blades of the scissors are applied against the skin. The sutures are then cut close to the skin by applying pressure against the skin and upward traction on the suture (Fig. 25-16, *E*). As the tension is released, the cut ends of the suture disappear beneath the skin; these are absorbed without causing tissue reaction. Silk or nylon sutures occasionally break, remaining under the skin causing tissue reaction, and in some cases, inflammation, suppuration, and absorption of the graft. One piece of cartilage may be adequate (Fig. 25-16, *F*); two pieces sutured to each other may be required; occasionally three segments of septal cartilage are indicated. The cartilage is shaped with a sharp scalpel to provide adequate contour.

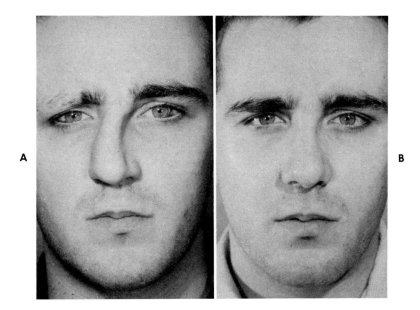

Fig. 25-17. Corrective surgery for malunited fracture of nasal bones. **A,** Severe deviation of nose as result of malunited fracture. **B,** Result obtained with technique illustrated in Fig. 25-18.

STRAIGHTENING THE BONY NOSE: EQUALIZATION OF THE LATERAL NASAL WALLS

The nasal pyramid in cross section is triangular in shape. The lateral walls in the undeviated nose form equal sides of the triangle, and the apex is in the midline, whereas the lateral walls of the deviated nasal pyramid are of unequal length, and the apex of the triangle is located to one side of the midline (Fig. 25-2). The equalization of the lateral walls is essential to straighten the nose. Because such cases usually require resection of the laterally situated hump, equalization is best achieved by resecting the hump along a beveled line; this technique is preferred to that originally advocated by Joseph, in which a triangle of bone was resected from the base of the lateral wall on the wider side. Straightening the septum is a prime condition to prevent recurrence of the deviation resulting from pressure of the septum against the lateral nasal wall.

CORRECTIVE SURGERY FOR THE DEVIATED NOSE THAT REQUIRES MODIFICATION OF THE PROFILE LINE

When the profile must be modified in the course of straightening the deviated nose, the order of procedure is similar to that followed in a typical corrective rhinoplastic operation: after exposing the framework, the profile line of the cartilaginous nose is first modified, the tip is remod-

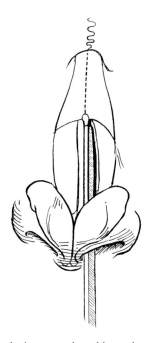

Fig. 25-18. Technique employed in patient shown in Fig. 25-17. Button-tipped osteotome is placed beneath septal mucoperichondrial flap on left side searching for lower border of nasal bones. Midline osteotomy is then performed. This osteotomy, along with necessary septal straightening procedures and lateral osteotomies, permits realignment of deviated nose.

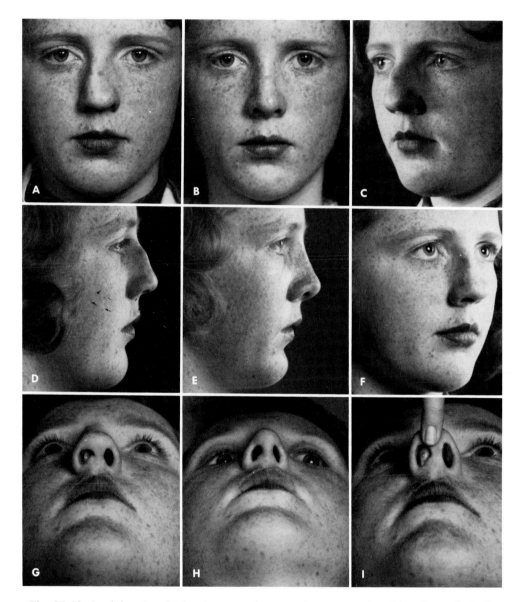

Fig. 25-19. Straightening deviated nose and concomitant corrective rhinoplasty. **A,** Full-face view shows C-shaped deviation, widening, and bifidity of tip (Fig. 25-3). **B,** Postoperative view. **C,** Preoperative three-quarters anterior view showing osteocartilaginous dorsal hump. **D,** Preoperative profile view. Note retracted columella. **E,** Postoperative view. Septal cartilage transplant has been placed in columella (Fig. 25-14). **F,** Three-quarters preoperative anterior view shows bifid tip. **G,** Wide tip and laterally dislocated septum. **H,** Preoperative view. **I,** Finger pressure on tip accentuates bifidity.

eled, and the bony hump resected. The septum is then straightened by one of the techniques that have been described (preferably a conservative technique), and the operation is completed by the osteotomy of the lateral walls of the nose.

CORRECTIVE SURGERY FOR THE DEVIATED NOSE THAT DOES NOT REQUIRE MODIFICATION OF THE PROFILE LINE: MALUNITED FRACTURES

The nasal framework is sometimes deviated from the midline in both upper and lower portions without a change in the profile line. Malunited fractures show this pattern of deformity (Fig. 25-17). A modified corrective procedure is used in such cases.

An incision is made at the lower border of the lateral cartilage on the right side, and the soft tissues are elevated from the lateral cartilage by sharp dissection with a sharp double-bladed Joseph knife. Another incision is made with the tip of the Joseph knife through the periosteum covering the nasal bone, and the periosteum is raised. Similar procedures are undertaken on the left side.

A submucous resection or a straightening procedure of the deviated septum is done. Osteotomy of the base of the lateral walls of the nose is performed.

A medial osteotomy is now required. A guarded, straight osteotome is placed between the mucoperichondrial flaps of the septum and is directed upward until the operator feels the lower border of the nasal bones in the midline with the tip of the instrument (Fig. 25-18). The line of osteotomy is in the midline at the junction of the nasal bones, using a mallet to tap the osteotome upward; the bones are thus separated and can be manipulated into a realigned position because they have been completely freed from the covering periosteum and musculature.

A horizontal incision through the mucous membrane at the base of the septum prevents septal hematoma. An external nasal splint is applied, and no intranasal packing is required.

COMPLICATIONS AFTER CORRECTIVE SURGERY FOR NASAL DEVIATIONS

In addition to the complications that occur after the usual type of corrective rhinoplasty, the major complication after surgery for the deviated nose is recurrence of the deviation. The most fre-

quent cause of the recurrence is inadequate straightening of the nasal septum. The inexorable pressure exerted by a deviated septum will press a lateral wall out of its alignment, cause the recurrence of an S-shaped twist to the nose, or deviate the nasal tip and lower cartilaginous nose to one side. When this complication occurs, the remedy is a secondary operation to straighten the septum and realign the nasal structures.

It is advisable to leave the dental compound or plaster nasal splint in position longer than for a routine corrective rhinoplasty, but this precaution does not obviate the essential requirement of straightening the septum and external nose by adequate surgical means. A successful result requires that every portion of the nasal pyramid be realigned and that symmetry be reestablished in the septum, the bony nose, the lateral and alar cartilages, and the columella (Fig. 25-19).

A major complication is collapse of the remaining dorsal portion of the septal framework, which, after resection of the caudal portion of the septum, remains in position as a cantilever. Fracture of the cantilever at the perpendicular plate of the ethmoid causes a collapse of the remaining septal framework, a loss of the contour of the nasal dorsum, and a resultant saddle-nose deformity. This complication is avoided by straightening the septum by conservative measures, thus preserving septal support.

REFERENCES

1. Converse, J. M.: Corrective surgery of nasal deviations, Arch. Otolaryngol. **52**:671, 1950.
2. Converse, J. M.: Deformities of the nose. In Kazanjian, V. H., and Converse, J. M.: Surgical treatment of facial injuries, ed. 3, Baltimore, 1974, The Williams & Wilkins Co.
3. Fry, J. H., and Robertson, W. B.: Interlocked stresses in human septal cartilage, Br. J. Plast. Surg. **19**:392, 1967.
4. Gibson, T., and Davis, W. B.: The distortion of autogenous cartilage grafts: its cause and prevention, Br. J. Plast. Surg. **10**:257, 1958.
5. Johnson, N. E.: Septal surgery and rhinoplasty, Trans. Am. Acad. Ophthalmol. Otolaryngol. **68**:869, 1964.
6. Kirschner, J. A.: Traumatic nasal deformity in the newborn, Arch. Otolaryngol. **62**:139, 1955.
7. Kravits, H., Driessen, G., Gomberg, R., and Korach, A.: Accidental falls from elevated surfaces in infants from birth to one year of age, Pediatrics (suppl.) **44**:869, 1969.

Discussion

Bingham: In his last statement, Converse said you should not correct a deviated nose without breaking the deviated septum. I wonder if the converse might be true. Is it possible, by a two-stage procedure working on the septum initially, for correction of the very severe deviation deformity, and then come back still another day to work on the external nose? It is yet another plan of management whereby you still manage to preserve your support and not wind up with a saddle deformity.

Converse: The obverse is true. You must do it in one stage. It has to be done in one operation. Sometimes you do a beautiful rhinoplasty, everything has worked out fine, it looks gorgeous, "Come on back and see me in a month." They walk in later and say, "My God, what happened? It was perfect!" You don't know this at the time of the operation, but what's happened is you've got a high deflection just below the straight hump. You take the hump off and you reduce the profile, but the septum is off, and you don't realize it at the time. The edema takes over. You put two straight nasal bones together with a crooked septum between them and all will look beautiful for about 2 weeks. At the end of 30 days, when the edema has subsided, it will be crooked again. My other remark refers to putting the septal strut back into the vomer groove. I tried to indicate in one of my drawings that it is not impossible to straighten this out by putting a 2 mm chisel alongside the crooked vomer and just scoring it along the side. Then if you put in the long speculum and open it forcefully, you might crack it open right in the midline so you can put your septum into it.

Dingman: Here is a word to you who might be covering emergency rooms. Any time that a small child with a possible fracture of the nose and a history of having a bloody nose comes in, you'd better look very carefully at the septum. You may not be able to see in there immediately because of the edema, but I think we all have the obligation to look at that child a week or so later. Many times he will have a fracture of the septal cartilage or the bony septum. If that child is permitted to go on to adult age, he will develop deformities that are very difficult to correct. I think we have the opportunity a week or so after the nasal injury in a child to put the structures back and avoid later complication. As Gorney would say to that patient as a legal defense a month later, "Damn it, now what have you done to your nose!"

Musgrave: One more question and then we'll get on. Al?

Ungaro: I caution you to remember that you may be able to see down the side of the septum. However, if the fracture is such that it deflects the air current transversely, you will have a physiologic obstruction even though you can see past it. It's a commonly used principle in stores, etc. There is a current of air going across to keep the heat in and the cold out. This does occur in the nose, especially the floor, so keep it in mind.

Musgrave: Ladies and gentlemen, we have had for the past 2 days here a very distinguished looking gentleman who has not been up to the mike or podium yet, and I'm going to let Ralph introduce him.

Millard: A New Zealander by the name of Gillies, Sir Harold Gillies, was knighted in 1930, and

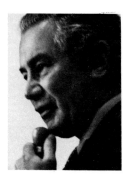

Dr. Dawson

240

about that time, Archibald McIndoe joined him. At the same time, a young fellow who had been working at Hammersmith Hospital by the name of Rainsford Mowlem had finished his general surgery house officership and was slated to return to New Zealand. Unfortunately, or fortunately for us, the house officer who was to take over for him choked on Christmas pudding and expired. Rainsford Mowlem stayed on temporarily to cover this position. About that time, Gillies began to take cases to Hammersmith, and he brought in a couple of forehead rhinoplasties. Mowlem noticed these and immediately became infatuated with plastic surgery, joined Sir Harold and McIndoe, and the two of them worked with

Gillies for a number of years until the Second World War. That's the first and second generation. Mowlem did great work as you all know, but he retired to live in an orange grove in Spain and left his dynasty to the fine gentleman that we're about to introduce, the president of the British Association of Plastic Surgeons. He not only became a chief plastic surgeon, but has had a very interesting history including careers as a successful male model, an athlete, a runner, good at rugby and cricket. He also has run a great show at his Mount Vernon unit, and that took some real skill, as his predecessor had been such a powerhouse. I take great pleasure in introducing Mr. Dick Dawson.

Chapter 26

Nasal bone grafts

the correction of acquired deformities

R. L. G. Dawson, M.B., F.R.C.S.

A common nasal deformity follows severe untreated trauma to the septum or hematoma and subsequent infection of the cartilaginous septum, where such hematoma has not been adequately drained. A complete loss of the cartilaginous septum results. Nasal deformity can also follow an overenthusiastic submucous resection of the septum.

In this type of deformity the nasal tip itself is maintained forward to a large extent by the alar cartilages, but the nostrils tend to be splayed out, and the tip is flatter than usual and completely lacks septal support. It can be flattened against the face by digital pressure.

The maximum deformity can be seen just above the alar cartilage domes, where, in profile, there is a marked saddle. This deformity may or may not be associated with fracture and displacement of the actual bony skeleton of the nose.

The deformities can therefore be as follows:

1. The deformity may be caused by septal trauma in adult life, with loss of septal support and overlapping of the cartilaginous and bony septal plates (Fig. 26-1). There is a flattened profile and a tendency to a wide front view, with the lower half of the nose showing a saddle deformity (Fig. 26-2). The actual tip is partially supported by the alar cartilages. The columella can be seen from the lateral view.

2. If the injury has been sustained in childhood before growth from the anterior nasal spine has finished, such growth may be affected, so that although the tooth-bearing segment of the maxilla is normal, there is a recession of the bone above the maxillary arch (Fig. 26-3,), causing a flattened profile of the central part of the face, with an upper lip curving backwards to meet retroposed

nostrils, just like a monkey's lip. No septal cartilage is left, the nostrils are rounded, and the tip of the nose is infantile. The columella may be slightly retracted inwards and not adequately visible from the side (Fig. 26-4). Bony septal displacement may occur with airway obstruction, but, alternatively, the airways may be so wide open that the air fails to take up moisture in passage, and atrophic rhinitis results.

3. A combination of severe trauma, untreated septal deformity, untreated septal hematoma, and subsequent infection results in a total loss of the cartilaginous septum with superadded fibrosis (Fig. 26-5). The final result is a fibrous contracture

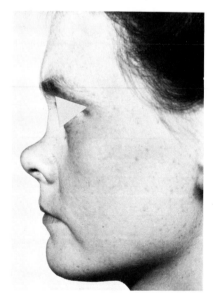

Fig. 26-1. Gross saddle deformity and columella visible from side.

242

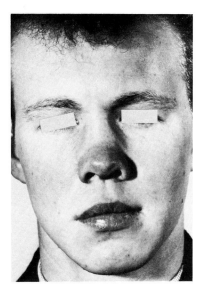

Fig. 26-2. Splayed-out nasal bones and flat nasal profile.

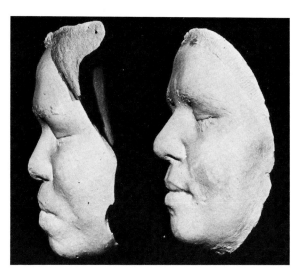

Fig. 26-3. *Left,* Retracted columella and recessed naso-maxillary complex. *Right,* Same patient after bone graft to nose, columella, and anterior maxilla.

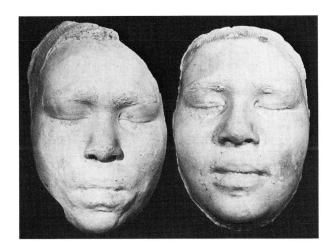

Fig. 26-4. *Left,* Small, flattened nasal tip. *Right,* Photograph taken after bone graft to nose, columella, and anterior maxilla.

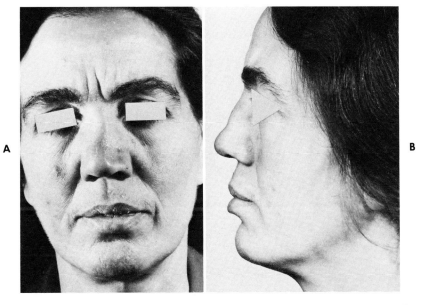

Fig. 26-5. A, Result of severe nasal trauma in childhood. **B,** Same patient, showing lack of development from anterior nasal spine with recessed columella, recessed anterior maxilla, and low saddle deformity but with nasal bones overprominent.

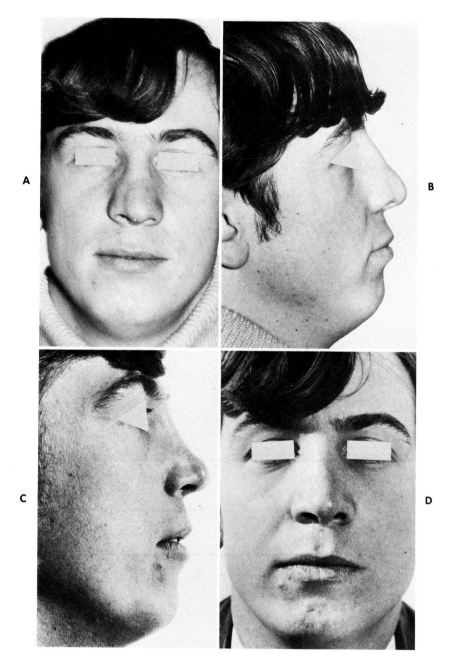

Fig. 26-6. A, Old nasal injury with Silastic that has been inserted into nasal tip. Note overprominence of tip, which is crooked because of misplaced implant. **B,** Same patient, showing overprominence of nasal bones in relation to enlarged nasal tip. **C,** Result of removal of Silastic, small nasal hump removal, and infracture. No bone grafting was necessary. **D,** Same patient after removal of Silastic, hump reduction, and infracture only.

of the mucoperichondrium, severe columella retraction, and a most ugly lateral appearance of the nose.

Frequently there is a combination of signs: a flattened tip with a saddle deformity, a retracted columella, round, infantile nostrils, a simian lip, and splayed-out nasal bones. However, in many cases the lower half of the nose is flat, and the bony bridge remains high.

OPERATIVE TREATMENT
Preliminary procedures

1. A good straight base must be obtained on which to place a suitable bone graft. This is achieved by preliminary infracture.

2. Adequate airways must be achieved, and a total submucous resection may have to be performed. The patient must be warned that the deformity will be temporarily increased.

3. A nasal hump, relatively prominent when compared with the saddle deformity of the lower half, should be removed to line up with the lower half (Fig. 26-6). About 50% of all my patients suffering from this type of deformity, and on whom I have performed this preliminary operation, have been happy with the shape and have not needed to have the bone graft.

These procedures are regarded as preliminary to the nasal bone graft operation, which is performed 6 months later. You must warn these patients that the second stage will be necessary, but in certain types of deformity just mentioned, about 50% will be satisfied with this preliminary operation.

Restoration of nasal contour and support

Some surgeons use rib cartilage instead of bone, but I prefer bone from the iliac crest. It does not bend, and one often needs more than can be supplied by the rib cartilage.

Other surgeons use implants and in the past have used ivory, polythene, even celluloid, and now Silastic. They all tend to be extruded, particularly if even minor injury is sustained (Fig. 26-7), and in my view the only real indication for a Silastic implant is for use in a child, where a badly collapsed nose needs temporary support to stimulate the forward growth of the center of the face. It is removed and replaced with a bone graft at about 16 or 17 years, when growth has ceased.

Cantilever type of bone graft. The cantilever graft is used for a simple saddle deformity of the bridge. The nose is cleaned inside and outside. The site of incision is marked in the center of the

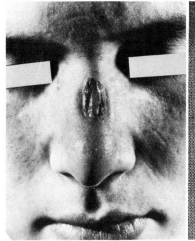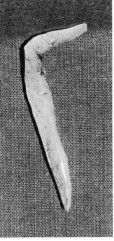

Fig. 26-7. A, Silastic implant with skin necrosis. **B,** Implant removed.

columella. I use this access in preference to an incision inside the nostril, since a direct approach is easier and more accurate. Normal saline is injected into the columella and the septum, expanding the two leaves of the septal mucosa, and then over the top of the bony bridge and on either side as far as the inner canthal region. This defines the tissue plane and aids dissection. Do not use any dilute epinephrine (Adrenalin) solution, since it will make the skin go pale, and you must always have a pink skin over the surface of the bone graft, or the skin will become necrotic. If the skin is too pale from epinephrine, you will not know if your graft is too large. Now incise vertically through the center of the columella between the domes of the alar cartilages, and, with small scissor dissection, split the two adherent leaves of the septal mucoperichondrium. Then pass the scissors, with spreading dissection all the time, up and over the nasal bones. With a larger pair of curved scissors, dissection down to the inner canthal region equally on both sides, but take care to stop just short of the angular vessels. Now you have the skin and subcutaneous tissues lifted off the nasal bones and periosteum. Note that the dissection is *superficial* to the periosteum and extends as far as the glabella region of the nose. No osteotomy cut is made into the nasal process of the frontal bone.

Pack the cavity with ribbon gauze and leave it while you are removing and shaping the bone graft. The bone graft is removed *after* you have made your nasal dissection, just in case you make a large hole in the septal mucosa and have to temporarily abandon the operation.

The operators change their gloves to avoid introducing nasal infection into the hip wound, and a different set of instruments is used.

An incision is made directly over the iliac crest, and I remove a block of bone incorporating the full width of the crest to the desired length and about 2.5 cm deep, avoiding the anterior superior iliac spine. I bevel off the bone edges on the crest and suture in three layers, always draining the wound. A firm spica bandage is applied.

The block of bone is now shaped using the compact bone of the crest for the dorsum of the graft. It is shaped on a cantilever principle with a short bevel to fit against the glabella and a narrow end to sit just behind the dome cartilages. The lower end of the graft must not lie between the alar domes, or the tip will be too wide. It is hollowed out on its undersurface so that it will sit on the curved surface of the nasal bones. It does not become fused with the nasal bones, since the periosteum is between (Figs. 26-8 and 26-9). It therefore is not liable to fracture if the nose is hit. It is maintained in place by the skin tension and by its shape. The bone graft must be a tight fit. It is no use having a small, loose graft. An antibiotic powder is sprayed over the graft before it is put into place. The dome cartilages are sutured together in front of the end of the graft, and the columella incision is closed with 5-0 silk.

To fix the graft I use 1-inch Elastoplast, split to incorporate the tip. You must never use a hard plaster of Paris fixation, since you will be sandwiching the soft skin between a hard bone graft and a hard plaster, and the patient will get skin necrosis.

The nasal fixation remains for 7 days.

L-shaped bone graft and bone onlay to alar bases and part of the maxilla. The approach for the insertion of these grafts (Fig. 26-10) is through a midcolumella incision that then branches at its lower end across the nostril entrance on each side as an inverted Y. The dissection, besides proceeding in the nose, must also free the retracted alar bases and nasal floor, and in these areas it is subperiosteal.

I use this type of grafting when I am operating on a nose with collapsed tip, retracted columella, and a simian lip. The graft, depending on the shape of profile required, either goes up, over the nasal bones to the glabella, or stops at the junction of the lower half of the nose, with the nasal bones, and the other part of the L sits in the columella incision, pushing it downward. The tip cartilage domes are sutured together in front of the graft (Figs. 26-11 to 26-13). The columella strut rests in the region of the hypoplastic nasal spine, usually on a cancellous bone graft placed across the nostril

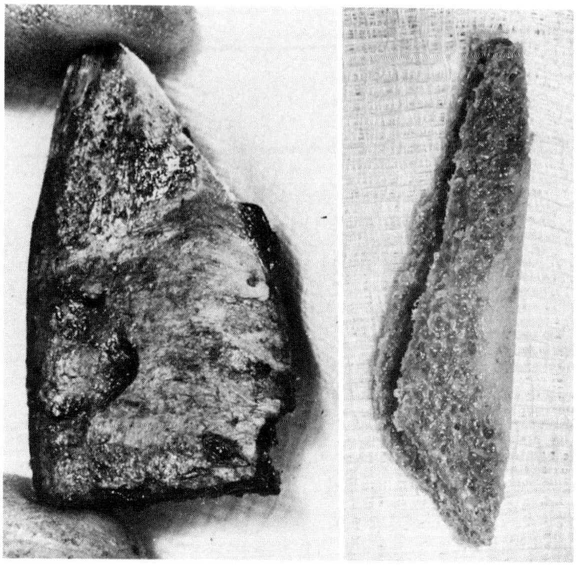

Fig. 26-8. A, Size of iliac crest bone that should be removed, for modeling: 2.5 cm × 5 cm. **B,** Modeled cantilever bone graft is given short bevel at upper end; cancellous bone is grooved out to sit on nasal bones. Narrow end lies just behind nasal dome cartilages.

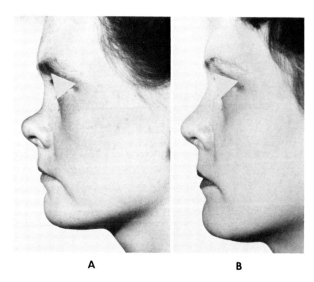

Fig. 26-9. A, Same patient as in Fig. 26-1 in great need of cantilever type of bone graft. **B,** Postoperative view of same lady. (Courtesy Stewart Harrison, F.R.C.S.)

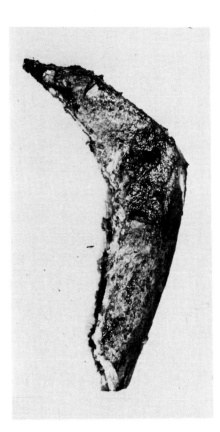

Fig. 26-10. L-shaped bone graft for correction of collapsed bridge and retracted columella. Note bevel at upper end to sit against nasal process of frontal bone.

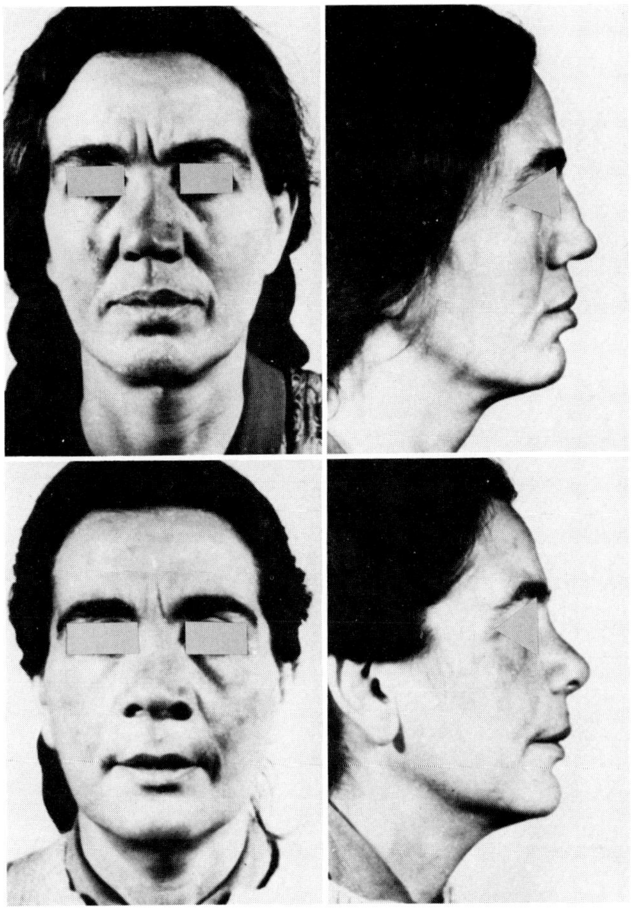

Fig. 26-11. Same patient as in Figs. 26-5 and 26-6. Lower two photographs show postoperative appearance after infracture, hump removal, and straightening, followed by L-shaped bone graft up to nasal bones only and bone graft onlay to anterior maxilla and beneath alar bases.

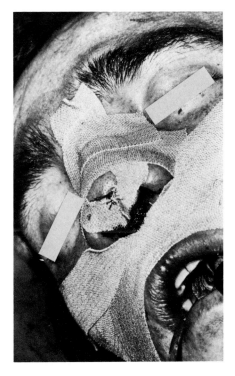

Fig. 26-12. Elastoplast fixation. No plaster of Paris must be used.

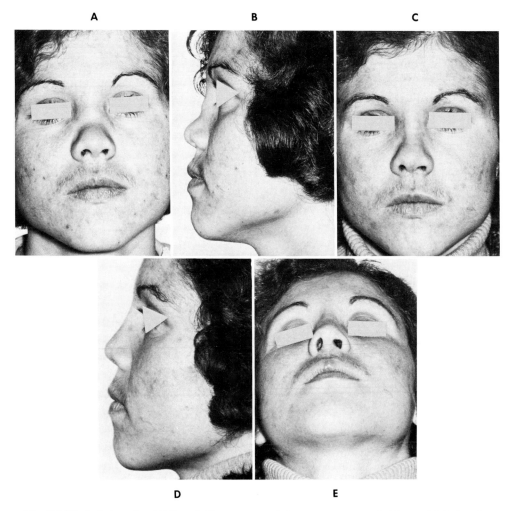

Fig. 26-13. A, Injury in childhood. Nose was straight, narrow across bridge, with infantile nostrils and rounded tip. There was no necessity for first-stage operation. **B,** Profile of same patient showing retracted columella and simian lip with flattened anterior maxilla. **C,** Five months after L-shaped bone graft up to glabella into columella and onlay grafts to maxilla and beneath alar bases. **D,** Profile shows good bridge line elevation. Columella, although not perfect, is just visible, and central part of face has been brought forward by onlay bone graft. **E,** Patient still has irregular nostrils, but tip is less rounded and alae are further forward. Central scar is still just visible.

floor. More bone chips are placed through the lower part of the columella incision into the pockets that have been prepared subperiosteally, beneath the alar bases and right across the upper part of the upper lip, so that the whole of this part of the nose and maxilla will be built forward. If atrophic rhinitis is present, the airways are reduced by laying cancellous bone chips subperiosteally along the nasal floor on each side.

Elastoplast fixation is applied to the nose and upper lip for 7 days.

AFTER OPERATION

The patient is nursed in the Fowler position. Ice is applied to the eyes for 24 hours. Routine parenteral antibiotics are given for 5 days. Physiotherapy and gentle ambulation are allowed on the second day. The hip drain is removed at this time, and the hip sutures are removed on the tenth day. The nose and face remain swollen, slowly decreasing over the next 3 months.

SUMMARY

I advocate the use of cancellous bone from the iliac crest to correct these nasal deformities. The bone will survive, even if it is placed superficial to the periosteum, since it is performing a *function*.* The advantages of this method are as follows:

1. Good, permanent restitution of contour is performed.

2. There is not the risk of loss of implant or absorption where a homograft is used.

3. Autogenous material is being used.

The disadvantages are as follows:

1. There is a hip wound, with pain, indisposition, and subsequent mild deformity and scarring.

2. Time of hospitalization is increased.

However, in my opinion, the advantages far outweigh the disadvantages.

---

*Mowlem, R.: Hunterian Lecture to the Royal College of Surgeons of England, 1941.

Chapter 27

Secondary deformities
minor, typical, and severe

D. Ralph Millard, Jr., M.D., F.A.C.S.

The popularity of corrective rhinoplasty continues to increase, and this would not occur if the majority of these operations were not successful. Yet, with the gradual increase in the total number of rhinoplasties, as might be expected, there has been a corresponding increase in the number of secondary deformities. As already noted previously,[5] the prognosis of a corrective rhinoplasty operation is influenced by several factors: (1) the condition and degree of difficulty of the original nasal deformity, (2) the training and skill of the operating surgeon, (3) the postoperative course and healing of the patient, and (4) unexpected or unknown circumstances, which, for lack of a better name, can be referred to loosely as luck. Actually, such may be explained as a late unexpected hematoma, a low-grade infection, necrosis of tissue in invisible positions, and other subtle and unusual reactions secondary to the surgery that result in unexpected deformities.

The nose is composed of a general skin and subcutaneous *cover,* an elongated tripod of bone and cartilaginous *support,* and two cavities of mucosal *lining.* Any occurring secondary deformity that is of concern will be reflected in the cover, support, or lining. It may involve only one, a combination of two, or it could include all three. Diagnosis of which of the three is involved deserves first priority. Once this decision has been made, then the standard techniques of reconstruction must be employed to achieve the correction.

MINOR DISCREPANCIES

Remember that this work is done by hand and eye. No matter how careful the surgeon may be when shaping three layers of living, bleeding tissue

along three planes, it is inevitable that minor discrepancies will occur. A difference in skin cover thickness may give a slight depression of contour. Residual loose pieces of cartilage or bone can give a visible interruption in profile or a roughness to the touch. Shortness of lining, misplaced interruption of cartilage intergrity, or the pull of one stitch can cause kinking along the alar rim. The lowering of the bridge without reduction of the alar bases can give a relative widening of the nostrils. Reduction of the nostrils can produce slight asymmetries. The mere process of narrowing a nose with an adequate airway can encroach just enough on the passages to become bothersome even in the absence of a deviated septum or enlarged turbinates.

Depending on the *degree* of these minor discrepancies, the amount of overall improvement already achieved, and the contentment and stability of the patient, action is determined. Under suitable conditions, whatever is not perfect deserves improvement, provided there is a maximum chance of correction with minimal chance of compounding the problem. For instance, a slight hump can be used to support the tip and fill out the moderately retracted columella (Fig. 27-1). Nasal reduction in this patient had resulted in a thickened nose, which was thinned and sculptured with alar margin resections in continuity with alar base wedge excisions[4] (Fig. 27-2).

THE COMMON THREE

There are three postrhinoplasty secondary deformities that are common enough to have earned nicknames. They are the ski jump, the parrot's beak, and the pig's snout (Fig. 27-3).

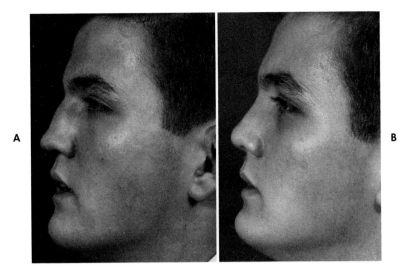

Fig. 27-1 A, Minor deformities are humped bridge and retracted columella. **B,** Hump is used to correct columella and support nasal tip.

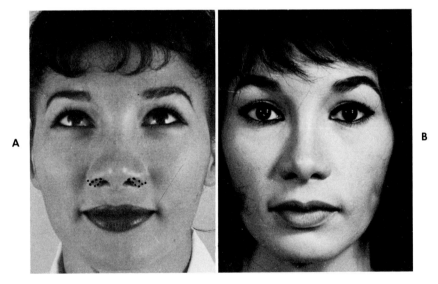

Fig. 27-2. A, This 26-year-old woman, after reduction rhinoplasty, had thick, broad, slightly Oriental nose. Design of correction involved marginal excisions in continuity with alar base wedge resections as marked. **B,** This marginal sculpturing gave more delicate thinning and shaping of alae without noticeable scars.

Ski jump

The character of a face and the pride of a nose depend in part on the graceful height and relative straightness of its bridge. Minor degrees of scooping the bridge to make it retroussé are sought by some and can be attractive in certain women. When carried beyond the ideal, the bridge lowering becomes a deformity requiring elevation and straightening. Regardless of whether the deformity has been caused by traumatic or surgical re-

moval of the bridge itself or is indirectly the result of loss by trauma, surgery, or infection of the septal support, the bridge will require additional onlays. Minor to moderate bridge correction can be achieved with an autogenous septal strut or tiered struts. If the discrepancy is minimal to moderate with no septal cartilage available, then, if the skin cover is in good condition, an auricular or costal cartilage may be necessary. Since this is an area where the implant lies quietly without a work

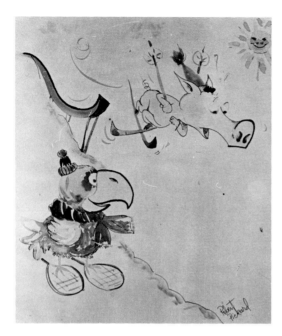

Fig. 27-3. Ski jump, pig's snout, and parrot's beak—all out in the cold.

load such as tip support, a suitable sliver of block Silastic will usually achieve the correct effect and lie there silently without serious reaction.

More severe depression and flatness may require the costal osteochondral hinge graft (Fig. 27-4).

Parrot's beak

The convex curve of the bridge and tip hooking like a parrot's beak is a rather common sequela of corrective rhinoplasty. Numerous causes of this deformity have been conjectured. The most obvious is the failure to carve the septal bridge correctly, leaving a curved hump. Another cause is the piling up in this area of thick dorsal skin when the nose is shortened. Aufricht[1] suggested extra scooping of the bridge in this area to accommodate this excess. Safian[9] blamed the overlap of the freed sidewalls on top of the septal bridge. Rees[8] accused the piling up of granulation and the following fibrosis in the supratip area. As the free

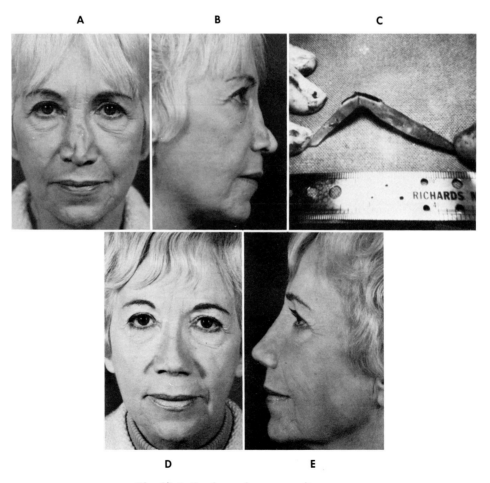

Fig. 27-4. For legend see opposite page.

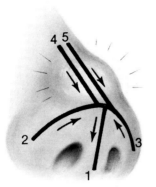

Fig. 27-5. Five incisions, membranous septal, *1,* anterior vestibular, *2* and *3,* and division of sidewalls from septum, *4* and *5,* all coverge in contraction toward supratip area.

edge of the septum can bleed severely, a postoperative hematoma[6] with subsequent fibrosis is also a possibility.

Yet, it is import to note that this supratip swelling rises at the exact point of convergence of five incisions, and this, indeed, may offer further clarification (Fig. 27-5). First, there is the vertical membranous septal incision, *1.* It diverges bilaterally as vestibular incisions, *2* and *3,* either anterior vestibular or intercartilaginous. The dorsal skin undermining is a proximal extension of the vestibular incisions, *2* and *3,* and, when the sidewall lining is divided on either side of the septum, incisions *4* and *5* are made. If, instead of two anterior vestibular incisions, *2* and *3,* the surgeon uses intercartilaginous and marginal incisions, he adds an extra two for a total of *seven* converging scars.

Whenever even five incisions meet at one point, the scarring is usually exaggerated. In this case, the incisions are at different angles, converging to a central point, and, with contracture of each inci-

sion, a humping at the center could be expected. The membranous septal incision contracts, pulling the tip down; the lateral incisions contract, pulling the sidewalls toward the septum; and the sidewall incisions with haphazard approximation add greater areas of humping granulation and subsequent fibrosis. Thus, several years ago, I began suturing the sidewalls back to the septum after trimming, and this seemed to help the healing. More recently, the mucosa of the sidewalls has been maintained intact when possible, and the septal cartilage of the bridge and upper lateral cartilages have been shaved and tailored. This not only ensures perfect approximation of the sidewall lining to the septum, but it also avoids two of the five scars. As a result of this modification, the early postoperative tip swelling seems to be less, and the amount of supratip swelling has been impressively reduced.

Once the parrot's beak deformity has occurred, then its correction is relatively standard. Through anterior vestibular incisions and a short membranous septal incision, the dorsal skin is undermined carefully and well beyond the specific supratip swelling to allow later draping. The thickened scar over the bridge is excised, and the thickened sidewalls are shaved of scar without being divided from the septum. Any rise of the septal cartilage bridge is lowered and in fact overcorrected by scooping, and any overriding of the upper lateral cartilages is trimmed (Figs. 27-6 to 27-8).

If the nose length is already correct, the lower half of the membranous septal incision can be avoided, reducing the converging vestibular scars to $2^{1}/_{2}$ in number. Healing without humping should be relatively consistent.

Text continued on p. 258.

Fig. 27-4. A and **B,** This 57-year-old housewife allegedly had basal cell carcinoma of skin of nose excised inadequately at time of reduction rhinoplasty. This was followed by complete excision and secondary rhinoplasty, including submucous resection of septum 3 months later. Finally, Silastic implant was inserted, resulting in infection, septal chondritis, cartilage dissolution, collapse of support, and furrowing of nasal skin. **C,** Piece of costal cartilage, with its perichondrium intact and including bit of bone on one end for nasal bone contact, is carved to shape, and wedge is resected up to perichondrium to allow bend at columella-tip angle. Advantage of this hinge graft over L-shaped type is smaller incision necessary for insertion. **D** and **E,** In first stage of reconstruction, through anterior vestibular incisions, lower lateral cartilages were reduced and skin was freed from sidewalls and septum, revealing large lining defect. This was filled with upper labial sulcus mucosal flap. One severe nasal skin furrow had to be excised directly. Bilateral osteotomy was also carried out. Eight months later, through vertical columella splitting incision, autogenous costal osteochondral hinge graft was inserted after further freeing of nasal dorsal skin. Alar marginal excisions sculptured sidewalls.

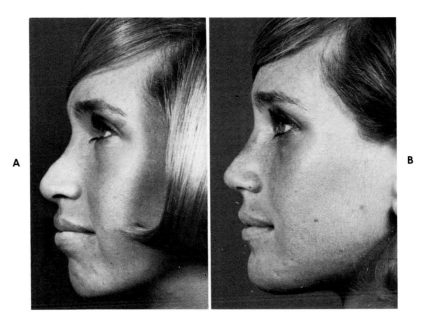

Fig. 27-6. A, This 21-year-old woman had postoperative parrot's beak, whicn was accentuated by receding chin. **B,** Secondary correction included removal of superior half of lower lateral cartilages, lowering of septum, triangular resection of anterior septum, alar base excisions, and insertion of Silastic implant to chin through 1 cm incision in lower labial sulcus.

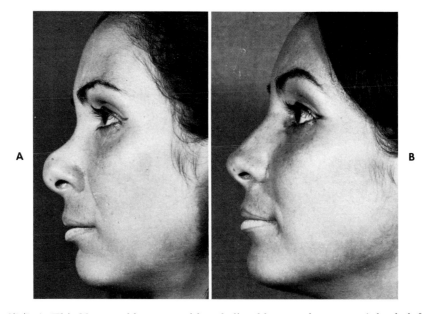

Fig. 27-7. A, This 28-year-old woman with unbelievable secondary parrot's beak deformity was first presented in Millard, D. R.: Plast. Reconstr. Surg. **44:**553, 1969. **B,** Her secondary corrections included reshaping her bridge by chisel at root and with scalpel along distal septal bridge. Resection of ellipse from anterior septum and from each alar base along with removal of superior three quarters of lower lateral cartilages completed her reshaping.

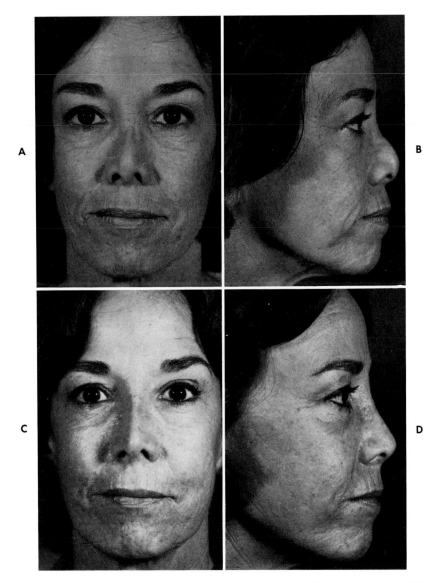

Fig. 27-8. A and **B,** This 49-year-old woman had had two rhinoplasties, a nasal injury, and radiation for facial acne. She revealed thin skin standing in three ridges, nasal bone and septum, in upper bridge. Her profile revealed severe parrot's beak with depressed upper bridge and flat, rounded tip, hanging alar bases, and retracted alar rims. **C** and **D,** Through columella-splitting incision, pocket was dissected over bridge, and through this exposure, septum was lowered, nasal bones were trimmed, and piece of Silastic sponge was slid over area to raise and smooth contour. Bilateral osteotomy with infracture only was followed with lower marginal rim excisions and alar base resections. Silastic block strut was inserted in columella to give moderate tip projection, a maneuver I almost never use and still do not advocate, but which has worked well for last 5 years in this specific case.

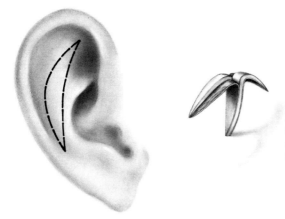

Fig. 27-9. This auricular composite banana-split graft can be used as a three-dimensional nose lengthener. (From Dingman, R. O., and Walter, C.: Plast. Reconstr. Surg. **43:**117, 1969.)

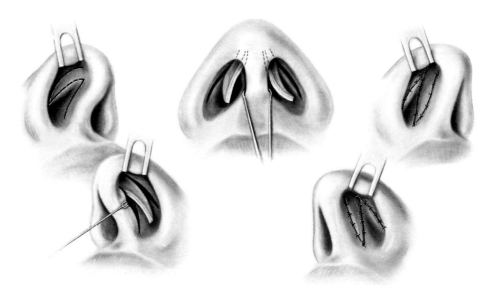

Fig. 27-10. Chondromucosal flaps based anteriorly are taken from lateral vestibules and transposed into membranous septal releasing incision with cartilage to cartilage. This bilateral action simultaneously corrects retracted columella as it lifts long sidewalls.

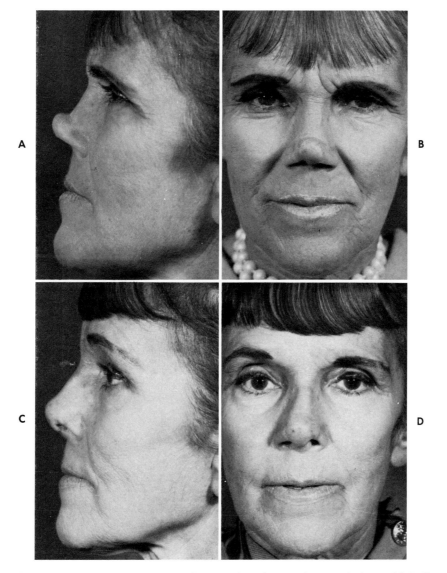

Fig. 27-11. This 49-year-old woman, after a series of operations, ended up with bulbous, snubbed tip, retracted columella, collapsed alae with knock-kneed sidewalls, and depressed nasal bridge. This case was presented in Millard, D. R.: Plast. Reconstr. Surg. **44:**549, 1969. Although there was much missing tissue, there was ample vestibular lining. Thus bilateral chondromucosal flaps based forward on septal tip were taken from upper lateral cartilages and transposed into membranous septal releasing incision. This lifted sidewalls and lowered columella retraction. Silastic block was inserted over bridge in specific pocket. Patient had suffered with this deformity for 20 years, and when splint was removed on seventh postoperative day to reveal dramatic improvement, she floored me with the comment, "But doctor, isn't one nostril a little different than the other?" **A** and **B,** Preoperative views. **C** and **D,** Postoperative views.

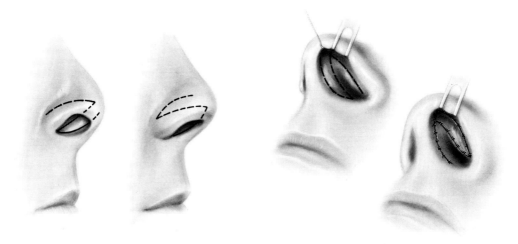

Fig. 27-12. Bilateral chondromucosal membranous septal flaps carrying sliver of medial crura or septal cartilage are transposed laterally into vestibular releasing incisions. This double action simultaneously lifts hanging columella and lowers retracted sidewalls.

Pig's snout

This is a secondary deformity that terrorizes the layman and is not particularly easy for the secondary surgeon to correct. It is usually caused during enthusiastic anterior septal resection accompanied by generous sidewall reduction of lining and cartilage. This not only shortens the nose but also tilts it upward, exposing the nostrils. Since septal shortening has the most direct effect on the nasal entrance, usually there is also a quality of columella retraction in the deformity. Regardless of whether the sidewalls were long and thick in the original nose or have become relatively long after septal shortening, the effect is a flat, double-barrel nasal entrance not unlike a pig's snout.

Here, again, diagnosis must direct the method of correction.

If the entire nose is snubbed, then there is shortness of the septocolumella component as well as the sidewalls; relief of this condition requires release of all three with the insertion of a free graft. It can be split-skin, full-thickness skin for the sides, but it will require a composite graft for the membranous septal defect. Dingman's auricular banana-split chondrocutaneous graft[2] seems to be the best to satisfy the entire three axes of the defect (Fig. 27-9).

When the columella is retracted but the sidewalls are relatively long, then the lateral vestibular chondromucosal flaps can be transposed into the membranous septal releasing incision[3,6,7] (Fig. 27-10). This corrects the front entrance tripod with more projection of the center column, and, at the same time, it lifts the long sidewalls (Fig. 27-11).

When the central column is long with what is sometimes referred to as a hanging columella and the sidewalls are pulled up short in retraction, then chondromucosal flaps[7] (Fig. 27-12) from the membranous septal area, carrying slivers of medial alar cartilage or septal cartilage, are transposed into lateral releasing incisions that pull up the hanging center column while letting down the retracted sidewalls and stiffening them if they flail (Fig. 27-13).

The third degree of secondary rhinoplasty deformities involves full-thickness losses. These are indeed rare and can usually be explained by a violation of principle with a sacrifice of blood supply, the occurrence of infection, and the overzealous or unwise use of foreign body implants. All three were involved in the case example in Fig. 27-14.

A   B   C

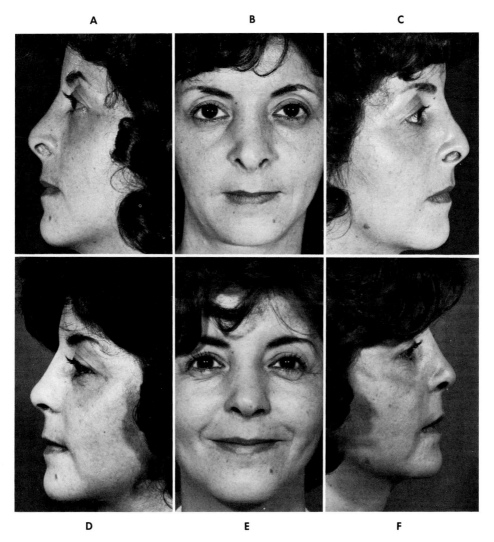

D   E   F

Fig. 27-13. A to **C,** This 35-year-old housewife, after rhinoplasty, had secondary postoperative deformities, including irregular bridge line and slight parrot's beak with retracted alae, flaring alar bases, and hanging columella. **D** to **F,** Simultaneous correction of retracted alae and hanging columella was accomplished by bilateral membranous septal chondromucosal flaps based anteriorly at tip and transposed into lateral vestibular releasing incisions. This pulled columella up and let alae down. Other refinements included bridge revision and alar base resections.

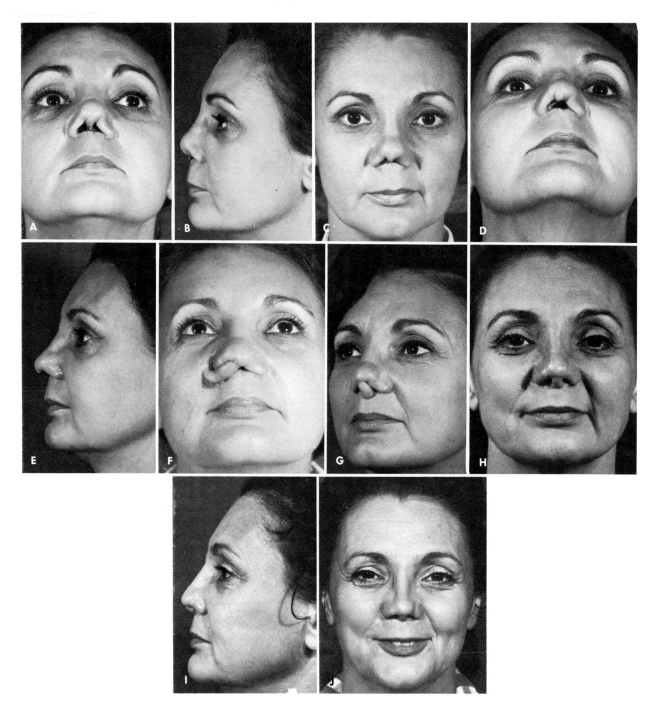

Fig. 27-14. A and **B,** This 42-year-old housewife, with history of trauma to nose 2 years previously and seven nasal operations thereafter, reported having had bone grafts, auricular cartilage grafts, and Silastic implants. She revealed broad, bulbous, foreshortened nose, severely lacking in lining. Between nasal tip and lip, there was nestled a dried, escharotic chunk of tissue wrapped in gauze, which she had been told would "granulate and heal." **C** and **D,** It was gently removed with forceps without evidence of bleeding and proved to be remnants of her original columella. There was also absence of anterior third of septum. **E,** Reconstruction involved opening airway, introduction of lining, and reconstruction of columella. First, submucous resection of remaining obstructive septal cartilage opened airway and produced a mucosal flap on one side to aid in lining. Bony bridge was corrected through paramarginal vestibular incision. Skin of nose was mobilized and lengthened 2.5 cm beyond its lining. Full-thickness inguinal skin graft was sutured as inlay into this defect, resulting in better length to nose. **F,** Four months later, a 1 × 6 cm right nasolabial flap was denuded at its end and inserted under nasal tip. **G,** Six weeks later, cheek attachment was divided and inset into defect in lip prepared by turnback flap. **H,** This attachment was revised by splitting and splaying lip end of columella 3 months later. **I** and **J,** Six months later, autogenous costal cartilage strut was shaped and inserted into new columella. Vertical elliptical excision of thickness of columella and reduction of its inferior cuff have been last minor surgical revisions.

REFERENCES

1. Aufricht, G.: Personal communication, 1958.
2. Dingman, R. O., and Walter, C.: Use of composite ear grafts in correction of short nose, Plast. Reconstr. Surg. **43:**117, 1969.
3. Millard, D. R., Jr.: The triad of columella deformities, Plast. Reconstr. Surg. **31:**370, 1963.
4. Millard, D. R., Jr.: Adjuncts in augmentation mentoplasty and corrective rhinoplasty, Plast. Reconstr. Surg. **36:**55, 1965.
5. Millard, D. R., Jr.: Corrective rhinoplasty. In Gibson, T., editor: Modern trends in plastic surgery, New York, 1966, Appleton-Century-Crofts, p. 300.
6. Millard, D. R., Jr.: Secondary corrective rhinoplasty, Plast. Reconstr. Surg. **44:**545, 1969.
7. Millard, D. R., Jr.: Versatility of the chondromucosal flap in the nasal vestibule, Plast. Reconstr. Surg. **50:**580, 1972.
8. Rees, T. D., Krupp, S., and Wood-Smith, D.: Secondary rhinoplasty, Plast. Reconstr. Surg. **46:**332, 1970.
9. Safian, J.: Fact and fallacy in rhinoplastic surgery, Br. J. Plast. Surg. **11:**52, 1958.

Discussion

Evans: Dr. Millard, I was very much impressed with your chondromucosal flap publication and had occasion to use this several times with great success. Except in the reverse! The reverse presented a problem for me in closure, and, though I know you had a little problem closing like you did today on one side of the donor closure, I wonder in the reverse flap, taking it from the midline out, whether you have had any closure problems? How do you treat them?

Millard: Thank you very much. I'm glad that you have had partial success. But no, I won't do it unless I have a really hanging columella that allows me to take quite a bit of tissue. Then I do it. Otherwise, I would rather merely take out expendable tissue in the midline, without trying to get flaps, and then release laterally and fill with full thickness grafts. It's only if you have enough to spare that you can dare it. Otherwise, you could get a retracted columella. In other words, don't drop one baby to pick up another!

Chapter 28

Finesse in rhinoplasty

Jack H. Sheen, M.D.

Rhinoplasty, as originally conceived, was directed toward those patients whose nasal configuration fell well outside the accepted norms of their cultural standard of beauty. Surgery usually involved the gargantuan hump with a low-hanging tip and a patient who would state, "I don't care what you do; anything would be better than this."

With the increasing popularity of rhinoplasty and the apparent need for physical perfection, patients consult plastic surgeons with noses that are close to being as good as their tissues will allow. These patients embody a new sophistication and discernment in their expectations, which challenges today's plastic surgeon to produce a result that is more subtle and artistic. They have little to gain and potentially much to lose. When the result is less attractive than the preoperative version, both patient and doctor suffer much distress. The finesse or minor correction is a relatively new concept. In 1904, Nalaton and Ombredonne published a textbook, *La Rhinoplastie,* in which they stated, "The surgeon cannot pretend to correct a slight malformation. If a nose be slightly deviated or humped, or show a slight saddle deformity, these are unfortunate defects, but we do not believe that the corrrection of such defects can be achieved by surgery."

The essence of rhinoplastic finesse is the surgical correction of slight aesthetic distortions in the relationship of nasal parts. In today's aesthetic surgical practice, the plastic surgeon cannot refuse the challenge of the minor distortion. However, in so doing, careful preoperative planning is most important, since the latitude is narrow. All of the routines for rhinoplasty must be put aside and each case approached as a special challenge.

The surgeon is constantly faced with form. This being subjective, I would like to briefly illustrate, from my point of view, the anatomic landmarks and relationships that are important to achieve a proper aesthetic result.

Fig. 28-1, *A,* shows a 16-year-old girl on whom I have done a primary rhinoplasty. The following landmarks and relationships are essential for aesthetic balance:

1. The nasion, or root of the nose, begins on a plane with the superior tarsal fold.

2. The dorsum is relatively straight, ending in a slightly projecting tip.

3. The tip is the highest point in the nasal profile.

Lateral preoperative and postoperative views (Fig. 28-1, *B*) show the following:

1. The line from the tip to the insertion of the columella is broken at the columellar-lobular junction.

2. The nasolabial angle is open or obtuse.

3. The subnasion is neither too full nor too sharp.

4. The columella is lower than and parallel to the alar rim.

Frontal preoperative and postoperative views (Fig. 28-1, *C*) show the following:

1. The nose flows in gentle, divergent lines from the root to the base.

2. The tip is well differentiated and has delicacy or faceting.

3. The nares are visible.

4. All parts of the nose have a subtle continuity.

Preoperative and postoperative basal views (Fig. 28-1, *D*) show the following:

1. The basal perimeter is softly triangular.

2. The nares are ovoid or tear shaped and incline toward the apex of the triangle.

This aesthetic concept applies to any patient seeking rhinoplasty, regardless of the physical proportion, and should be an important part of the preoperative plan.

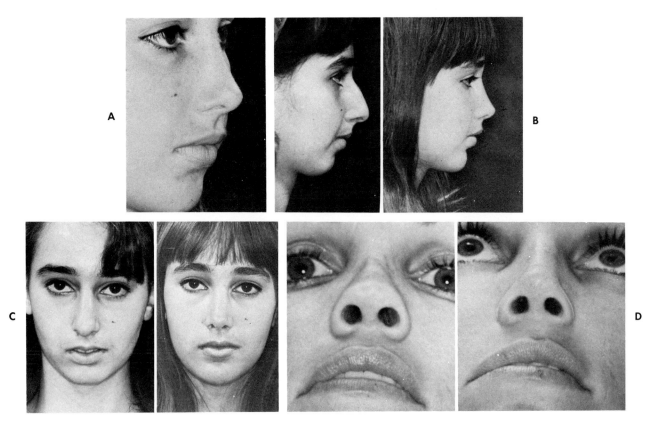

Fig. 28-1. A, Three-quarters profile of primary rhinoplasty, illustrating my concept of proper nasal relationships. **B,** Dorsum begins in line with superior tarsal fold and is relatively straight, ending in slightly projecting tip (highest point in nasal profile). Line from tip to insertion of columella is broken at columellar-lobular junction. Attention is paid to prominence of subnasion and to slightly receding chin. **C,** On frontal view, there must be enough dorsal height to give visual effect of separation of eyes in white people. Radix is not overly narrowed and flows in gradually diverging lines to base of nose. There is good tip differentiation, and nares are visible. **D,** Basal perimeter should be triangular with nares ovoid or tear shaped and inclined toward apex of triangle.

The following series of cases demonstrate the need for modification or departure from the general technique of rhinoplasty in the correction of the slight or unusual nasal deformity—the rhinoplastic finesse. The aesthetic concept just outlined will be used as a frame of reference in the following cases, which progress from the simple to the more complex in the approach to the rhinoplastic finesse.

Case 1. The first patient (Fig. 28-2, *A*) illustrates a simple finesse in that the only part involved is the tip configuration, and yet all parts of the nose are involved with the correction. The dorsum is straight, ending in a tip that is the highest projecting part in the nasal profile. The nasolabial angle is a bit sharp, and the relationship of the alae with the columella is slightly off. On frontal

projection (Fig. 28-2, *C*), the dorsum ends abruptly at the area of tip differentiation. The tip is too full and without delicacy. The hypertrophied lobular cartilages form visible bilobed masses in the tip, which give the tip a *down* look in spite of a fairly good nasolabial angle.

PROCEDURE (Fig. 28-2, *D*). The initial incisions were intercartilaginous with limited skeletonization. The membranous septum was incised to only the lower third, with a resection of a triangle of superior caudal membranous septum. The tip cartilages were delivered through a rim incision. The cephalic portion was trimmed. The dome was transected, and 2 mm was resected from it to allow the lateral crus to settle more medially, changing the basal configuration slightly to a more triangular perimeter. Lateral osteotomy only was needed

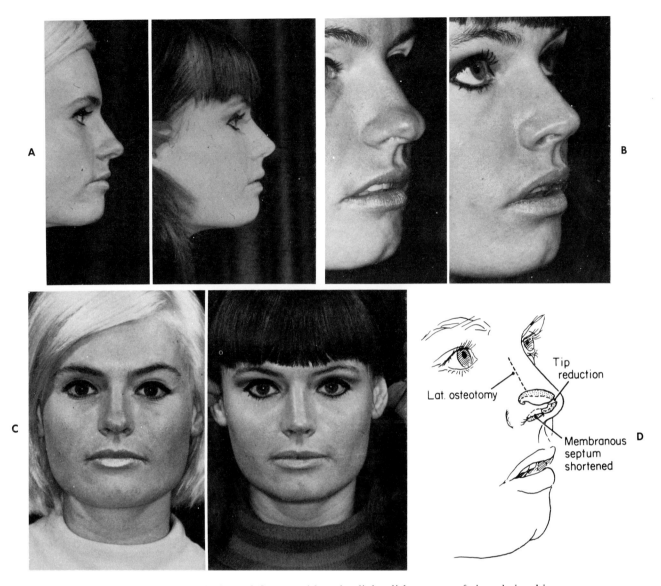

Fig. 28-2. A, Lateral view of finesse with only slight disharmony of tip relationships, yet all parts of nose are involved with correction. **B,** Three-quarters view showing disharmony of tip relationships. **C,** Front view illustrating illusion of lengthening and thinning of nasal configuration by way of tip refinement. **D,** Schematic representation of surgical correction.

to move the inferior caudal portion of the bony vault more medial to narrow the frontal contour and complete the procedure.

Case 2. On lateral and frontal views (Fig. 28-3, *A* and *B*), this young patient has excellent relationship of her nasal parts. The tip is a bit full, and the relationship of the columella to the alae is slightly off. On three-quarter projection (Fig. 28-3, *C*) the disharmony can readily be seen. The caudal borders of the bony vault project laterally, forming a sharp line of demarcation with the relatively de-

pressed upper cartilaginous vault, which exaggerates the already hypertrophied lobular cartilages.

PROCEDURE (Fig. 28-3, *D*). Limited skeletonization of the upper cartilaginous vault was accomplished through bilateral intercartilaginous incisions. The skeletonization of the bony vault was limited to just expose the lateral bony projections. A transfixing incision was made to the lower third, with resection of an ellipse of membranous septum at the superior caudal septum. A coarse rasp was used to reduce the lateral projections of the nasal

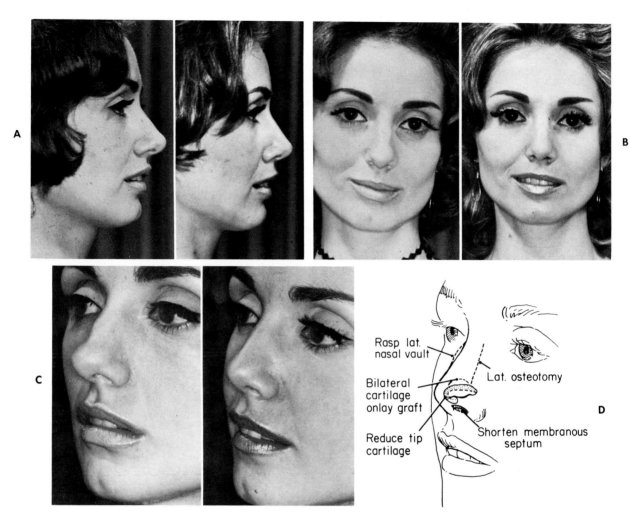

Fig. 28-3. A, Lateral view: minimal disharmony of nasal parts. **B,** Frontal view: lines from root to base are broken and irregular due to hypertrophied lobular cartilages. **C,** Three-quarters profile shows striking irregularity of nasal line. **D,** Schematic respresentation of surgical correction.

bones, opening up the roof laterally. The tip cartilages were delivered through a rim incision, and a generous cephalic portion was resected. (A minimum of 5 mm of the caudal part remained to make up the new lateral crus.) This was followed by resection of 2 mm from the area of the dome, changing the basal configuration from a square to a slightly triangular perimeter. A lateral osteotomy was done, and the bones were gently repositioned. To augment the upper cartilaginous vault, the two fragments of lobular cartilage from the cephalic part were trimmed into a triangular shape and sutured in place over the upper lateral cartilages with a percutaneous suture of 6-0 nylon.

Case 3. This young male patient (Fig. 28-4, *A*) has a high dorsum that elevates the tip up and

out and an unusually prominent nasal spine that distracts it down and in. The distorting influence of the nasal spine can be seen in the frontal projection (Fig. 28-4, *B*) with the nares forming an ellipse down towards the philtrum. The added flare to the alar lobules gives the patient's face a built-in snarl. On lateral close-up (Fig. 28-4, *C*), the line from the tip to the insertion of the columella is almost a straight line. The relationship of the columella to the alae is poor, diverging at about 45 degrees instead of being parallel to the alar rim.

PROCEDURE (Fig. 28-4, *D*). Intercartilaginous incisions were made to widely skeletonize the upper cartilaginous vault and limited skeletonization carried out over the bony vault. A deep transfixing incision was made to the base of the spine, expos-

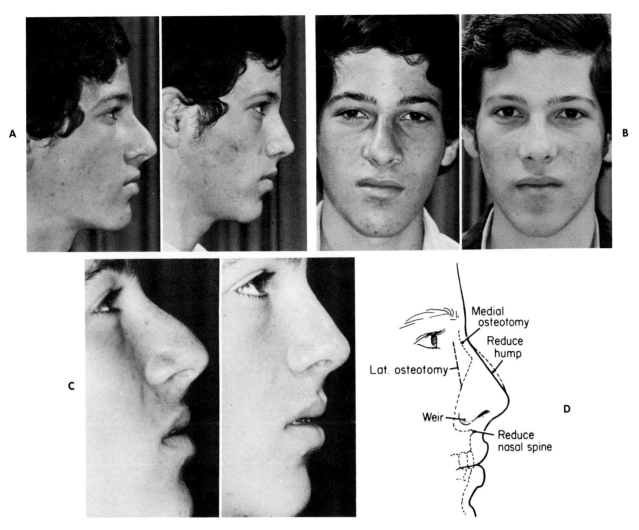

Fig. 28-4. A, Lateral view illustrates two opposing forces on nasal tip: dorsum and prominent nasal spine. **B,** Frontal view. Prominent spine brings nasal floor toward philtrum. This slightly downward curve medially toward philtrum plus flaring nostrils gives patient built-in snarl. **C,** Close-up lateral view. Line from tip to insertion of columella is almost straight. Relationship of columella to alar rim is poor. **D,** Schematic representation of surgical correction.

ing the prominent spine and inferior caudal septum. The dorsum was reduced approximately 70% of the estimate, followed by a resection of the nasal spine and inferior caudal septum.This was done using a double-action bone-biting rongeur.

After both of these distracting forces were softened, a more accurate assessment of the amount of the dorsal reduction could be made. The tip cartilages were delivered through a rim incision, and a simple cephalic trim was done, leaving 4 or 5 mm of the lateral crus intact. Final adjustments of the dorsum and lateral osteotomy completed the procedure.

Case 4. This very attractive young lady (Fig.

28-5, *A*) has excellent facial planes and relationships, and yet the lack of delicacy of her nose gives her a less feminine look. There is a slight dorsal hump and poor tip differentiation. The tip has no projection but forms a semicircle from the supratip to the insertion of the columella. The nasolabial angle is good, but the subnasion is too full for the short columella.

On basal view (Fig. 28-5, *B*), the tip is almost square instead of triangular, and the nares are perpendicular to the base instead of inclining towards the apex of the tip.

On frontal projection (Fig. 28-5, *C*), there is no differentiation of the nasal parts; the nares are

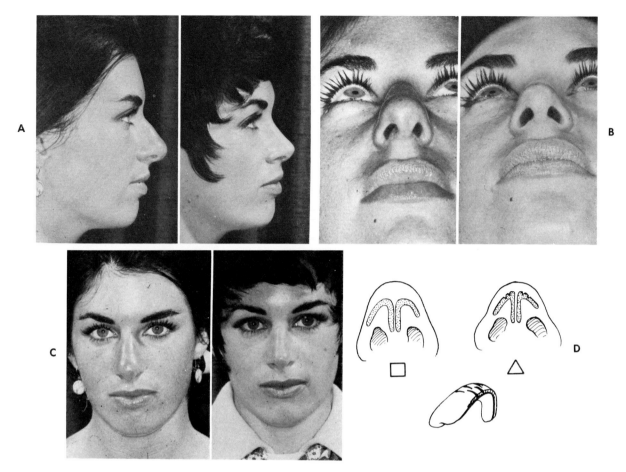

Fig. 28-5. A, Lateral view. Slight dorsal hump, poorly defined tip, and full subnasion give nose masculine appearance. **B,** Basal perimeter is almost square, with nares perpendicular to floor of nose. **C,** Frontal view shows broad nasal pyramid with poor tip differentiation. **D,** Schematic diagram of tip cartilage attenuation at dome to change configuration from square to more triangular one.

not visible, and the tip is bulbous. (The nasal tip that has proper definition produces a light reflex that is a small three-point equilateral triangle.)

PROCEDURE (Fig. 28-5, *D*). Limited skeletonization through bilateral intercartilaginous incisions gave adequate exposure to those parts involved with the correction. A transfixing incision was carried to the base of the spine. Resection of part of the nasal spine and 3 or 4 mm of inferior caudal septum was followed by resection of only membranous septum over the superior distal septum. The tip cartilages were delivered through a rim incision, the cephalic portion was trimmed, and the area of the dome was attenuated by interdigitating crosshatches as shown. Lateral osteotomy was done, and a gentle realignment of the bony pyramid completed the procedure.

Case 5. This young lady (Fig. 28-6, *A*) had a

primary rhinoplasty peformed 2 years ago, and although she was not unhappy with the result (which certainly falls within the acceptable aesthetic range of postsurgical noses), she hoped that more could be done surgically. Critical evaluation reveals a radix that begins a bit too caudad because of a slight (2 or 3 mm) overreduction of the dorsum. The tip has no differentiation or separation from the dorsum. The supratip area is the highest point in the nasal profile. The columellar-alar relationship is poor, the nasolabial angle is open, but the subnasion is too sharp because of a slight retraction of the maxilla.

On close lateral projection (Fig. 28-6, *B* and *C*), there is an overall retraction of the middle third of her face, exaggerated by virtue of a low nasal dorsum and a retrusive maxilla.

PROCEDURE (Fig. 28-6, *D*). Because there was

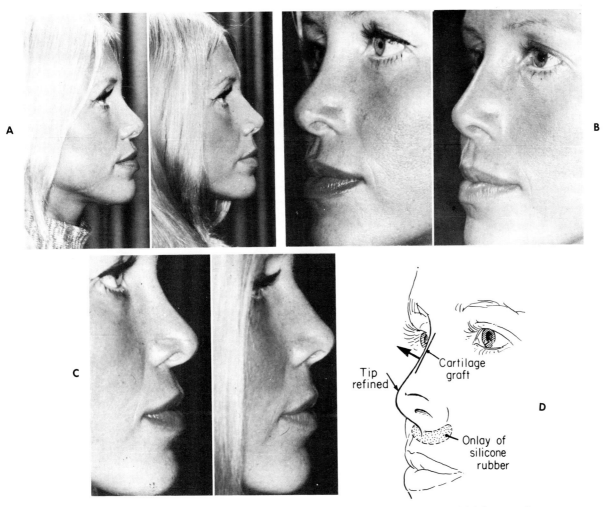

Fig. 28-6. A, Lateral view shows low dorsum, poor tip differentiation, and high supratip. **B,** Three-quarters profile. Due to slightly high supratip, tip has a *down* look. Columellar-alar relationship is poor. **C,** Close-up lateral view. Retrusive maxilla and low dorsum give middle third of face pushed-in look. **D,** Schematic representation of surgical correction.

no need to shorten the nose or involve the caudal ends of the upper lateral cartilages, incisions were made as one would for a cartilage-splitting incision, gull-wing shaped, just 4 or 5 mm cephalad to the caudal border of the lower lateral cartilages. This was followed by modest supratip thinning. After resection of a triangular portion of scar tissue over the distal superior septum, a pocket was developed to the root of the nose just large enough to accommodate a single graft of septal cartilage (obtained from the patient's septum). This graft, carefully shaped to reduplicate the normal anatomic roof or dorsum, was slipped into the pocket and secured with a mattress suture of 6-0 nylon. A transfixing incision was made down to the maxilla, where a wide periosteal elevator was used to

elevate tissues lateral to the spine, just large enough to accommodate a hand-carved silicone rubber prosthesis, which curved over the anterior maxilla, going laterally to a point just beyond the alar lobules.

Case 6. This young patient was concerned about the differences between her touched-up black-and-white photos and the color photos, which seemed to exaggerate her deep retroussé (color photos cannot be retouched). The touched-up photo was interesting in that the artist had effectively reduced the saddle deformity, rotated the lobule caudally, and reduced the flare of her nares.

On lateral projection (Fig. 28-7, *A*), the deep saddle and the cephalic rotation of her tip is obvi-

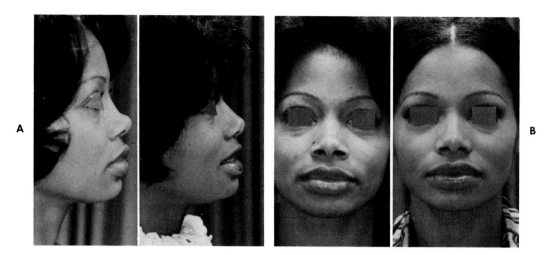

Fig. 28-7. A, Lateral view. Deep retroússe has effect of rotating lobule cephalad. **B,** Frontal view. There is poor separation of eyes. Nares are overly flaring and have almost horizontal attitude.

ous, and this is made even more pronounced by the long, arching, thin alae. On frontal view (Fig. 28-7, *B*), there is poor separation of the eyes because of the low dorsum, and the tip configuration is flattened with the nares almost horizontal. Because of the cephalic tilt of the nasal tip, the nares are visible. The problem, then, is to narrow the flare of the nostrils and retain her racial characteristics. In planning alar wedges on this patient, any error in judgment as to placement or amount could be deforming and irreversible. I know of no procedure that would not leave notching in the area of resection, instead of preserving the soft curve of the lateral floor of the nostril—the so-called nasal sill.

Alar sculpting as originally described by Weir has gone through many modifications by Joseph, Aufricht, Seltzer, and others, indicating that there really is not a single procedure that can be universally applied. Alar sculpting has to be as judgmental and individualized as rhinoplasty. However, the point I am directing your attention to here is the notching that frequently occurs from resection of tissues, by whatever means, from the floor of the nose. The narrowing of a flare at the base of the nose should be more; it should be a preservation of all of the normal anatomic landmarks, with a reduction of the aberrant part.

I would like to introduce and briefly illustrate a simple procedure that can be helpful in preserving the continuity of the nasal floor (Fig. 28-8, *A*). After the planned excision has been marked with ink along the alar base, an incision is made with a no. 11 blade in the usual fashion, carrying it me-

dially along the alar base until the final 2 or 3 mm or so have been reached. It is at this point that a back cut is made (Fig. 28-8, *C*), preserving a small triangular flap that I shall refer to as the medial flap. The superior cut is made in the usual manner and the resected material is removed (Fig. 28-8, *C*), leaving a small flap, the medial flap, at the edge of the inferior wound (Fig. 28-8 *D*). This is a diagrammatic representation of the usual wedge resection, which produces an unnatural angulation at the base of the nostril instead of a soft, uninterrupted ovoid. After the preservation of the medial flap, the proper contour can be seen in the patient shown in Fig. 28-8, *E*, before suture placement. Fig. 28-8, *F*, is a schematic representation of the preservation of the medial flap, which results in a soft ovoid floor of the nostril. Fig. 28-8, *G*, shows the same patient after completion of suture placement with good continuity of the sill and an ovoid floor.

Returning to the patient for further analysis, Fig. 28-9, *A*, is a basal view in which can be seen the thin alae, which are horizontal, in continuity with the sill of the floor of the nose, and with no lobular portion to the alae. The basal perimeter is too broad-based even for this race.

On three-quarter projection (Fig. 28-9, *B*) the deep retroussé is apparent with a cephalic tilt to the lobule. The augmentation of the dorsum was planned to be less than that amount that would eliminate the natural retroussé expected in this race but enough to correct the saddle deformity and rotate the lobule caudad.

PROCEDURE (Fig. 28-9, *C*). A single incision was

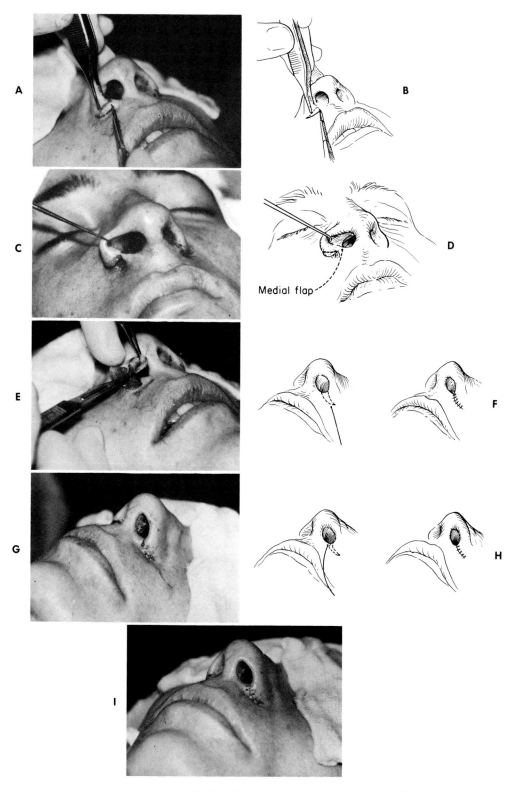

Fig. 28-8. A, Preservation of medial flap for improving contour of nasal sill. **B,** Schematic drawing. **C,** Unsevered inferior incision illustrating area referred to as medial flap. **D,** Schematic drawing. **E,** Completed excision of wedge, showing medial flap. **F,** Diagrammatic representation of usual wedge resection resulting in sharp angle along area of resection. **G,** Patient with medial flap retained, showing soft curve of nasal sill before suture placement. **H,** Schematic representation of retained medial flap resulting in smooth nasal sill. Compare with **F. I,** Patient after completion of suture placement.

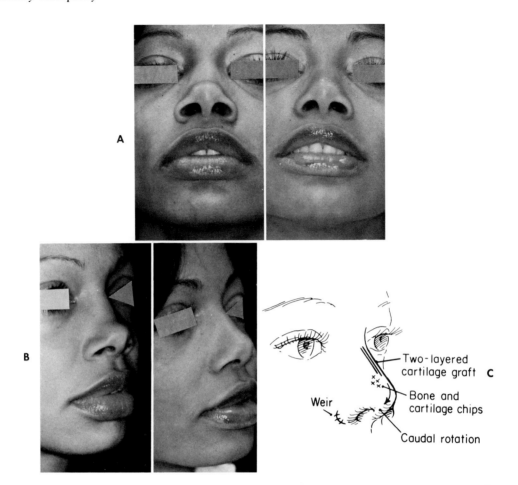

Fig. 28-9. A, Basal view. Basal perimeter is flat and broad. Improper resection of nostril could be deforming and irreversible due to cephalic tilt of lobule and thin alae. **B,** Three-quarters profile view. Augmentation was planned to preserve some retroussé and enough to rotate lobule caudad. **C,** Schematic representation of surgical correction.

made over the left reflection of the caudal edge of the upper lateral cartilage, and a pocket was developed to the radix. A radical submucous was done to obtain as much autogenous material as possible—always deficient in the black. A two-layered cartilage graft was placed over the dorsum, and the caudal end was shored up with excess fragments of cartilage, vomer, and perpendicular plate. Alar sculpting as just described completed the procedure.

Case 7. This model (Fig. 28-10, *A*) was always happy with her nose except for the way it photographed over the past several years. Because of her height (5 feet 10 inches) she wanted to retain the look of elegance or strength her nose gave her.

The nose on lateral projection appears only slightly high, with the middle third the highest point in the nasal profile. The tip is dependent by less than 1 mm, but enough to give the nasal

configuration a *down* look. The nasolabial angle is open, but the break at the columellar-lobular junction is flattened, which gives the illusion of tip droop. The relationship of the columella to the alae is improper in that the alae inserts lower than the columella, which gives the illusion of displeasure. On frontal projection (Fig. 28-10, *B*), the nose is slightly broad, and the nares are barely visible. On close frontal examination (Fig. 28-10, *C*), the bony vault is slightly broad, flowing into a narrower upper cartilaginous vault and finally a broad lower cartilaginous configuration. This serves to give the frontal projection an irregular line, which is difficult to camouflage. The nose, by virtue of the exaggerated lower lateral cartilages, appears shortened. The tip is flattened without delicacy.

PROCEDURE (Fig. 28-10, *D*). Because the nose was to be shortened (by rotation of the lobule cephalad), the approach was through wide inter-

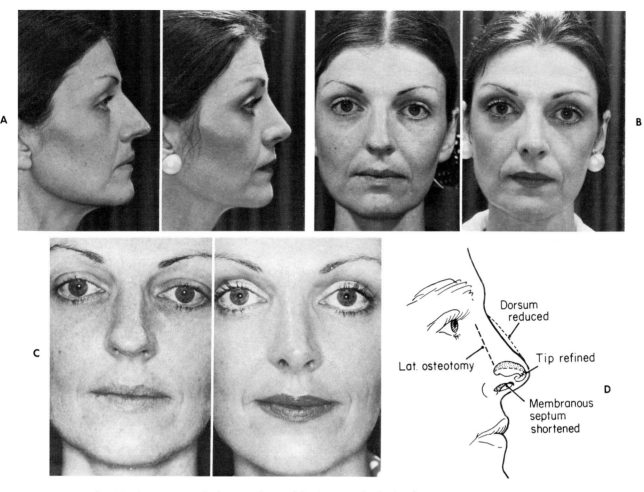

Fig. 28-10. A, Lateral view. Patient wished to retain look of elegance or strength her nose gave her as professional model but wanted coarse features modified. **B,** Frontal view. Nose is slightly broad with irregular lines from root to base of nose. **C,** Frontal close-up view. Nose appears shortened due to flat, broad nasal tip. **D,** Schematic representation of surgical correction.

cartilaginous incisions, skeletonizing the upper cartilaginous vault to the malar groove. The skeletonization over the bony vault was limited. A transfixing incision was made down to the middle third of the membranous septum, and an ellipse of membranous septum was removed from the superior caudal septum. A Fomon rasp was used to lower the slight prominence of the bony vault. The tip cartilages were delivered through a rim incision, the cephalic excess was trimmed, and a 2 mm segment was removed from each dome area, which allowed the lateral crus to settle more medially, changing the basal perimeter from a square to a more delicate triangular one.

Later osteotomy was done to gently reposition the nasal bones.

CONCLUSION

The subtle change in the relationships of nasal parts, the rhinoplastic finesse, can only be learned through experience and attention to detail. The presentation of a series of representative cases can hopefully suggest some guidelines and patterns of thinking in the approach to this most interesting surgical challenge.

REFERENCES

1. Aufricht, G.: A few hints and surgical details in rhinoplasty, Laryngoscope **53:**317, 1943.
2. Aufricht, G.: Rhinoplasty and the face, Plast. Reconstr. Surg. **43:**219, 1969.
3. Benton, C. D.: Chemical cauterization of the inferior turbinate, Eye Ear Nose Throat Mon. **45:**90, Oct., 1966.

4. Cole, P.: Nasal turbinate function, Can. J. Otolaryngol. **2:**259, 1973.

5. Converse, J. M., et al.: Reconstructive plastic surgery, Philadelphia, 1964, W. B. Saunders Co.

6. Fry, J. J.: Judicious turbinectomy for nasal obstruction, Aust. N. Z. J. Surg. **42:**291, 1973.

7. Gonzales-Ulloa, M.: Quantitative principles in cosmetic surgery of the face (profileplasty), Plast. Reconstr. Surg. **29:**186, 1962.

8. Hinderer, K. H.: Diagnosis of anatomic obstructions of airways (abstr.) Arch. Otolaryngol. **78:**660, 1963.

9. Fomon, S., and Bell, J.: Rhinoplasty—new concepts, Springfield, Ill., 1970, Charles C Thomas, Publisher.

10. Littell, J. J.: Partial decortication of the inferior turbinate body, Trans. Indiana Acad. Ophthalmol. Otolaryngol. **45:**57, May, 1962.

11. Little, S. W.: Management of enlarged turbinates, Va. Med. Mon. **90:**484, 1963.

12. Millard, D. R.: Columella lengthening by a forked flap, Plast. Reconstr. Surg. **5:**454, 1958.

13. Millard, D. R.: External excisions in rhinoplasty, Br. J. Plast. Surg. **12:**340, 1960.

14. Millard, D. R.: Alar margin sculpturing, Plast. Reconstr. Surg. **40:**337, 1967.

15. Millard, D. R.: Secondary corrective rhinoplasty, Plast. Reconstr. Surg. **44:**545, 1969.

16. Peer, L. A.: The fate of autogenous septal cartilage after transplantation in human tissues, Arch. Otolaryngol. **36:**696, 1941.

17. Peer, L. A.: The neglected septal cartilage graft, Arch. Otolaryngol. **42:**384, 1945.

18. Rees, T. D., Krupp, S., and Wood-Smith, D.: Secondary rhinoplasty, Plast. Reconstr. Surg. **46:**332, 1970.

19. Rees, T. D., Krupp, S., and Wood-Smith, D.: Cosmetic facial surgery, Philadelphia, 1973, W. B. Saunders Co.

20. Rogers, B. O.: The importance of "delay" in timing secondary and tertiary corrections of post-rhinoplastic deformities. In Transactions of the Fourth International Congress of Plastic and Reconstructive Surgery (1967), Amsterdam, 1969, Excerpta Medica Foundation.

21. Safian, J.: Corrective rhinoplastic surgery, New York, 1935, Paul B. Hoeber, Inc.

22. Seltzer, A. P.: Inferior turbinate surgery: a new technique, J. Natl. Med. Assoc. **64:**476, 1972.

23. Sheen, J. H.: Achieving more nasal tip projection by the use of a small autogenous bone or cartilage graft, Plast. Reconstr. Surg. **56:**35, 1975.

24. Sheen, J. H.: Secondary rhinoplasty, Plast. Reconstr. Surg. **57:**137, 1975.

Discussion

Musgrave: The thing that bothered me most in the final pictures was the appearance of the very Negroid lower lip. You never work on the lower lip? You work on chins or noses; have you ever done this, and have you had any luck with it?

Sheen: Since I did this rhinoplasty, I've done work on her upper lip and her lower lip. And she looks quite satisfactory!

Musgrave: I was just worrying about this because I recently did this on one patient and I didn't know if any body else had. I know Dr. Aufricht has written about the cartilage in the lip and in chin contour, and sometimes even with putting in a chin, they still have too much lip tissue. I wondered if you ever combined it with your rhinoplasty.

Part III

Rhinoplasty forum
an open discussion of problem cases

Millard: I know some are going to have to leave early, so just drop off as you tire out, have to catch a plane, or whatever. First, there have been a few requests for discussion of special items that have not been included in the faculty presentations during the symposium. We will deal with these first. Then we are going to show a few cases that have had solutions, since they are different than what has been shown so far. Finally, we will turn to problem cases that have been submitted by participants and faculty. Last night, my residents and I went through all the problem cases, grouping them and picking representatives of different problems. We will take a certain problem, and since we have the experts up front, they will go first, but any of you that have an idea are invited to contribute. Let's see what we can do to solve some of the problems.

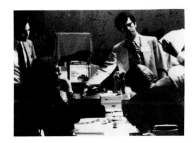

Dr. Millard and staff

I want to take this opportunity to thank the faculty for taking their valuable time to tell us their secrets. I'm sure that everybody here has gotten a lot out of it. At first I was discouraged to hear one surgeon say that when he goes back to do a nose, he is almost afraid to go into the operating room. After all this! But, on second thought, maybe that's the best thing we've done for him. Caution can lead to better work. Now, Dr. Converse has a few points he would like to make.

APPROACHES TO RHINOPLASTY

Converse: I have just a few things that I would like to speak about. Some of them have not been discussed, but I've taken a considerable interest in them. The first is the problem of teaching

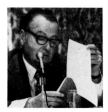

Dr. Converse

residents how to do corrective rhinoplasty. I think I mentioned yesterday this is the most difficult operation to teach. Now, as a result of that, our group is pretty much doing the same type of procedure, and what we are teaching is a system of approach—systematic approach to the problem of rhinoplasty. First is the uncovering of the framework, and one of the problems that we encountered constantly with our residents was the teaching of the modification of the profile by the saw technique, in other words, the Joseph technique. We have had to get away from the Joseph approach in order to make it easier for the residents to achieve an acceptable result. So, the first is the uncovering of the framework, and that is done by an intercartilaginous incision. Now, stage 2 is modification of the profile line of the cartilaginous portion of the nose. This involves modification of the tip, modification of the dorsal border of the septal cartilage. When this has been achieved, this being the most difficult part of the procedure, then you know how much of the bony hump to remove. Now, I'm not saying that this is something that needs to be employed by experts, but certainly for the beginner it does help him. At this point, if the septum needs modification, this can be done, and it is preferable to do the septum after you know where you stand. Next is the resection of the hump. That's done with an osteotome. After the entire profile has been made and prior to the osteotomy of the lateral walls, the septum is taken care of by excision or by conservative methods and if necessary, more radical methods prior to the osteotomy. This is done at this time because you don't want to mobilize the lateral walls by an osteotomy, and you want to know how much of the septum you have left after its removal along the dorsal border because in the case of the large hump, you remove a great deal of cartilage. Then comes the stage 4, the osteotomy of the lateral walls. We have modified the dorsal border of the septal cartilage by resection, and we have done the tip operation. Now, we are removing less and less alar cartilage than we did before. At this point, you see, the bony hump becomes evident and how much to take off. So here we remove the bony hump with the osteotome and then we do the osteotomy. You can see the progressive changes in the nose. Now, the only thing is that if you only modify the septal border up to the level of the lower nasal bone and then take your hump off, you sometimes get a little irregularity in the dorsum, so it is preferable that you make these cuts through the septum and the amount you want to remove, and then put your osteotome in and take off the hump along with the septal cartilage. Then make the necessary minor modifications. So much for this point.

EXTRAMUCOUS APPROACH

Now, the next thing I want to talk about is the extramucous approach. As you know, this was described recently by—I don't know who described it, I think an otolaryngologist, and now I've forgotten.

Millard: Anderson described this about 1958.

Converse: But the method has become quite popular in other countries and in Europe it is being extensively used. Dr. Mitz over here from France was telling me that he thinks the biggest advantage for the beginner was that it gave a very good exposure, and it made the teaching of rhinoplasty easier. Here is the approach (Fig. 1). At the septal angle, you start peeling the mucoperichondrium, and it is dissected right up to the nasal bone area. If you want, raise the

mucoperichondrium, which is dissected right up to the nasal bones, and some even raise the mucoperiosteum from under the nasal bones. I don't know if that is necessary or not. I think all this is interesting, and it is to be interpreted. Then, of course, the separation of the upper lateral cartilage from the septum is done without cutting through the mucous membrane. You can, at this point, after having modified the septal cartilage, remove the hump. Now this no. 12 osteotome is helpful, and this actually was developed by Dr. J. L. Robin. It is helpful because you avoid the possibility of an oblique resection of the hump by lining up the osteotome with the level of the eyes. Also, the cross prevents the osteotome from obliquing away. This is, I think, very helpful.

INTERNAL OSTEOTOMY

Now, the last thing I want to talk about is internal osteotomy. That has not been discussed at this meeting, and this is also an interesting approach (Fig. 2). Instead of doing the osteotomy from the outside, you do it from the inside. A small incision just at the medial edge of the pyriform aperture gives entrance for the Joseph elevator to raise the mucous membrane from the

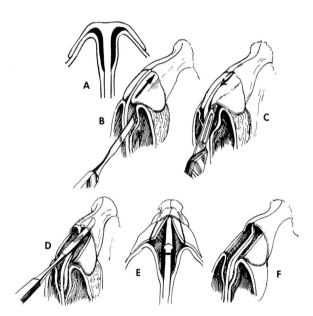

Fig. 1. Submucous approach for extramucous resection of skeletal structures to modify nasal profile. **A,** Front section through septum and lateral cartilages; black areas illustrate raising of mucoperichondrium from septum and lateral cartilages. **B,** Raising mucoperichondrium along dorsal portion of septum and at junction with lateral cartilages. **C,** Severing attachment of lateral cartilage to septum. **D,** Raising nasal lining from undersurface of nasal bones. **E,** Broken lines illustrate incisions for resection of septal and lateral cartilages. **F,** Appearance of cartilaginous dorsum after correction.

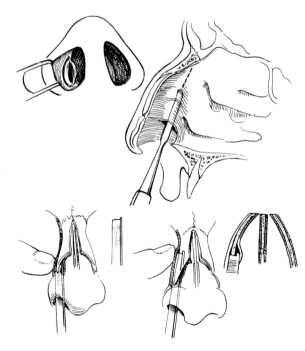

Fig. 2. (From Converse, J. M.: Deformities of the nose. In Kazanjian, V. H., and Converse, J. M.: Surgical treatment of facial injuries, ed. 3, Baltimore, 1974, The Williams & Wilkins Co.)

side of the nose. Then, you take an osteotome
with the button on the outside; you can feel the
button as you go up, and you do your osteotomy.
This technique I've been using now just to try
it out, and the remarkable thing is that there
is no ecchymosis around the eyes. Dr. Sheen
does a high osteotomy, and because of the fact
that he doesn't transgress the front tier between
eyelid skin and nose skin, he says that he doesn't
get ecchymosis either. Now, what happens here
I don't know. I can't interpret it. Maybe the
bleeding goes inside the nose; it doesn't seem
to interfer at all with nasal physiology; I haven't
used it long enough to be absolutely sure that
this is the best way to do an osteotomy.

Millard: Any questions?

Participant: Much of this comes from a fellow
named Jack Anderson, an ENT man, who mentioned the use of the osteotome to do this internal osteotomy. He used a curved one that goes
wide as it gets closer to the radix. I wonder if
you'd comment on that?

Converse: I don't know what to say. I've always
used the straight one, and I've just gone straight
up, and I've been using the button one about
3 months, so I really can't say. I'm just bringing
it up for the possible discussion. Does anyone
else have experience?

Participant: Anderson described this some time
ago; well over a year.

Converse: No, Anderson didn't describe the internal osteotomy. A man from Minnesota, an otolaryngologist did, according to my literature!

Participant: Okay, whoever. I just wanted to endorse it, that's all. We notice remarkably less ecchymosis doing it this way. We use the curved
osteotome, and it works very well. I just thought
I would endorse it.

Rogers: I wonder how many people in the audience use an antihistamine? I've been using one
since I was with Dr. Peer; 50 mg of tripelenna-
mine (Pyribenzamine), qid, for 5 to 7 days
postoperatively. Number 1, to dry out the nose
internally, but number 2, I sincerely believe that
it cuts down remarkably on ecchymosis. I have
been so satisfied with it that on several occasions
when the residents failed to order it, I've been
astounded by ecchymosis that my patients have
had. An American surgeon in the American
University of Beirut, about 8 or 9 years ago,
reported in our journal the routine use postoperatively of an antihistamine in a controlled setting and the amount of ecchymosis in the eyes,
and the swelling was remarkably reduced. I was

pleased to hear John Lewis say the other day
that he gives diphenhydramine (Benadryl) during surgery and afterward.

Millard: I'm afraid to let John Lewis get started
with his bag of patent medicines!

Lewis: This is not a rebuttal to Dr. Converse but
just to throw a curve at him to see what he has
to say about it. I have tried this internal osteotomy years past and still do it occasionally. Basically, I do a modified internal osteotomy using
a little elevated chisel and slip it in without any
undermining as I did in the operating room on
the left side the day before yesterday. Incidentally, her eye is swollen more on the right side,
which I did undermine and use a saw; I saw
her this morning. But the reason I don't use it
routinely is that I want the nasal bone to be attached to the mucosa, and I want it to be supported there so that it doesn't drop down inside
the maxillary ledge. My skin is not widely undermined, and my mucosa is not widely undermined. Therefore, I have support and when I
narrow the nasal bones, as Rogers said yesterday, I do get raising of my nasal bridge, and
I have to allow for that. It doesn't drop down.

In a wide nose with a low bridge, after the
narrowing, the bridge level will be a little higher
than in the original profile. Again, if you leave
your mucosa and skin attachment, they do help
support your nasal bones upward when you put
your splint on. The packs help to support it further by keeping the mucosa pressed against the
nasal bones.

Converse: I don't know how to respond to this.
I know that many of you may recall Dr. Aufricht
wrote a paper quite a few years ago in which
he emphasized the cutting horizontally, avoiding
any obliquity in the cut. In his article, he felt
that it was important to have bony contact con-
solidation of the lateral osteotomy.

Participant: Does anyone in the audience know
of good general literature to be sent to the patient who is a prospective rhinoplasty patient for
their general information before they are seen
in the operating room? Is there anything generally available that's good?

Millard: John says he wouldn't send it to them
before. Bob Pool, take the microphone and talk
to the participants.

CASE 1

Pool: This is a 23-year-old girl who had a submucous resection by a very competent otolaryngologist, and over a period of approximately 4

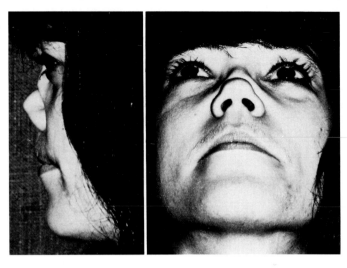

Fig. 3

months, she had gradual absorption and contraction of her entire nasal pyramid. She had a huge perforation in the septum with almost no membrane left. This is her presenting appearance. She had no other cartilaginous configuration, no evidence of any triangular cartilages left, and the alar cartilages were partially destroyed (Fig. 3). Is there a suggestion from the panel?

Millard: Would anybody raise his hand? We're going to take first offers and then we'll pick experts. Is Dick Dawson down there? Come on up front; we want you up here—there's room in the front two rows.

Participant: I would like to see the front view again. Could we see the preceding slide, which would be the front view?

Millard: What's the interval between this point and the surgery? How long did you wait?

Pool: My surgery was done approximately 3 years after she developed this full-blown collapse. I did not see her for 3 years.

Millard: Is this just before surgery?

Pool: This is just before surgery. The lining was very contracted.

Sheen: What was the interval in time when she was relatively normal till the time she developed this deformity, and what was done prior to this?

Pool: A submucous resection was the only surgery she had. According to her, she had noticed approximately 6 weeks after surgery a progressive collapse. It has been reported in the English literature that enzymatic absorption of cartilage can occur. She did not have a septic course, no drainage of a septal abscess, but by the time I

saw her 3 years later, she presented this picture of collapse.

Millard: Was there any cocaine or other drugs used by the surgeon?

Pool: She herself was not a drug user at all. The surgeon used the usual premedications. She had no evidence of chondromalasia of the trachea or bronchi, or degenerative cartilaginous disease.

Millard: I think we've dragged this out long enough.

Pool: My goodness, Ralph, isn't your panel going to make any suggestions?

Millard: At least they have asked some good questions.

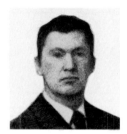

Dr. Pool

Pool: Well, this patient was treated as Dawson had suggested with a bone graft, and it was an L-shaped graft. It was put in through the mouth in the manner of Schmid, and the big problem here is the smallness of the columella. The bone graft stayed in good posture. It was viable, but the swollen columella here still gave it a peculiar look, and because of this, it was still the pig's snout nose, and she was deficient in both membrane as well as support in this area (Fig. 4). The solution that was used is not particularly new, except perhaps the slightly different variation of donor site. The inferior crus of the triangular fossa was utilized as a composite graft to augment the columella in the lower portion. It is a double-backed double cartilage composite graft that has the shape necessary to augment the columella either superiorly or inferiorly (Fig. 5). The donor site is very accessible and leaves very little problem in that you get about 8 mm by about 11 or 12 mm, and you can extend it up if you need (Fig. 6). This was reversed, and an incision was made to open the defect, and the graft was sutured into the distal substance of the bone graft and then inserted to fill out the columella-philtral angle (Fig. 7).

Millard: This is a very nice result. Thank you, Bob. Here are some cases that Dr. Aufricht has kindly offered to show us, as he said, with very minor problems with possible solutions.

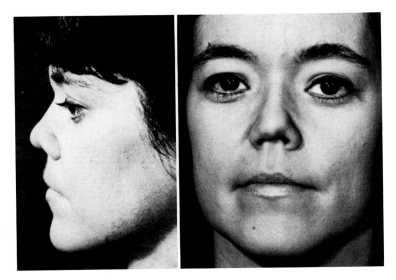

Fig. 4

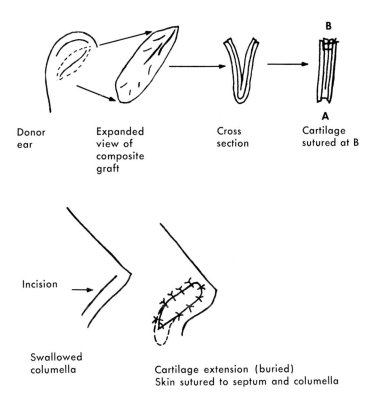

Donor ear

Expanded view of composite graft

Cross section

Cartilage sutured at B

Incision →

Swallowed columella

Cartilage extension (buried)
Skin sutured to septum and columella

Fig. 5. Cartilage sutured at *B* gives a graft that is (1) double cartilage and (2) adherent to double skin lining. Side *A* is put to distal septum. Skin is trimmed as needed. Excess cartilage may be used to bolster columellar philtral area.

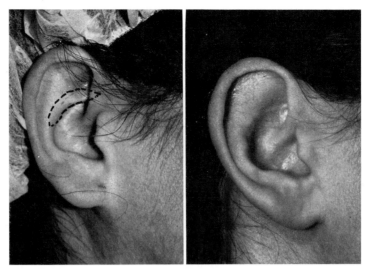

Fig. 6

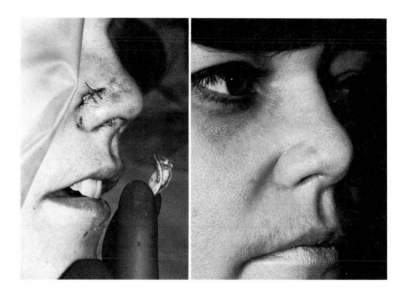

Fig. 7

CASE 2

Aufricht: This 32-year-old patient had had two accidents and three rhinoplasties revealing irregular bony dorsum with indented, firmly ad-

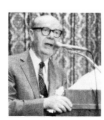

Dr. Aufricht

herent skin, high radix, pinched, abnormally pointed nasal tip, deviated septum (Fig. 8).

My secondary operation consisted of undermining of the dorsal skin from the routine intercartilaginous incision; careful sharp dissection of the adherent skin from the bony dorsum. The radix nasi was lowered by superficial application of Joseph's saw, followed up by rasp. The bony sides were refractured by lateral osteotomy and digital pressure. Minimal shaving of the cartilaginous dorsum. Through marginal incisions, the lower lateral cartilages were exposed. The cartilage was divided with transverse incision to

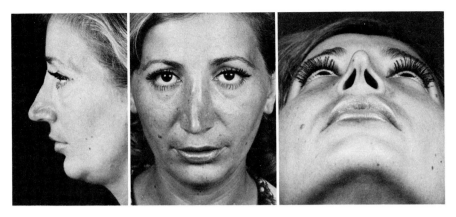

Fig. 8

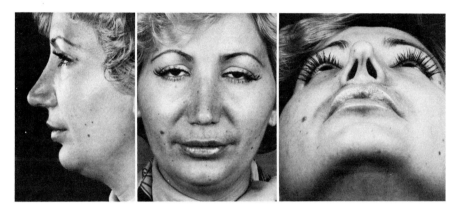

Fig. 9

upper and lower half. The upper half was removed, preserving its lining in form of a bipedicled flap. The cartilage of the lower half was cut vertically through at the dome in five places, but leaving the lining intact, one incision through the center of the dome and two incisions to each side, about 1.5 to 2 mm apart. Thus two cartilaginous blocks were created from which a broader convex dome was reconstructed. The convex shape was maintained by light mold of Vaseline gauze in the vestibulum and gentle adhesive strapping externally. The dressing was left in place for 1 week. The surgery included a submucous septal resection (Fig. 9).

Millard: We're going on now to problem cases that you have brought along with a request for solutions. Whoever sees a quick solution and can explain it without a total history, let's get with it. Otherwise, we'll be here until the day after tomorrow. I will give you an idea of what we have, and you can raise your hands if you want to attack the general problem. We have a few

long, thick noses, one bifid tip, short noses with pig's snouts, short and artificial looking. I suppose you'll want to see somebody attack those subjects. The retracted columella we've dealt with pretty well. Hanging columella, retracted alae, we've discussed that enough. The black nose? A lot of hands up. All right. Wide bridge with the nasal bones splayed quite widely? Supratips, do you want to deal with that some more? Yes, okay. Secondary, deviated septums? Are you fairly happy with septums now? Good. How about the pinched nostril? Yes? Okay. Put on a long nose and let's start. Let's see that profile.

THE LONG NOSE

Now, this is a nose with moderate length (Fig. 10). Most long noses that are thick are difficult to reduce gracefully. Here is one that is relatively wider than it is long (Fig. 11). Now, here's another one that is deviated but is reasonably long in the bridge. It is slightly thick, but the deviation makes the problem a little more

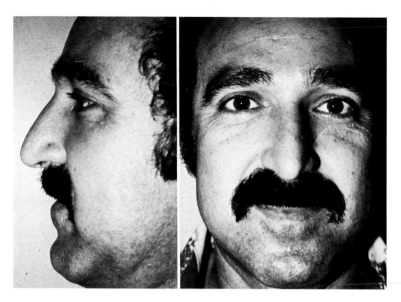

Fig. 10

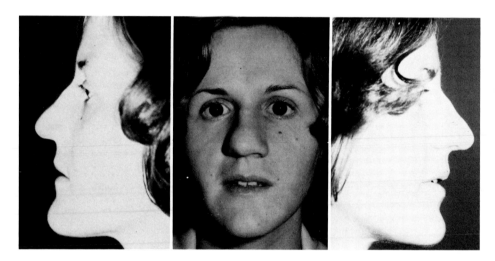

Fig. 11

difficult (Fig. 12). I think this is more of a problem of deviation than length. There is one classic long nose that looks like the face backed off and left the nose out in front alone. Here she is, but not actually a great problem to correct (Fig. 13).

Sheen: I think I have the nose that the face dropped away from (Fig. 14). The point I thought I'd make with long noses is not to try to reduce it too much; in other words, a large nose that is anatomically correct. Now, this is what I call a projecting nose (Fig. 15). The front view is broad, the tip is very sharp, the alar cartilages are projecting and very, very sharp. I took just a little bit of the hump down, trimmed the caudal septum, delivered the cartilages, and they were very thin, transected the bony part leaving about a 5 mm ridge, took out about 5 to 6 mm at the dome to allow the tissues to accommodate down and to shrink down as much as I judged, or that it was possible for them to shrink, and removed the dome of the lower cartilages.

Millard: With or without lining?

Sheen: I leave the lining intact; I always do. I shortened more of the caudal septum because I want this thing to be shortened a little bit—not a chunk of caudal septum. Through the open route, 2 or 3 mm of dorsum was removed. I did my osteotomies and took off more of the inferior caudal septum. Then I adjusted it. Here is the reduction in the projection (Fig. 16).

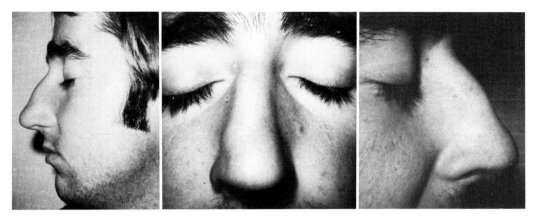

Fig. 12

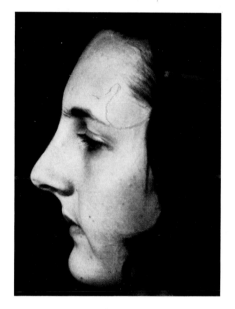

Fig. 13

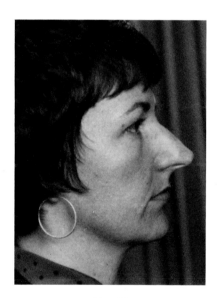

Fig. 14

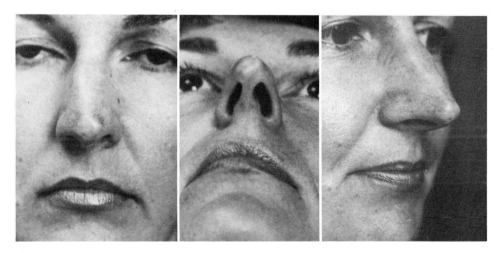

Fig. 15

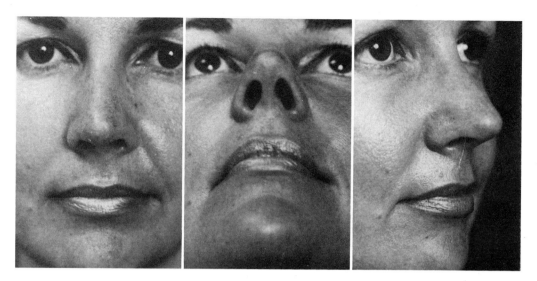

Fig. 16

She has the normal anatomic nose. I haven't really given her anything great. This is only about 2 weeks postoperatively. She has exactly the same nasal configuration with the reduction of the projection of the tip, so the most objectionable part of this nose has been reduced by resecting about 5 mm of the dome and doing a very conservative nasal reduction.

Millard: Thank you, Jack. Let's have the lights up. Blair?

Rogers: I'd like to warn the audience to start with the tip in a nose like this. A great mistake can be made assuming that the dorsum can be reduced, and you proceed under this assumption first. When you reduce the tip, you find that you have corrected some of the protrusion of the tip, but the nose will look extra long because you've taken too much dorsum away, producing actually a worse deformity than when you started.

Millard: How about the really long nose with strong medial crura and strong feet splayed a bit and not a lot of alar cartilage? Does anyone want to discuss the way they handle this?

Converse: There is a technique for what I call the plunging tip, that is, a long nose with the tip going down almost to the upper lip. Although it sounds antiphysiologic, I suggest you shorten the septum, the central portion, and the lateral walls also. A technique that has given me very good results in these cases, which tend to reoccur, is to overlap the lower lateral cartilage, denuded of its mucosa, on top of the lateral cartilage, and in this way, you get a firm fixation of the shortening of the lateral walls.

Peck: You all have probably read the article of the Pinocchio nose that was in the journal (*Plastic and Reconstructive Surgery*), and I wrote a rebuttal on that and said I have a technique, a lateral rotation of the alars, and this is going to be a paper this coming summer at the international meeting. I'd just like a few minutes to describe this. I like to do the technique as I described, but in the high projecting tip, after I'm sure that I'm down 2 or 3 mm of alar cartilage and I still feel that my tip is too projecting, more action is necessary. I dissect the alar cartilage out of its bed and crosscut it at the medial crura. Now you're creating a new dome. As you do that, the lateral crus will now bend down and of course become longer because you've now made what was originally dome to become lateral crus. You have to excise a little segment of the lateralmost part of the lateral crus. Then you put this back in its bed and tape it in position. I'm going to give this summary in Paris and show two cases with a mother and daughter with real high projecting tips. The reason I've done this again is because it might preserve continuity. Now, it might very well be, Ralph, that the rimming incision and deliverance of the alar cartilage in a high projecting tip where we can see it and do this type of procedure under direct exposure might be a better approach.

Participant: How do you do it without blood supply?

Peck: Well, you don't have to have blood supply to the alar cartilages. That's for sure.

Millard: Oh!?

Gorney: I'd like to endorse the idea of conservative resection of the long nose, which is also the answer to the overall too-large nose. Now, in addition, I'd like to stress the medical/legal importance of warning your patient ahead of time that you're going to do a conservative reduction. I always say to the patient, and this is a metaphor they can understand and what I can impress them with is, doing this nose is like walking through a tent and reducing the framework and expecting the tent to shrink around it. If you have a thin nylon tent, it will shrink around it nicely, but if you have a boggy old canvas tent, it's not going to shrink around it very well. So I warn them ahead of time, their nose is not going to be as small as they'd like it to be.

Lewis: Well, first I'd like to agree with what's been said, but I would also like to add that I prefer that the nose has been reduced a little more and looks a little prettier as long as it's been done safely. I think that the tip could be reduced in the method that George has described and which I have used. I think that if you reduced the nose in other ways, you can have better success. When you've got the very prominent medial crura in the tip, you can even go in and chop it off. Oh, I don't do this routinely, but I have done it in unusual instances. Usually, I thin the top of the medial crura laterally and then do a lateral alar base resection.

Millard: I agree with the principle of going for the best you can get.

Musgrave: I hesitate to get up and talk in front of all these experts. Part of our problem I think always is in what I talked about, perhaps ad nauseam, the other day: communication with the patient. It is very difficult for them to understand the anatomy of the nose no matter how much you talk about the septal cartilages. But they all know McDonald's golden arches (Fig. 17). So I explain it like that. You have different kinds of

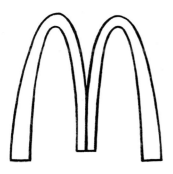

Fig. 17

skin draped over your McDonald's arches. Some people have them sticking out more and some people have them sticking out less. John, just what you've said. We've all seen columella extension of the alars that are very unattractive sticking out. Quite frequently, I go in and not only dissect them out, but I very carefully measure and take off 3 or 4 mm. There is too much of an arch. Robin Beare made the point many years ago when he visited us. You can drop your whole arch back as George does or very many people do. I think we're all taking it off in the same general way, trying to keep it even. You cannot correct by stitching or doing anything if you leave the middle tent vault too high. The only way I know is to either take out a wedge, or, if you have a bad angle, make a pocket and like Gustie showed years ago, you put cartilage in there. Otherwise, you're ignoring the principle of building bridges. Architects know all about arches. So if you do this, you must come out to the side here and detach this little overlap where your alar goes up over the top of your upper laterals. You let it float free and then get all the sesamoid and all this junk out of here, and you've lowered the whole McDonald's golden arch.

Millard: I think when you're lowering a high tip, there are several actions. There are the alar wedges, there is amputation of the feet of the medial crus, sliding the columella and medial crus down, and transfixing to the septum with a suture. Then if you want to take medial wedges out of the crural angles, this will also help to lower an excessively projecting nasal tip.

Musgrave: I must say that almost always you will have to do a complete Weir wedge with this.

CASE 3

Aufricht: I don't know what is the problem. Here you have a lower lateral cartilage that is too prominent. You resect as much as you want from the lower lateral cartilage and the skin will follow it. After reduction, you crosshatch the lateral part, reconstructing the dome of the lower lateral. You can reduce a tip any amount; just resect a sufficient amount of dome.

This patient suffered injury to the nose and two rhinoplasties, resulting in a columella somewhat hidden by the alae. In front view, the bony sides were wide. The lower dorsum and upper tip were extremely narrow, pinched. The tip was irregular, asymmetric. There was an angular prominence on the left side due to a defective,

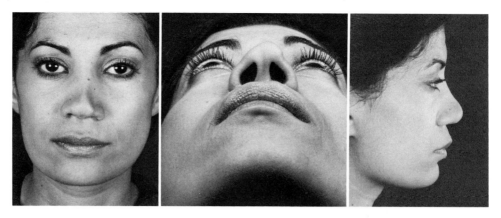

Fig. 18

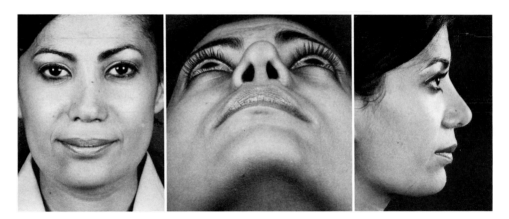

Fig. 19

hooklike lower alar cartilage. Same irregularity was noticeable in the nostril view (Fig. 18).

The operation consisted of narrowing the bony nose. The adherent skin was carefully undermined through the routine intercartilaginous incision. The back-to-back adhesion of the pinched skin was separated with special care. The right half of the tip of the nose was narrowed by cutting through the lower lateral cartilage and its lining at the highest point of the dome. Besides the narrowing effect, the separated crura straightened up, adding to the prominence of the tip.

The left half of the tip was a different problem. The upper half of the cartilage was missing and so was the distal third of the crus laterale. This gave a short, narrow hook effect to the remaining cartilage that manifested itself in an angular prominence of the tip.

Through marginal incision, the cartilaginous dome was exposed and divided at the center of the dome with a vertical incision, whereupon the hooklike distal end of the cartilage bent down, and the angular prominence of the tip subsided.

Secondary septum resection was performed. The septal cartilage so gained was placed in a retrolabial pocket in front of the maxilla to correct the acute nasolabial angle. This process at the same time forced the columella into a downward convex position by shortening the distance between the upper lip and the tip. The perforation in the septum was closed by refreshing its edges and carefully suturing the mucuous membrane flaps on both sides.

Finally, the nostrils were narrowed by excisions from the inside of the alar base. The nose was packed lightly with Vaseline gauze. Adhesive strapping of the tip followed. Special attention was paid to the loose undermined skin over the lower dorsum and upper part of the tip in order to prevent pinched healing. (It had a tendency to do so.) The loose skin was flattened under mild pressure with several transverse adhesive tapes. The central part of the tape was lined with reversed adhesive tape to prevent it from sticking to the skin and to allow even distribution of the undermined skin (Fig. 19).

I really don't know what the problem with the prominent alar cartilages is; but just like your McDonald's—I don't go there; I like other hamburgers better!

Musgrave: Dr. Aufricht, as you know, I learned most of my rhinoplasties from Milton Dupertius, who learned most of it from you. But I found that I was doing more secondaries when I had those cartilages either overriding or where I had broken the continuity of the arch. I've had many, many fewer secondaries to do to the tip when I leave that arch, no matter how big the nostrils, intact.

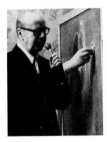

Dr. Aufricht

Aufricht: Thank you. Dr. Sheen makes mention that he never removes the lining. Well, I think during radical reduction, the lining should be reduced too.

Hook: I am filled with admiration for the techniques shown by Dr. Sheen and Dr. Peck. One of the things that worries me, and I am sure my colleagues agree, that when you delivered the alar cartilages away from the lining to mold them and to model them, and also when you make them very thin after you've returned them, there's a danger of disintegration. Also, if you take out some of the dome, the great danger or great fear we all ought to have is the asymmetry and the twisting of the tip that follows. Of course, this is the reason why most of us have been afraid to do it. Can somebody give us some ideas on how to avoid that twisting and asymmetry?

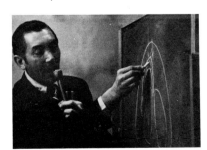

Dr. Peck

Peck: I have tried not to remove any wedges from the dome, and that is the point of my lateral rotation. After we have made our intracartilaginous incision in the high projecting tip, and we now have in essence an inverted view of approximately 2 or 3 mm of cartilage, when you dissect that from its bed and put it back in its bed a little shorter by excising a piece most laterally from the lateral crus, in many instances it will accommodate without even any crosscutting in the dome. Now, the point that I am trying to make is that after we have made our intracartilaginous incision and we have now converted the cartilage rim to 2 to 3 mm, I then deliver this cartilage in a high-projecting tip from its bed. If we leave it thick in the bed and crosscut, we still have the full length of cartilage, so it is difficult then to lower the projection. But if we deliver it from its bed and excise a segment of cartilage from its lateral end, we are now shortening the cartilage and when we put it back, this cartilage can now move down in the bed in this position and effectively lower the projection of the height of the tip. Now, in the bulbous tip, almost the same thing is true except that instead of dissecting out to the medial crura part of the dome, you only dissect to the dome, to where your broadness is, excise a piece laterally, and then as this is put back into the bed, it is shorter and will accommodate to the bed so that we will get rid of the bulbousness. If you've got a thick, rigid cartilage that when it's put back in its bed, it wants to maintain that curvature, then you would have to crosscut. In the real high projecting tip, where the lobule hangs down below the level of the columella and there's nothing you can do with the skeleton and the septum, even though you shorten the septum, I've found that an external excision, a little ellipse of skin in this area, will bring it up.

Millard: Bill, what are you burning about over there?

CASE 4

Conroy: I would like to show a picture while we're not doing anything. Would you put on the slides of mine (Fig. 20)? I just want to make the point that I published an article about 10 years ago, and the name of the article was "Simple Nasal Tip Set-Back." I disagree with George as he works on the premise that you have to leave the rim of the alar cartilage in continuity. I think he boxes himself in. I like what Jack Sheen does because I think this means keeping all your

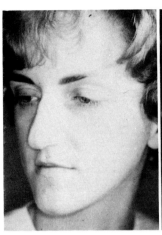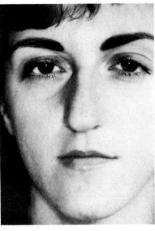

Fig. 20

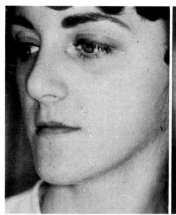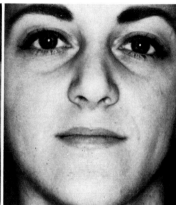

Fig. 21

options open. This is simply excising across the dome and shortening the nose. Let me see the next picture, please. This little lady is very happy, and she's been happy for 10 years. And she's always going to be happy (Fig. 21). But that is what I call a long nose.

Ungaro: The first three photographs that were shown to us at the beginning of today's symposium at the angle I was sitting at, did not really look long to me. They looked like the columellar/lip angle was too acute, almost a retracted columella base. Therefore, I could create the illusion of normal length by merely lowering the base of the columella with a strut in there. I was wondering what the panel felt on that? I think it was a relatively normal-length nose that looks long and you shorten it, you tend to get the effect we don't like: the pig's snout.

TIP REDUCTION

Lewis: About reduction of the tip, since I can't show you on my own, I shall demonstrate on Dr. Aufricht's nose (Fig. 22, *A*). If you look from the front, the rim of the alar is quite a bit lower than the dome of the alar. So often you don't have to go through the very rim of the alar cartilage to lower it. You see, if you come across this way with your lower lateral cartilage resection, you can lower the tip that much and still have a rim. You can see from the side we still can keep a rim of alar cartilage even in Dr. Aufricht (Fig. 22, *B*). He's already made an appointment, by the way.

Aufricht: I'm planning already to sue you!

Participant: Does anybody ever trim the caudal edge?

A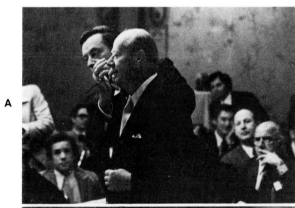

B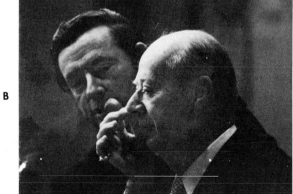

Fig. 22

Millard: As for trimming the caudal edge, you do it when you need it. There are certain cases in which you need this reduction and certainly should do it.

Peck: It is irregularities of the caudal end of the alar cartilage that must be avoided.

Millard: It already has been said a few times: you want to keep the alar arch intact. It's only when you've got unusual problems that I'm willing to interrupt it. You can have a safer chance of breaking it if it's a secondary case where the scar sticks things into position and you don't take quite as much chance of notching or pinching; in the original reduction rhinoplasty, I think it is important not to break the integrity of the midlateral arch. You get a midalar collapse with pinching. Other deformities appear if you also shorten the lining too much.

Kaye: As a teaching symposium, we've had excellent treatment of four or five standard ways of treating the projecting nose. I think just for the sake of completion perhaps two other techniques can be mentioned. One is a method that Dr. Safian has advocated all these years. It is a type of chondrocutaneous flap procedure in which he amputates the medial portion of that flap to lower the tip of the nose. Lipsett later adapted this and put his name to it, but I'm sure Dr. Safian is the originator of it. The second method is to make the Brown-McDowell's so-called double break where the inferior line of the nose is changed so that you have a slight angle upwards and a slight angulation posteriorly that takes away from the appearance of projection. Otherwise, I think today we covered the projecting nose quite well.

THE BIFID NOSE

Millard: Shall we go on to the bifid nose now? Here is one slide with a bifid tip (Fig. 23). This is a reasonably simple problem, but let's have the lights and someone describe how he deals with it.

Sheen: I think maybe you have too much arch in your lower lateral alar cartilages. I personally would just deliver these through a rim incision, take out the dome, and let them collapse together.

Millard: And if it didn't, you'd be willing to suture them?

Sheen: I personally feel suturing the lower cartilages is bad because you never are sure of how they're going to reset. I'd rather just put them back in and model them.

Millard: And if you have soft tissue between them and a groove down the columella?

Sheen: I slide cartilage in there.

Millard: Yes, of course that's an important part of the correction. Reduce the cartilages to smooth the contour as much as possible, take out the subcutaneous tissue between the two cartilages, and then you can either suture them together, if you have faith in your stitching, or insert little slips of cartilage in to build out whatever grooving remains as a deformity.

Sheen: We're talking about reducing the nasal framework all the time. Have you ever had any problem with the skin accommodating to that framework?

Millard: Does anybody have any trouble with the skin accommodating to the framework?

Sheen: Rex Peterson talked about that yesterday.

Millard: Well, that's one way. But wide enough undermining in these noses will let the skin slide into the cheeks. Any other suggestions? Some excise it one way or another. Vertical or lateral,

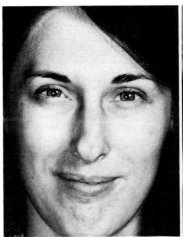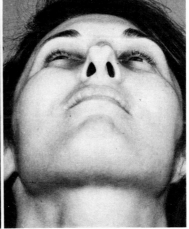

Fig. 23

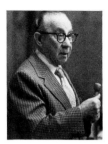

Dr. Safian

alar base excisions, and Weir wedges take up some from the sides. Any other suggestions? Abrasion from on top? Hardly!

Safian: The long nose is never a problem at all. I have three ladies who really had long noses that came right over the lip. You can shorten that type nose, but you must keep every structure, all the eight structures, in proportion. The important thing is never to touch the lower lat-

eral cartilages before you shorten the nose. The lower lateral cartilage becomes an entirely different problem than you faced when it was pendulous. This is a family, quite personable, the mother and two daughters. The important thing is to concentrate on the shape of the tip. Making the tip smaller in an adult is not sufficient. Each tip has to be reshaped to keep its own character, some individuality, and it must correspond properly with the newly corrected nose as well as the shape of the face. Each face is different and has a different shaped tip, and it is important to keep each feature in proportion to all the other features. One daughter had a prominent nose with a definite convexity (Fig. 24, *A*). You could shorten it and straighten it. It was a long nose but not the longest I've had. I've had them all. This one has irregularities, and one side of the tip is entirely different from the

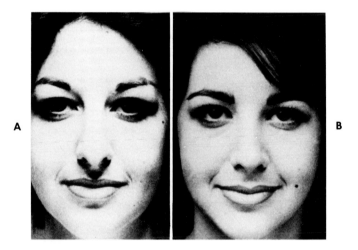

Fig. 24

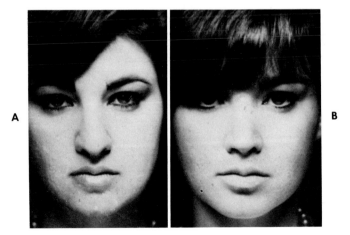

Fig. 25

other. Therefore each alar cartilage had to be treated separately and match the two of them up when they were finished. She also had a hanging columella, which was corrected (Fig. 24, *B*). Now, this is a long nose (Fig. 25, *A*). You can see it reaches almost down to the upper lip, and it's been shortened and the tip has been corrected, reduced in size, and reshaped completely. It is in proportion to that girl's face, and it does not look like an operated nose (Fig. 25, *B*). The mother had a long nose (Fig. 26, *A*). There is no difficulty in shortening the nose, but the important thing is that when you turn the tip up, it no longer is a long nose but it is a prominent tip that sticks up like a sore finger. I may tell you that I have transsected every alar cartilage I ever operated on, and I have had no trouble whatsoever (Fig. 26, *B*).

I once had a male patient who asked for his nose to be a little shorter than I usually make them, but he distinctly asked for it. He was a comedian, and he wanted to change his entire routine. He wanted to change the shape of his face and the expression, and everything else, so we made him a Swede! Now, there are noses in good proportion with a tiny bridge elevation, and to remove that small cartilage, it is only a convexity, it can be done with a saw just as easy. I never use anything else but a saw to take off a hump or a lateral osteotomy. It is not difficult to take off a small elevation on the bridge of the nose with a saw if you know how to use it!

THE SHORT NOSE

Millard: Let's go to the pig's snout—the overly short postoperative nose. They all have the same

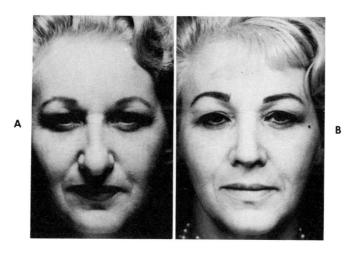

Fig. 26

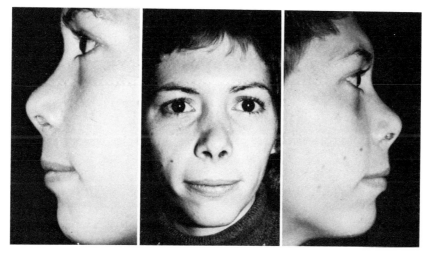

Fig. 27

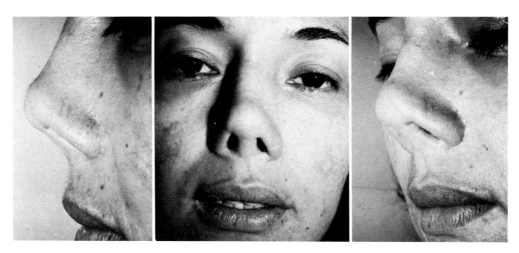

Fig. 28

sort of artificial look (Fig. 27). Weir wedges have put those alars straight down into the cheeks. That's going to be tricky to correct. But it has to be done. We have another snubbed nose that was shortened too much and the lining reduced severely (Fig. 28). Dr. Dingman has a solution to this that works beautifully. I've used it in one case, and it went well.

Dingman: There are cases in which too much lining has been removed and there is little probability that you're going to find anything intranasally to lengthen the lining with. So we have to bring in tissue from outside. The operation that I have used two times, which Ralph facetiously terms as the "banana split" operation, consists of removal of a full-thickness section of skin from just anterior to the rim of the ear, incorporating cartilage and the skin on both sides. Then, by selective splitting, you take half of the cartilage on each side and actually get a lot of tissue that will augment the length of the septum and also the lateral sides of the nose. You can get wide amounts of cartilage and skin with a very minimal deformity to the ear. When you need a composite graft to replace the missing tissue that is cartilage and lining, this is a very excellent method.

Millard: It fits in just perfectly where you divide your membranous septum and then do anterior vestibular releasing incisions, free up the skin, the nose comes out, making an anterior septal hole, and into that hole fits the "banana split" graft.

Dingman: I wasn't going to say anything more about this, but Rex Peterson came up and drew two sketches, so I think I may take advantage

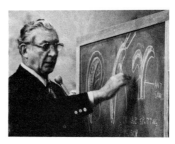

Dr. Dingman

of them. The full-thickness graft is taken from the ear. Take skin, cartilage, and skin on the back. That gives us a banana-type piece of tissue with skin on both sides and cartilage in the middle. The skin on each side is peeled halfway down, taking half of the split cartilage with it. So we end up with a half of the graft as a composite skin, cartilage, and skin, which fits into the septal defect. The two peeled skin and split cartilage fit into the lateral releasing incisions in the lining of the lateral walls.

Participant: Which journal was that in?

Dingman: *Plastic and Reconstructive Surgery,* 1969.

Participant: I'd like to reinforce that we use Dr. Dingman's operation for this snub nose both in bilateral cleft lip and palate cases. You combine it with a little cartilage graft like Dr. Sheen, but more in the Minerva Helmut design described by John Pauley in the May, 1972 *Plastic and Reconstructive Surgery* journal.

Millard: There are several variations of what can be done with this banana split graft. You can take the cartilage on one side and not on the other for a unilateral cleft lip, which I have used, or you can split it as a pure banana split.

Dingman: Ralph, can you show that next case? I

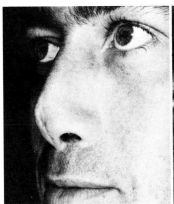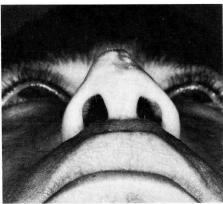

Fig. 29

need a little help (Fig. 29) because this man came to me 3 months ago and he's a hairdresser. He's had four operations, the first of which was a Silastic implant, which was positioned badly, and he lost the skin of the tip of the nose. It is obvious that he started out with one of those short columella–flat tip noses. Now, in addition to that, he has lost the skin of the tip of the lobule, and he also has a bone graft in the dorsum of the nose, which is moving around from one side to the other. It is obvious that he needs additional skin at the tip of the nose, and he needs some lengthening of the columella. How are we going to get tissue there? We're trying to work out a plan that will give us some possibility of success. Would you go back on the front view again? I wonder if we can move in flaps from the nasolabial area to augment the dorsum?

Millard: Go back to the first one of that series.

Is Dr. Berkeley up close? Oh, good. Bill, have you seen this tip? This is an external scar that isn't working out too well, and as you like external scars, I just wondered if you wanted to say anything about it?

Berkeley: No, I don't want to say anything about *that* scar because it is a different problem, and of course this does not occur in the average cleft lip nose. Here you're dealing with a Silastic graft,

and I think Silastic grafts are dangerous things to use.

Millard: But now that we're here, what would you suggest?

Berkeley: I think you're going to have to get some good tissue here, and I would be inclined to use a composite graft. I have used a full-thickness graft in this area. Later, you can free it up sufficiently to lengthen the nose.

Aufricht: Could I see the profile again? Well, all right. Reduce the bridge and then take a flap from the nose itself and turn it down as nasal skin. I think there is enough profile there to reduce it and take a flap and add it to the tip. I think you'll have a little bit smaller nose, but a good-shaped nose could be made out of it.

Millard: Gillies' leather cutter flap, too.

Sheen: I agree with Dr. Aufricht because I think that before you do anything, try to get the nasal parts to better relate to each other. First of all, take out whatever it is that is moving around; I don't know what it is, silicone possibly. Remove that. I would also pull the columella up a little bit to give a better relationship to the alar rim. So, as Dr. Aufricht said, we can have a smaller nose but one that would be in better relationship to its partner. However, eventually, after you're sure what you have in the tip, you can make

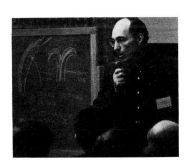

Dr. Berkeley

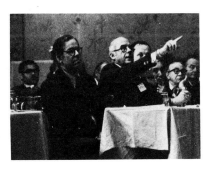

Dr. Rogers and Dr. Musgrave

a judgment as to what you can do to fill out that tip and perhaps ultimately augment it with a septal cartilage graft to give it projection.

Musgrave: This looks, if you were to see it from no history at all, very much like it might even be a basal cell, and in this area, we use a very lovely composite graft with a fairly high percentage of take. Just excising this and moving tissue forward, you're adding more scars; you're limiting the total contour, and I would use a composite graft very carefully even if it meant throwing away a smidgen of good tissue. I would make this composite graft either a hexagon or maybe even a pentagon with the points aimed down into the columella. If you put in a circular or oval composite graft, contracture of the periphery is going to give you a biscuit. This is suggested in all composite grafts. This is something no one ever wrote about, but we make them all with the hexagon or pentagon shape. I think you can get a symmetric composite graft with a good take, sandpaper the edges, and wait. Later you can reduce the framework. Then too, instead of using a single composite graft, it is possible in a male patient where you don't mind getting a little chiseled tip contour, to put two composite grafts in, one at a time: one on the right side, let that take with a little bit of angularity, and then close to it on the other side, another composite graft. We've done that in several cases at our clinic and have been satisfied with it.

Lewis: Well, this is what I was going to say, just pretty much what Ross has said. There is another possibility: a graft and then overgraft it as a second procedure if you can't get a composite take, but I prefer the composite graft when possible.

Musgrave: I don't think that gives us a good

enough blood supply for subsequent undermining.

THE BLACK NOSE

Millard: Now you have a choice between the black nose and the wide bridge. Black nose? Okay, here is one (Fig. 30).

Rogers: I'd like to ask a question. In New York, we have a large black population that comes to our clinic. Many blacks who have wide, oily noses seem to have a very bad sebaceous condition of their skin which looks like an early rhinophyma. Have any members of the audience treated the black nose the way we treat a white nose with rhinophyma? Have you deeply abraded it or shaved it?

[Boos]

Rogers: I know, I know. The reason I ask that question is that many of the black patients coming now will go to the Academy of Medicine, read the white literature, and say, "If you do this in a white nose, why can't you do it to me?" I've not had the experience. Has anyone else had it? Can you dermabrade the black nose?

Millard: One thing you can do, and that is give them a white nose!

[Much laughter]

Lewis: I would not abrade the black nose for the thick oily skin, but when you've got multiple scarring of the nose with a lot of depigmentation already, you talk it over frankly, get good pictures, and lightly abrade the area and then go back later and lightly abrade again. You can get them to blend and eventually the pigment returns. But a deep abrasion—well, you get depigmentation.

Conroy: It takes you about 2 years to get the color

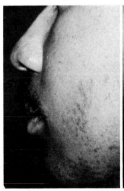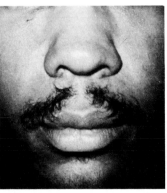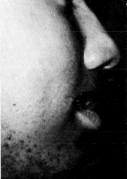

Fig. 30

to come back. The color first of all, after you abrade it, looks red just like in a white person. Then, it gets that dark color to it—hyperpigmentation—and it takes 2 years till that blends back in. You're not worrying about keloids here. This is going to heal poorly, a dark color, and don't believe that the black person doesn't object to hyperpigmentation strenuously. They don't love this one bit!

Millard: That's the problem. Now, we know pretty well that marginal and certainly alar base excisions don't give a lot of trouble. At least they haven't keloided so far, and there has been literature from predominantly black population areas where the surgery has been carried out in all parts of the body and the scars noted. The nose has been free of keloid. So I think from that point of view, we're not greatly concerned. In the black nose, the osteotomy of course is important, and the reduction of the rather diminuitive alar cartilages is helpful. Remember that the septum in a flat nose is smaller and offers less tissue, but there is some there, which you can use as supporting structure. In general, I think the literature has covered this subject to some degree, but if anyone has anything else to offer that hasn't been mentioned, please feel free. This is a problem we may see more and more. All right, a question?

Block: This is my case. I'm asking a question because I'd like to know what you say to these people. How much do you offer; how much do you promise? What is your approach? You said that you use the same approach surgically, yet you're not supposed to accomplish the same thing surgically. Do you just turn them down?

Millard: Who wants to answer that?

Berkeley: I have treated these noses with scar tissue excision. I've also treated a case with a nevus of the nose that involved the entire face of a boy. You must be honest and fair with them. Tell them the difficulty of the problem; you're going to get some degree of smoothness by shaving abrasion, but you're going to get some hyperpigmentation. They must know it and if they don't want this, they can refuse. Explain carefully that it is going to take them 2 years for this to settle down. If you're honest and fair with them, I think they may make up their minds, and in many cases, they will go ahead.

Millard: Thank you. That was a good point!

Participant: I want to make a point here that I feel it is easier to handle the black nose than it is to handle the Asiatic nose.

In regard to the black nose, as Dr. Block said, there are many respects in which it is quite similar to the Central European Slavic nose, which we see quite often. You have to talk to the patients about their aims. The patient with a heavy, thick-skinned, Slavic nose is no different from the black who comes to you for a rhinoplasty. Explain to them that they will never have the slender, aquiline, thin-skinned English or Scottish-type nose. In the blacks, there is a special problem and I think you have to speak very squarely to them. Find out if they are attempting to change their nose into a whitelike nose, or will they be satisfied to maintain the characteristics associated with their race. I think if you can determine this, then you can safely operate on them.

Participant: I'd like to hear who has essentially gotten more tip projection and how they did it for the black nose.

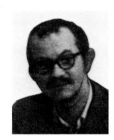

Dr. Gorney

Gorney: I think you recall a short time ago we published an article on taking the concha out in the form of a jai alai basket, split the top part of it as a gull wing to produce the exact anatomic reproduction of the alar cartilages. If you put this in subcutaneously, you will get good tip projection.

Millard: Also, with the septal cartilage, we can get good tip projection. Tessier splits the end of the septal strut to soften the tip projection.

Let's turn to the flat, thick nose which has lost its septal support (Fig. 31). There is usually enough lining and cover, but thin septal struts will not be sufficient. In this type, I turn to a modified Gillies autogenous costal osteochondral hinge graft inserted through a vertical columella splitting incision. Then there is the depressed bridge that requires a costal strut but does not need columella support (Fig. 32). Tip reduction and a bilateral osteotomy will be of benefit here.

Let's turn to the pinched nose and dimpled scarring (Fig. 33).

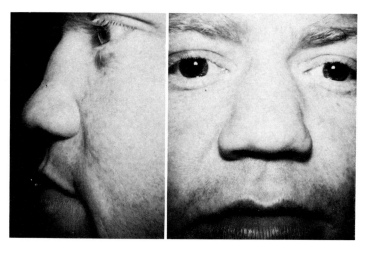

Fig. 31

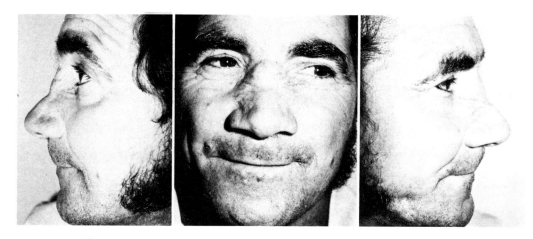

Fig. 32

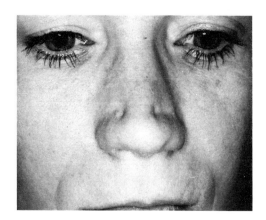

Fig. 33

PINCHED NOSE AND DIMPLED SCARRING

Sheen: On these, I have had a fair amount of success by very carefully pulling up the dimple and then getting a piece of perpendicular plate, which is the most fantastic reconstructive material I can imagine. I've used this in a rim, and if you place the perpendicular plate just above the mucosal/vestibular side, then sandwich on top of that or augment on top of this platform of perpendicular plate little progressive layers of cartilage, you can elevate that dimple enough to be quite acceptable. I have had several successes with it.

Millard: Thank you, Jack. Dick Dawson, what do you feel about bone, ethmoid plate bone from the nose, floating in a free pocket in the soft tissue of the tip or under a scarred dimple? You've said that bone on bone is okay, but how about bone floating is soft tissue with a good blood supply or not any at all like in this scarred dimple here?

Dawson: I said yesterday that bone in soft tissues survives as long as it is performing a function. Now this bone would be performing a function; therefore, it would survive.

Millard: I'm not so sure that bone here is performing a bony function!

Dawson: I just wonder if you tried the cartilage split very finely put in here, instead?

Sheen: I haven't tried it only because the cartilage is so curled and the perpendicular is so firm and so flat, and so beautiful for this purpose. And Peer has proved, I think, that this material does survive without contact with bone.

Millard: I think the principle of replacing what is lost is important. Bone is so flat. If you took a little piece of postauricular cartilage with soft tissue on the posterior side, it seems to me that would fill under the dimple and then the cartilage would hold it up. So I would go for something like that rather than tiered layers of bone and cartilage. But as you know, one man's meat is another man's poison. Oh, there is another point. If you elevate that scar deep so that you've got backing under it to start something with rather than just thin, scarred skin, you are on the right track. Then what you put under it isn't that important, really.

Someone asked about the medial crura feet, narrow airway, and what's done for this. I think Welsh was interested in this. All right, that starts

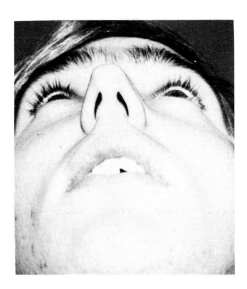

Fig. 34

the subject, and let's get on to it a bit. Airways are almost closed as seen in this case (Fig. 34).

Aufricht: I do these corrections routinely. The base of the columella is thick. I just invert it and remove the soft tissue, some septum, and if it is necessary, even the tip of the lower crus medial of the lower lateral cartilage. And then they're put together with a master suture.

Millard: With a master suture—right! All right, John.

Lewis: Plus the lowering of the tip is going to help the airway.

Millard: Right! Lowering the tip will flare the airway!

Peck: I think just one word of caution with that: the foot of the medial crus is adherent to the skin in that area. As you dissect the skin from the cartilage foot, you've got to be very careful or it will buttonhole.

Millard: And if you do, you stitch it.

Peck: You always have to be careful.

Millard: Did you hear that, Dr. Aufricht? You alway have to be careful as the thin skin is tightly attached and very difficult to dissect. You're looking right on it, so you do have a chance to do it without buttonholing. Blair?

Rogers: John Conley, our good friend in the otolaryngology field, has a very nice operation for this. Unfortunately, he hasn't reported too many cases after describing it in the *Archives of Otolaryngology*. But what he does is to take the septal cartilage as grafts, and he carves two new alar margins, lower lateral cartilage margins, that fill out this depressed area. I've tried it once in a clinic case and once privately, and I haven't had very good results. I know it is described in the literature, and I wonder if anyone else has tried the Conley maneuver?

Participant: What's the cause of this problem? Can we see the pinched tip again (Fig. 35)?

Millard: As Gillies once said, find out the cause, and the solution should follow very easily. Anybody want to say right off what the main causes of collapsed alae and airway obstruction are? Removal of lateral crus? Transsecting it? Removal of inferior portion of the upper lateal cartilage?

Conroy: My experience is that these are all wrong. I save the rim in most of the noses I do. I don't have any compunction when I see it's indicated, of removing the entire lateral crus.

Sheen: I would just like to say that we had a fellow in California, name of Holden, who in every single nose he did, transected about the midportion of the lateral crus. I think you can recognize

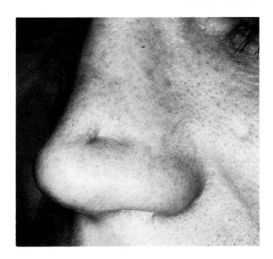

Fig. 35

a Holden nose across the street, and it has the collapsed alae.

Rogers: One other cause is that in the routine rhinoplasty, a lot of men do not reapply the bipedicled mucosa in the alar cartilage region after they've removed a great deal of cartilage. As a result, they casually pack the nose, and the bipedicled mucosa rumples upon itself and heals with an intranasal stenosis, which causes this pinching and because of this, I recommend to our residents that they very loosely apply plain catgut sutures and do not tie down tightly, just one or two, so that in the packing maneuver, there is no likelihood of the lining to contract on itself. A lot of this is due to missing lining—not because lining has been taken away, but because it has contracted on itself.

Millard: But basically, we say that this pinching is mucosa attached to skin. Whatever has happened in between, we've got mucosa attached to skin in an abnormal position. It has to be freed and filled. Where you are going to get what you use to fill the defect is up to the individual.

Participant: How is this different from the old pinch suture? Just a little bit lower? It was deliberately put in, in a number of cases, to give what was thought to be an aristocratic pinch. What does it look like on the inside? Is there any connection between the mucosa of the lateral wall and the mucosa of the septal area?

Millard: No, I don't think so. I don't think there is any attachment across the gap.

Aufricht: Dr. Safian mentioned that full-thickness tissue must be removed from the dome, both lining and cartilage. I remove it also when neces-

sary. In this case that you present us, in all probability the dome was removed. So you have to make a new dome. In order to do this, you deliberately expose the remaining cartilages and make a cross-section cut through the very edge of the cartilage, leaving the lining intact. This will make a new dome; it will be rounder, and it might recess the projection of the tip a certain amount. Therefore you must be ready to revise that supratip area of scar and cartilage.

THE THICK NOSE

Millard: Thank you. Thirty thousand noses between Dr. Safian and Dr. Aufricht! Isn't that something! Well, shall we go on to a thick nose (Fig. 36)? Here he is after one operation with some improvement (Fig. 37). Let's have some suggestions! Lights. No hands? I thought the whole front row would put up both hands!

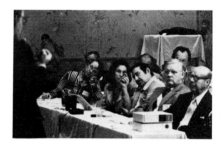

Dr. Rogers speaking to Dr. Peterson, Dr. Sheen, Dr. Natvig, and Dr. Aufricht

Rogers: I'm sorry to be talking so much. I have a lot of male patients in New York, and lots of them have thick tips like this. Most of them are Italian/American or Jewish/American. I cannot see how George Peck or Jack Sheen can say that this type of nose can be corrected without sacrificing or taking out a wedge of cartilage and mucosa. I do it routinely. I take out a wedge in the apex to narrow it, and you can get considerable improvement. I want to discuss an unusual patient. He is a very famous male dancer in New York, but there was a very interesting aspect about his request. In his three-quarters view, he was somewhat deviated. The thickness of his tip was markedly reduced; a lot of it was cartilage and a lot of it was skin. But he asked me something which I think has not been discussed at this meeting. He said too many dancers are too effeminate looking. "Leave my nose a little irregular." I wanted to fracture his nasal bone in keeping with the deviated septum, and he had talked me into not doing it. I think this is very important, especially in male noses.

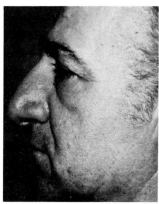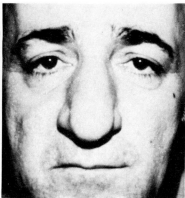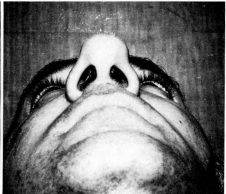

Fig. 36

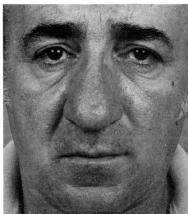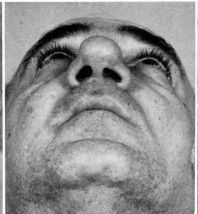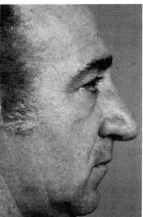

Fig. 37

There is too much of a tendency on the part of rhinoplasty surgeons to use their personal aesthetics in the female nose and transfer it to the problem of the male nose. A male doesn't look so bad if it is slightly deviated in the nasal bridge, and it doesn't look so bad if it is a little aquiline.

Millard: That's a very important point. Sheen and Peck both want to speak. Why don't you two sit together!

Peck: Come on over here, Jack.

Sheen: If you think that Peck and I agree on a tip, Blair, you haven't been listening!

Rogers: No, you've only been saying that you don't touch the mucosa when you're doing the reduction—you say you don't even do a wedge!

Sheen: I've been commenting long and hard on resecting the cartilage. I feel the vestibular lining accommodates very nicely, and it is a matter of policy. I have not had any problems and I have

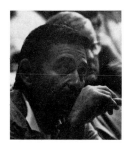

Dr. Sheen

not removed any vestibular lining, even with a forked flap that we've resected. But I am a firm advocate of the resection of the dome of the alar cartilage, so I think perhaps you must have misunderstood me. Now, you can talk to Dr. Peck!

Peck: Yes, I think one of the problems in the thick, heavy nose is that we've got to preserve the architecture of the alar cartilage, and if you cut across the dome, then you're going to destroy that architecture, and it's that architecture that is holding up the nasal tip. I think in this case and especially in the heavy-skinned nose, you want to try to get some leveling of the discrepancy with your sculpturing incision. One thing I might add, with this last patient, I would consider external dermabrasion as an adjunct for the tip. This was published in *Plastic and Reconstructive Surgery*.

Aufricht: George, Joseph remodeled the tip or sculptured the tip with two actions. He removed from the upper part of the lower lateral cartilage both crus medial and lateral. You can see in his diagram that he cut through the dome as far as necessary, and when you say you are not changing the architecture of the vestibule when you leave a rim there, I am afraid you are mistaken. The tip cartilages are just like an umbrella. When you leave only a very narrow rim, with stress the umbrella collapses and the vestibule becomes very much smaller. This has, I'm sorry to say, been a routine operation with Joseph, with myself, and with Safian. I think where you recess the tip only a small degree, you remove only from the upper part of the lower lateral cartilage. I hope I have made myself clear without making an enemy!

Participant: On this man we have just seen with the long nose, I guess that was a postoperative view, it looked to me like he had globular rhinophyma with a thick, subaceous tip and a lot of excess skin. If he's well informed, this is an ideal case for a long, vertical, midline elliptical excision of skin and repositioning the alar cartilage in a higher position.

Millard: So, you'd do a lift and then you'd take an ellipse out of the center too?

Participant: A vertical ellipse. If the patient is informed about the scar and the possibility of dermabrasion. Midline ellipse.

Participant: With that case, he needs a little more reduction of cartilage just as an ellipse on each side of the midline to take care of the bulge on each side.

Millard: Yes, but he's still awfully long. It's true; you may have to do a transverse elliptical excision of the skin and everything.

Rogers: I think Dr. Converse recommends undermining between the dome and the thick tip after you've done all your other contouring in order to allow the dome to come medially into a subcutaneous pocket.

Millard: I suture the alar cartilages together occasionally and if the stitches pull them out of place, take them out. In the very thick tip, I think we just have to go back and thin as much as you can and do alar margins. It's too long and too thick, so you can thin it on the sides with that. You just have to reduce it as much as you can with thinning and keep the integrity of the skin with a little protective subcutaneous tissue, or you'll get dimpling. Of course there is the danger of little irregularities as this is only a human hand and eye procedure, half blind, and the patient must understand this.

There's one real classic, a truly thick secondary postoperative nose (Fig. 38)!

Peck: I think you should handle that, Ralph. That's a Gillies and Millard!

Millard: Let's get a little history on this case. Does the gentleman who offered it—it's not his result, but he may have to deal with it now. If he'd like to add any light on the subject?

Finger: There is no mention of any lateral osteotomies. In this case, I feel certain there is probably still some cartilage left. This case is 6 months postoperative, but it's still not mature.

Millard: It's still not mature. Do you know any-

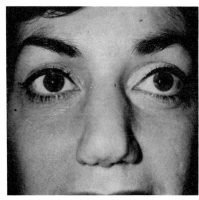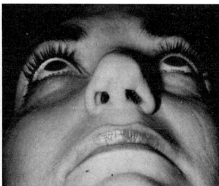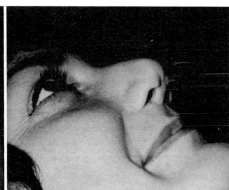

Fig. 38

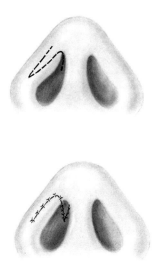

Fig. 39

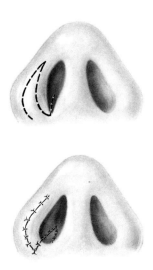

Fig. 40

thing about the tip? Dr. Sheen wants to know.

Finger: I have no preoperative photos, but I know there was a dorsal hump.

Participant: She has hanging sidewalls there, and I wanted to ask you if in this kind of a case, you'd consider that composite chondromucosal flap?

Millard: No, I don't use the method primarily for this type of sidewalls; I would just do a marginal excision of those sidewalls. It's the columella that's short here. But that's a long nose, I feel. It's not really overly long, but I wouldn't want to lengthen it.

Participant: It looks to me that her alar sidewalls are too long.

Millard: Yes, as I just said, I'd take those off. I wouldn't put them somewhere else in this case. Incidentally, alar margin excisions can be kept as flaps—either at the top of the arch of the alar and introduced into the vestibule to take a sharp angle out of the arch (Fig. 39) or, if it's contracted at the bottom, base it at the bottom and turn in to open the airway at the bottom (Fig. 40). So your alar margin need not be thrown away. It can be put in below or above if you need it. In other words, never throw anything away until you are certin you do not need it.

Lewis: This nose is short in the columella and tip, and I think using a little graft just as an adjunct in the shoulders would be worthwhile in this tip. But the alar webs could be handled either by an elliptical resection—just simply dividing the skin as lining to approximate, trim to the edge of the cartilage, elevate the opening of the nos-

trils—or it could be done as a three-dimensional Z-plasty as Straith described about 25 years ago, trimming the cartilage and folding the skin in on one side and the lining out on the other, so as to line the columella and the alar.

Millard: Is there webbing on the inside too? No airway? Adequate airway? Web? Does the profile have the funny look that the underview seems to indicate?

Aufricht: There is an operation that Joseph used regularly in connection with extensive narrowing of the tip of the nose. After resecting a wide vertical strip from the dome of the lower lateral cartilage and its lining, he cut away a triangular piece of skin in front of each nostril (Fig. 41).* He sutured the skin edges with horsehair. The scar was inconspicuous. The circumference of the nostril became a bit smaller. I have used this method for a few years in the beginning of my practice, but haven't used it later. Namely, I found that small protrusions of skin usually disperse and smoothen along wide enough marginal undermining. If there is marked protrusion, I remove small transverse slivers of cartilage (sometimes with lining) from the lower edges of the bisected crura. This depression will provide a place for the surplus skin to sink and smoothen. Secondary marked skin protrusions in this area might be eliminated by Joseph's triangular excision or apparently with Sheen's cartilage transplant.

---

*Joseph, J.: Nasenplastik und sonstige Gesichtsplastik, Leipzig, Germany, 1931, Curt Kabitzsch, p. 128.

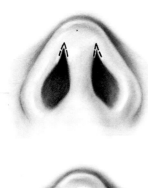

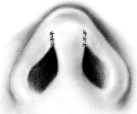

Fig. 41

Sheen: I think this deformity is caused by a complete collapse of the tip of the columella. I think those irregularities you see on the alae are probably remnants of the lateral crura. And although I object strongly to the siphoning out of tissue on the secondary patient, I think I would make an incision at the columella-lobular junction with the anticipation of lifting the tissue up to erase some of those wrinkles. At the same time, I would dissect out the cartilages to remove any adhesions to the skin in the hopes that in elevating the tip tissues with my graft, they would smooth out and ultimately, in the postoperative viewing, give you a better, smoother result.

Rogers: Jack, do you think that she's not a problem of first restoring a better airway? Do you think you can accomplish this just by a Z-plasty?

Sheen: Well, I think this doctor has, first of all, transected or cut the attachment with the upper lateral to the septum, and then he's taken out an enormous triangle. This gives you the synecular web that closes off the airway. On the basal view, I thought what I saw was enough airway to certainly make the nose functional. At this point, we are treating the aesthetic. I really can't evaluate the functional part without seeing what degree of airway is present. If it is in fact completely closed, obviously it has to have something done.

Rogers: Would you do that first before you do the aesthetic?

Sheen: I would do the thing that bothers the patient most.

Millard: Just a minute, Dr. Peck.

Taylor: Last summer, I had a case exactly like this with the projecting alar web, and I performed procentric excision of this and injected silicone into the columella to bring it out, in divided doses, once every 2 or 3 weeks. It came out very nicely.

Millard: Well, all of these suggestions, I think, are pertinent. Incidentally, that little curl there is what I was trying to show you on the nose I was doing yesterday. Only it is a little more exaggerated here. In that case, when I had filled out the columella in front and freed up the membranous septum, it more or less disappeared. It would not in this one. Let me start from the beginning. First, we must set a plan. Look inside and see how much lining is missing. If there is contracture in the lining, you have to add skin as a free graft. At least, get sufficient lining. Then we look at the cover, and I think probably the cover is adequate; it is collapsed because of the lack of support and possibly missing lining. I think we've got to put in new support between skin and lining, and this can be done after the deep scar has been excised. It may be like that crushed, crinkled nose that had collapsed with grooves that I showed yesterday. Whereas, if you free up the skin, you can get your understructure into position to make something that would be more ideal. In other words, set it up so that your lining and your cover are adequate. You can separate the two and thin at the same time, and then more or less do whatever you have to do, and I mean, by separating, whether it's just a small pocket or whether it is undermining the whole bloody thing. It's a matter of dealing with each case at a time. Then you can go ahead with marginal sculpturing of the edges or whatever. This is an extremely difficult problem, and until you actually sit down and go to work on it, you just don't know what you're going to find or what the solution will be eventually. At least that's the way I work. All right, I know everybody's getting tired but . . .

Finger: One last comment. I asked her about her airway, and she said she'd be happy with a tracheotomy if I'd just get augmentation of the tip.

Millard: Well, I hope you'll be able to save her the need of a tracheotomy and still improve her nose.

SNUBBED NOSE

Sheen: On the point of the snubbed nose—this is the problem of the high, raised, contraction of a snub tip. I just wanted to tell what I do with a tip that is actually contracted down.

Millard: Does everybody understand what he's talking about?

[Consensus: No.]

Sheen: I make an incision like I did yesterday, at the columella-lobular junction. Then it's just anterior to the medial crus, carry it around in the septal triangle, and carry it around the anterior part of the lateral crus. Then create an actual specimen of cartilage that's carved out to form the dome of the crura.

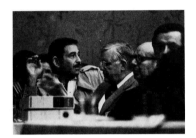

Dr. Sheen and Dr. Natvig

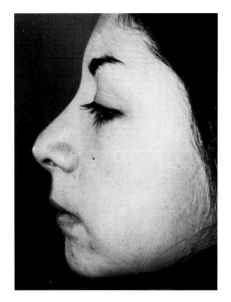

Fig. 42

Millard: Is that a centimeter wide?

Sheen: Yes, and notched for lateral stability. It's slipped into the pocket, and placement is at the base of the columella-lobular junction. These do get projection at the tip and the other part of the projection at the columella-lobular junction.

Millard: When you're going for tip support, if you make the pocket the exact size you wish, you can support the tip from any point. You don't have to give up because you can't get a long enough piece of cartilage that will reach from the nasal spine to the nasal tip. Incidentally, do not try to shove the cartilage in from the back of the columella with a posterior splitting incision. It does not work well. When you've made a pocket with the bottom of that pocket fixed, then from that point on, you're pushing up, and insertion of a strut of cartilage in this confined limit will give definition to the tip.

Here is a profile offered as a postoperative problem (Fig. 42). She has a raised supratip and in addition has a projection at the tip suggestive of too much alar crus. If this projection is a cartilage strut inserted too close to the tip skin causing blanching over its prominence, there is not only the unattractiveness of the point, but the danger of perforation. Note that in spite of this tip push, the patient has a polly-beak that requires septal lowering and scar excision.

Anyone want to offer a suggestion for this

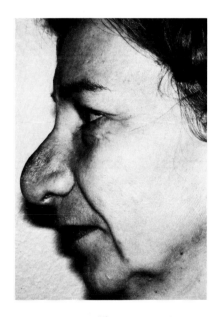

Fig. 43

other postoperative supratip (Fig. 43)? Dr. Sheen has warned that without sufficient support, one cannot carve a correction in a tip. In this case, I would think the skin would have to be elevated from the lining, excising the excess scar, and then a new support would have to be inserted so that the cover could drape upon it. There is a possibility here that external skin excision may be necessary.

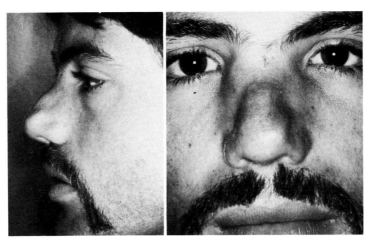

Fig. 44

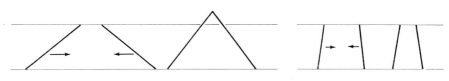

Fig. 45

LATERAL OSTEOTOMY

Bass: Can we get the panel to comment on the lateral osteotomies? Here is an example problem (Fig. 44).

Ashley: Front view shows the bones are wide. I'd like to see that profile one more time. There seems to be enough elevation. There is what looks to be septum making the supratip hump. The lower laterals will have to be dealt with some more. I use a—we haven't talked about this much and I don't know whether it's in order now—but I happen to like to use a 2 mm osteotome through the external route to do my osteotomy because it is easier for me. I know people object to that, but the scars haven't been any problem. I'm sure someday I'll get a keloid, but I haven't so far. That's what I'd do in this case and get a good, complete osteotomy, narrow those bones, take down the supratip hump, and then deal with the lower lateral cartilages.

Millard: Thank you, Frank. How many would go in medially and take off the bone on the medial side and let those bones move together? They look very broad and thick to me.

Ashley: I think you should do that in almost every case. You have to take out that wedge up at the apex that Dr. Aufricht talked about so much in

order to get it together, but I think that is just a routine thing.

Millard: Well, this is a little bit more than the usual, so I didn't know if you would want to shave the bone.

Aufricht: This is a very wide, bony nose, and I think I would remove those two pieces at the side of the septum, and I would do a basal osteotomy whether you do it with a chisel or a saw; it doesn't matter. But it has to be where the frontal process of the maxilla emerges from the maxilla. Then as you mentioned, reduce a little bit the septal cartilaginous hump, and do some correction at the tip of the nose.

Millard: How many think that when you do a lateral osteotomy you get a rise in the nasal bone? Just very little? Isn't it all the angle of the bone? If you've got wide spreading, you're going to get a rise. If the bones are more or less in straight up-and-down position, then they will move over without a rise (Fig. 45).

Sheen: The question is, if I would do a high or low osteotomy. Obviously, you'll find a wide base here. I would obviously do a low osteotomy. But 80% or 90% of all noses, I feel, are proper width at the base.

Rogers: Dr. Converse, following Dr. Aufricht's

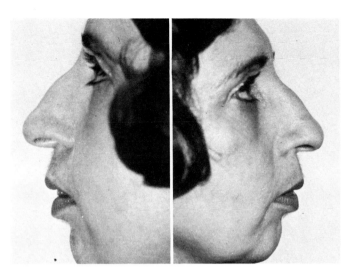

Fig. 46

suggestion, would take a rongeur in a case like this and cut out a very thin sliver of bone to create the space into which he can easily move these rather widely spread bones. I don't recommend that routinely.

Millard: Let's wind up now with this final profile (Fig. 46). Of course she can be improved a lot, but someone suggested a Dale Carnegie course for her! Anybody want to go further?

Participant: Well, this lady doesn't need Dale Carnegie. She's my patient. I was wondering if you were going to show her. I didn't bring too many slides because I thought you'd have enough. She's a 55-year-old woman who is very active in the business world without a husband, who has what you can see, but is a very personable individual. I spent a long, long time operating on this nose as obviously no external incisions will be tolerated, and she does have very thick skin.

Millard: Of course you can deal with this problem like all the others. She's got quite an underbite, and it's going to take a pretty good chin implant unless you want to do an osteotomy and move that jaw into occlusion. The nose is not all that difficult!

Aufricht: This is a typical case that I tried to describe the other day, the tri-feature aesthetic syndrome. She has a humped nose, a high labial columella angle, and a receding chin. I think this lady could be made very attractive. Reduce the nose and build out the receding chin, and bring out the acute angle of the upper lip. I think then she will be a very attractive lady.

Millard: We have taped the entire symposium and hope to record as much as comes through well. I hope we can get most of it verbatim.

THE OLDER PATIENT

Participant: One thing that hasn't been mentioned in the symposium is the operation on the older, aged person. We find many older persons, who because of changes due to their age, they have a long nose and a thick tip. In my younger days, I was always afraid to operate on these patients, fearing that the skin would not adapt to the rearranged framework. I don't feel that way any more, and I have a number of older patients that I've operated upon. I think you have to be careful not to overoperate them to give them a nose like an 18-year-old girl. But a modest operation does help these patients quite well. I find that they heal just as well generally as the younger patients do. Skin does adjust itself very well to the dome. I had a very delightful lady come to me just recently; her husband was the president of a small university down where we were, and she was 73 years of age. She said, "I just can't stand it any longer! He's been calling me hawk nose for 45 years and not only that, he ran off with a younger woman!" Here was a 73-year-old woman that was really in distress. I operated upon her, she healed very nicely, and I've given her a new lease on life. I wonder if anyone has anything to say of operations on the older-aged patient.

Millard: I'd like to add a story to that which I heard from Dr. Straith. A 76-year-old lady came in for a rhinoplasty consultation and when asked why she had waited so long, she said, "I have wanted my nose reduced all my life and my husband was against it. I buried him yesterday!" During consultation, I tell this story to the husband who is sitting belligerently with his mouth hanging down, obviously against his wife having corrective surgery. Then I turn to him and say, "You see, she'll get it done sooner or later!"

THE MALE PATIENT

Participant: How about some discussion on male patient selection?

Millard: That's a good question. What is your other question?

Participant: Do you ever operate on hypertensive patients when they have the hypertension controlled?

Millard: Does anybody fear doing a hypertensive patient under control? Not with it under control? And your other question? Male patients? Good question. Dr. Aufricht, on a male patient, how do you—what is your guide to us about which male you would take? That's a whole book, I know, but. . .

Aufricht: In male patients, you have to be more careful. First, I believe it should be a young person. If an older male comes in and complains about his appearance, you have to be a little bit suspicious. But if the nose is very bad and you have operated on the rest of the family, the wife and children, you can do a very good operation. But one has to be more careful. I just had a recent case, Ralph, a secondary operation, on a 56, no, I'm wrong, on a 60-year-old man. He had a very bad nose before, and his reaction was similar to your case, of the woman who did not appreciate fully her improvement.

Millard: As for the male patient, I think in general the principle is the same as in all of plastic surgery; that we have to try to evaluate the size of the problem as well as the degree the patient is concerned about this problem. If they come in with a tiny hump and they call it a tremendous hump, and express hate of it, look out! If they come in with a great big nose and they say this little hump, look out! On the other hand, if they come in and say I hate this *great big hump* which is a *great big hump,* then the surgeon and the patient should be able to get together quite happily.

Aufricht: I had a patient, a hairdresser, and he came in to the office with the typical side motion of the effeminate. He wanted to have his nose tilted. So I told him that would make you feminine, and he said that's beside the point!

Millard: Did you go ahead and do it for him?

Aufricht: I did not!

Conroy: I think probably the most important point is whether or not you're dealing with a schizophrenic or not. In most instances, you won't pick it up. In those instances where you think there might be a problem, I think you should ask the patient if he has been under therapy. If so, then I think you probably shouldn't operate on him. I don't feel that the fact that his psychiatrist says that it would be safe to do this or that is totally dependable. I still think it is possible he shouldn't be operated on. If you suspect psychologic problems even after being screened, if you have the impression that he may be schizophrenic, you should not operate on him.

Rogers: We talk about male patients as if they come from another planet! I don't think there is anything different in male patients than in female patients. There is going to be that small proportion of patients whose sense of vanity is going to make them very difficult. But we also have female patients who give us postoperative problems. I think the clue in evaluating a male patient is, number one, the routine use of preoperative photographs so that when the patient comes into your office and you go with him over two or three consultations to learn what his own body and physical image is, when he prefers on your marking of the photographs something that is effeminate, I would say immediately cancel him out because his body image is not going to be anything like your approach to him as a patient. But there are many male patients, and I've just thought over, sitting here, the last ten male patients I've had. About five of them are married men, two of them are college students, one is a physical education teacher, and one is working for the Peace Corps. These are patients who are normal. You may have different patients in California, but we have a very healthy bunch of male patients in New York City. Yes, we get the occasional bizarre one, but I think the use of preoperative and postoperative photographs will rule out the problems because you soon learn of any peculiarities in their desires.

Millard: I had a pilot on whom I made a straight, masculine nose. He kept trying to get me to scoop his bridge to give him a more feminine appearance. I just refused to do it. But I wonder how right we are not doing what they want instead of what we think they should have?

Rogers: I think the mistakes we've seen in New York and in the malpractice cases, and I've sat on the malpractice mediating panels, the majority of them have been when the surgeon does do what the patient wants when he innately knows it is wrong for a male face. These patients are never satisfied. And they are the most dangerous patients. They don't want to be male; they want to be something else. And they are the ones who are the biggest postoperative problem.

Millard: Of course, in the transsexual, we have to change them all the way.

Participant: A few years ago, in the New York Regional Society, they had a panel on rhinoplasty that included a psychiatrist interviewing a patient. And something came out of it that I have watched very closely, and it seems to be true. In those borderline patients where you're not sure, you suspect schizophrenia and you cannot elicit a humorous response from the patient during the primary interview, please run. The pro-

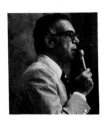

Dr. Millard

fessor of psychiatry gave us a real clue which I thought was a very valid truth: no humorous response—don't touch the patient!

Millard: That about does it. Thank you all for your contributions. First, the patients who cooperated so well in the operating room and especially their *noses;* the members of a superb faculty who have been at their best; and you who have come to listen to the faculty, to stimulate them, challenge them, and get more out of them than you ever expected. Corrective rhinoplasty is one chicken we have picked pretty clean to the bone. I thank you all and wish you many more, happier noses!

Postscript

Throughout the entire symposium, there was an atmosphere of excitement and anticipation. The faculty and the participants both seemed to become ignited. This, of course, extracted the best possible out of the faculty, each attempting to top the other not unlike the Emperors of Rome, each leaving architectural masterpieces better than the ruler before him. This competitive teaching seemed to be sustained well past our planned schedule, which was set to end about 5 PM each evening. On Thursday, January 16, we ran until after 6 PM and on Friday, January 17, to nearly 7 PM. On Saturday morning, set for 9 until 12 noon and mostly devoted to problem cases, there seemed to have been such a thorough handling of these aspects the previous days that the subject and the problem cases had been exhausted by 11:45. At the end, Dr. Aufricht admitted that this symposium had rejuvenated him to such an extent, that it frightened him. I requested he put that in writing, and this is an excerpt from his note, written January 31, 1975:

> The symposium was most successful. The enthusiasm of both registrants and faculty was extraordinary. It stimulated me also to such extent that I was surprised myself. I almost felt as if I could go back to full-swing practice of 5 days surgery and all the rest!

Index